Six Group Therapies

Six Group Therapies

Edited by

SAMUEL LONG

Empire State Poll, Inc.
New York, New York

Plenum Press • New York and London

Library of Congress Cataloging in Publication Data

Six group therapies.

Includes bibliographies and index.
1. Group psychotherapy. I. Long, Samuel. [DNLM: 1. Psychotherapy, Group. WM
430 S625]
RC488.S55   1987   616.89'152   87-7187
ISBN 0-306-42642-0

© 1988 Plenum Press, New York
A Division of Plenum Publishing Corporation
233 Spring Street, New York, N.Y. 10013

To my parents

Contributors

Raymond J. Corsini • Department of Psychology, University of Hawaii, Honolulu, Hawaii 96821

John Grimes • 3480 Dixiana Drive, Lexington, Kentucky 40502

Sheenah Hankin • Cognitive Psychotherapy Associates, 68 East 91st Street, New York, New York 10128

Robert L. Harman • Counseling and Testing Center, University of Central Florida, Orlando, Florida 32816

Melvyn Hollander • Department of Psychology, Queens College, City University of New York, Flushing, New York 11367 and the Center for Behavioral Psychotherapy, White Plains, New York 10605

Frank Johnson • Department of Training and Management Development, Ethyl Corporation, 330 South Fourth Street, Richmond, Virginia 23217

Katsushige Kazaoka • Late of the Greer-Woodycrest Children Services, Pomona, New York 10703 and the Center for Behavioral Psychotherapy, White Plains, New York 10605

Samuel Long • Empire State Poll, Inc., 154 East 29th Street, New York, New York 10016

Richard L. Wessler • Psychology Department, Pace University, Pleasantville, New York 10570

Preface

Five basic objectives were set for *Six Group Therapies* when it was conceived. It was to be limited to the presentation of six of the most prevalent group psychotherapies practiced today, reflecting a diversity of orientations, including personal growth, improvement of interpersonal relations, cognitive restructuring, and habit change. This resulted in the choice of Adlerian, encounter, transactional analysis, cognitive, Gestalt, and behavior group therapies for inclusion in this volume. Second, each chapter was to be original in content. A common outline was to be followed in the writing of each chapter. Authors were to be actual practitioners of group therapy. Finally, the book was to be written for an audience composed of professionals, as well as upper level undergraduate and graduate students enrolled in courses in clinical psychology, psychotherapy, counseling, and related subjects. These objectives have been met.

The common outline followed by all authors in *Six Group Therapies* was designed to structure the discussion of the group therapies and to facilitate comparisons among the group therapies. Following a brief introduction, each chapter offers a definition of the group therapy under discussion, especially from the vantage point of its philosophy, theory, and system of techniques. A history of the group therapy is then presented, in which the group therapy's precursors and development are elaborated. Then the primary and secondary goals of the group therapy are outlined, particularly as they compare to the general goals of psychotherapy.

The theoretical rationale section in each chapter is comprised of four components. First, the central concepts, unique to the group-therapy orientation, are presented and discussed. The philosophical underpinnings of the theoretical system, as contained in the therapy's fundamental assumptions regarding human nature, are then presented. The theory of personality associated with the group therapy is described. Finally, the theory is compared to other theories of group therapy.

Three aspects of each system's conception of therapy follow. The system's theory of the etiology of psychological disturbance and how this disturbance can be modified is first stated. Second, the actual process of therapy and the reasons for its effectiveness are then discussed. Third, specific therapeutic mechanisms contributing to the amelioration of clients' disturbances are also considered.

Elaboration of four factors in the practice of each group psychotherapy follows. Frequently encountered problems in therapeutic practice, as well as typical solutions to these problems, are presented. Methods of psycho-therapeutic evaluation and assessment are then outlined. Various treatment formats and approaches are discussed by the authors. Management issues, particularly those relating to the group therapist's role and responsibilities, conclude this section.

The application section of each chapter focuses on seven issues common to the six group therapies. Processes of group selection and preferences regarding group composition are examined. The setting and physical structure of the group session are considered. Parameters of group size are weighed. Each author describes factors relating to the therapy's frequency, session length, and duration. Space is devoted to the various media used by each group therapy. The qualifications and skills required of a group therapy leader are explored. Finally, ethical issues unique to group psychotherapy are detailed in each chapter.

Both process and outcome research germane to each system of group psychotherapy are cited and evaluated.

To better convey the essential nature of each group psychotherapy described here, a hypothetical group therapy session is illustrated.

Each group therapy's fundamental strengths and weaknesses are also addressed.

In order to aid the reader, a glossary of key concepts concludes each chapter.

A number of individuals have played an especially important role in the development of my thinking about, as well as contributing to my appreciation of, group psychotherapy. Members of this group would include Delton Beier, Vincent Harren, Kenneth Heller, Leon Levy, James Miller, Thomas Mitchell, Gordon Rader, David Rimm, and Thomas Schill. Sheenah Hankin was also quite helpful in arguing and illustrating the benefits of the cognitive school with me.

The authors of the following chapters were very cooperative, helpful, and patient in the preparation of *Six Group Therapies*. I have learned much from them. And I have greatly enjoyed working with them on this project.

SAMUEL LONG

Contents

4   **Rational–Emotive Therapy and Related Cognitively Oriented Psychotherapies   159**

Richard L. Wessler and Sheenah Hankin

5   **Gestalt Group Therapy   217**

Robert L. Harman

6   Behavior Therapy Groups   257

Melvyn Hollander and Katsushige Kazaoka

1

Adlerian Groups

RAYMOND J. CORSINI

INTRODUCTION

Every system of psychotherapy has a number of unique elements distinguishing it from other systems, and the same is true for what is known as Individual Psychology or Adlerian Psychology. Unless these basic uniquenesses are known right from the very beginning it is highly likely that the reader of this essay may start and even end with incorrect concepts. Consequently, we shall be begin with a number of short statements intended to correct misconceptions and to set the stage for the specific subject of this chapter.

1. The single most important feature of Adlerian Psychology is what is absolutely unique among all other personality theories: its philosophy of *Gemeinschaftsgefühl* (Adler, 1962).

2. The personality theory of Adlerian Psychology, in contrast to most other systems, especially those of the time of its origin, Freud's Psycho-analysis and Jung's Analytical Psychology, is of the commonsense type (Adler, 1927); and in decided contrast to Freud's theory, Adlerian Psychology in the 50 years since Adler's death has not changed.

3. Although the philosophy and the theory are set and well established and held by all Adlerians, the methods of evaluation, training, and treatment differ substantially, to the effect that it can be said there is no Adlerian method of treatment. There are instead Adlerian methods of treatment, which may run into the thousands, because every Adlerian tends to operate according to his or her perceptions of the best ways to achieve desired results. This feature contrasts strongly with some other preestablished methods of treatment, for example, Carl Rogers's (1951) procedure, which is so strongly structured.

4. Even though Adlerian philosophy and theory are simple, the typical person in the field of psychology has either inadequate or incorrect understandings of Adlerian Psychology (Silverman & Corsini, 1984), believing for example such untruths as that Adler extolled the importance of power, that Adler was a disciple of Freud, or that Adler was a psychoanalyst.

Raymond J. Corsini • Department of Psychology, University of Hawaii, Honolulu, Hawaii 96821.

In view of the above, it is of greatest importance to understand Adlerian group procedures that there be an understanding of the philosophy and the theory of Adlerian Psychology and, having that, understanding group procedures as done by Adlerians will be a relatively simple matter.

DEFINITION

Adlerian Psychology may be best understood in terms of its basic concepts, and these add up to a definition. We shall present three different versions of more or less the same ideas in this section. This amount of repetition is considered crucial, because the evidence is that the typical well-educated psychologist or psychiatrist (Silverman & Corsini, 1984) has a fund of misinformation which must be corrected in order to allow him to comprehend procedures. The writer suggests that if the reader go over these next several passages carefully, he or she may learn that he or she already is an Adlerian!

> Individual psychology is a psychology of growth (rather than instincts or drives) in which each individual is seen as striving for maximum personal competence (motivated by feelings of inferiority) to achieve fictive goals, in a unique creative manner, within the limits of possibility established by biology and society, moving in a unitary holistic manner, the individual thereby establishing a unique life-style based on personal assumptions and conclusions developed over time, which becomes natural and useful when in accord with the needs of others.

Let us now repeat the information on the masthead of the *Journal of Individual Psychology* which will be more-or-less a duplicate of what you have just read, but using different language.

> Individual psychology is devoted to a holistic, phenomenological, teleological, field-theoretical and socially oriented approach to psychology and related fields. This approach is based on the assumption of the uniqueness, self-consistency, activity and creativity of the human individual; an open dynamic system of motivation; and an innate potentiality for social living.

And we shall now make a third attempt to define Individual Psychology by presenting twelve major concepts modified from Ansbacher and Ansbacher (1956):

Twelve Basic Propositions of Individual Psychology

1. People move in terms of perceived minus and expected plus.
2. Each individual has a unique fictional goal.
3. The final goal is not known to the individual. It is unconscious.
4. This goal is the final cause of behavior.
5. The person operates in terms of a consistent life-style toward the goals.
6. The person is a unified whole.

7. Objective determiners (heredity and environment) provide possibilities only.
8. The apperceptive schema determines all behavior.
9. Social conditions determine one's individuality.
10. All problems are social problems.
11. Social interest is a human potential to be developed.
12. Maladjustment is due to exaggerated personal uncooperative goals of personal superiority.

HISTORY

The history of Adlerian Psychology is relatively simple. Around 1902, Alfred Adler, then a physician in private practice working on a book that appeared eventually in 1907, *Study of Organ Inferiority and its Psychic Compensation*, became aware of the work of another Viennese physician, Sigmund Freud. Adler had already conceptualized what was to be an important part of his own psychological thinking: the importance of compensation. When, for example, a lung or a kidney is lost, and a person has only one of these organs remaining, there comes a compensation in the form of the remaining organ enlarging. The theme of Adler's book was that if a person actually had a physical inferiority that this knowledge motivated the individual to do better in either that particular area of deficit or in another area as a compensation for the deficit.

In 1902 Freud invited Adler and three other scholars to meet at his home to discuss the general matter of "psycho-analysis." These five scholars were interested in the general problem of neurosis, trying to understand human nature. They were interested in general psychology and as analysts of the psyche they were all "psycho-analysts" but *not* "psychoanalysts." For them, in those early years, the term *psycho-analysis* was not a propriatary name of one system, but rather was the general term for understanding the psyche. At these meetings, Adler, according to the memoranda that have been preserved, was one of the most vocal, and indeed as far as can be told, Freud, the host, never presented any of his ideas formally. From the very beginning it was evident that Freud's ideas and Adler's were contradictory. Freud believed that sexual repression was the cause of neuroses while Adler believed that sexual elements were only a small part of the problem of human adjustment, and that the real problem was the desire of people to *become*, that is, to grow and develop and improve and become more competent.

Eventually, after 9 years of uneasy association, Adler decided to break away from Freud's group and start his own. This was a year after Freud had nominated him to be president of the Vienna Psychological Association and while he was the coeditor of the group's journal.

Adler by 1911 was doing quite well in his medical practice. Between 1898 and 1909 he became the father of four children, two of whom as of the time of this writing (1987) are psychiatrists in New York City. Between 1904, the year of his first publication, and 1917 when he entered the Austrian army as a general physician, Adler had 31 publications. In addition to the already mentioned book on organ inferiority, in 1912 he published his masterpiece, whose title translated in English is *The Neurotic Constitution.*

After the end of World War I, during the dreadful period known in Central Europe as "The Hunger," Adler combined his social interests and his concern with the personality by becoming, in effect, an educator. He established family education and child-guidance clinics in schools, and he lectured and demonstrated to teachers, psychologists, physicians, parents his ideas about the proper treatment of children. He helped establish a school on Adlerian principles.

The fact that Adler never formally did group psychotherapy in the sense we know it now is important relative to the development of the group method. Nevertheless, he is one of the pioneers of the group movement as a result of the activities he started in 1922 in the schools of Vienna (Corsini, 1957). He did something that was then considered shocking, and possibly even unethical. He interviewed adults—teachers and parents—in front of a group, and then he interviewed children, also in front of the group.

The whole tradition of secrecy implicit in the relationship between a patient and a doctor was overthrown by Adler. None of the other physicians and psychologists of the time were doing anything out in public of this kind. Adler was a pioneer in this aspect of his professional behavior.

Then something very unusual happened, the same thing that happened to another physician as of 1907 in the United States: Joseph Pratt. Pratt, an internist interested in pulmonary diseases, gave a lecture at Johns Hopkins University in which he reported that he found that if he lectured to his patients about hygienic means of dealing with tuberculosis, they did not tend to pay much attention to his advice, but if they heard the same information in a group they were likely to follow directions. This was the same phenomenon that many years later, during World War II, Kurt Lewin would rediscover: that American housewives were more likely to change their food-buying habits if the information given them was discussed in a group. Adler noticed that members of the audience not only learned what he was lecturing and demonstrating, but that they also were being personally affected by the group process. There is no evidence that he paid any great attention to this phenomenon; however, one of his students and colleagues, Dr. Rudolf Dreikurs (1960) did notice this, and became the major impetus in the group procedures of Adlerians when he came to the United States in 1939.

GOALS

Of the various schools of psychology, none of the other early ones have ever shown any great interest in the group process. And of all the major current ones, probably only Transactional Analysis and Gestalt Psychotherapy emphasize groups to the extent that Adlerian psychology does; but, as will be seen, the range of use is much greater for Adlerians than for the other schools which, after all, is only to be expected of a system that is social in its nature.

We may as well mention at this point that the word "Individual" in the term Individual Psychology does not refer to individuals. Individual Psychology is a social psychology. Why then the word "Individual" in its title? This is another story: the word *Individuale* in German means about the same as Gestalt, and refers to the concept of the person as an indivisible unit. So what Adler called in German *Individuale Psychologie* would most accurately be translated into English as *Gestalt Psychology* and perhaps even better as *Holistic Psychology*.

The goals of Adlerian Psychology are the same as the goals of any of the major psychotherapeutic systems, except that they are wider in scope, and, consequently, Adlerian uses of groups are more varied than in any other system. We need not dwell too much on what the usual goals are: to help people be more comfortable with themselves and to help them make a better adjustment to the social world by acting in a more "reasonable" manner, all this through having better and more accurate concepts of self and of others. In short, they are the usual goals of psychotherapy; and, in a sense, this is the least important part of what Individual Psychology is all about. Individual Psychology is a philosophy of life (Adler, 1962). Adler was a social reformer in the same sense that his friend Abraham Maslow was: Adler was out to create a better world, and he believed in essence that if the world was composed of angels, it would still not be heaven. In other words, the perception of Adler and of Adlerians is that they have as a major purpose in their professional life to do good; to help others; to do what we call "social-interest work," or what may be called volunteer work, with the intention of changing the world by changing people.

THEORY

Basic Concepts

We have already mentioned some basic Adlerian concepts in the first part of this chapter, but they were not defined in any depth. This will be our purpose here. The major Adlerian view is that the individual is a responsible, creative person, with control over personal destiny—not fortune's fool. Or, putting it more accurately, the way an individual develops personality is a function of givens—heredity and environment on one side, and on the other, the person's own decisions.

Another basic concept is that Adlerian psychology is phenomenological, an ideographic rather than a nomothetic science: its concern is the single individual functioning in society rather than the group itself. We do not think in this manner: "about 9 percent of children are underweight"—that would be nomothetic thinking—but rather, "this particular child is underweight." There is nothing wrong with nomothetic science—and as a matter of fact nomothetic thinking is seen as entirely legitimate—but Individual Psychology is interested in individuals, how they individually cope in society. So, Individual Psychology is a subjective rather than an objective science. Our point of departure is the individual.

Still another important general position has to do with the separation of powers of the individual. In psychology there is a tendency to divide the individual into at least two parts: intellect and emotions; and possibly more: cognition, behavior, volition, affection, and so forth. Adlerians take a rather simple view in terms of this type of thinking: although the person is a unitary and indivisible unit, nevertheless (for heuristic purposes) we can divide the individual into three parts: cognition—behavior—affection; that is to say overt actions, thinking, and feelings. However, the order of precedence is what is important from an Adlerian point of view.

In dealing with anyone in therapy our first concern is the intellect: to try to understand the person's thinking. We are not so concerned with the feelings or with the behavior, seeing these other two aspects as dependent on thinking. Consequently, Adlerian psychology is a cognitive personality theory. We say, putting it simply, that as one thinks, one feels and acts. We believe that if we can change a person's thinking, we can then change that person's feelings and behavior.

Still another concept which we have already alluded to is the importance of the view of the person relative to others. Adlerians see the world in a horizontal manner: we are each different from one another, but no one is better than anyone else. Adlerians make a big issue out of the concept of feelings of inferiority, which in essence means that a person has some sort of concept that he or she should be better than others, and feels inferior relative to others. So, no matter how small or how young, how smart or how stupid, how strong or how weak, one should accept oneself as what one is, and strive to do better and to cooperate with others. The desire to be better than others, and to look down on those inferior or up to those superior, is the cause of most problems. We should think of ourselves on spaceship earth as having the obligation to do our best to help others and to provide also for future generations.

Assumptions about Human Nature

Adlerians take an unusual position relative to human nature: unusual in terms of other personality theories, but strictly common sense. The two formal positions that most theorists take are determinism and indeterminism. In a sense Adlerians reject both points of view, but in another way, accept both. Let us try to see the two extremes and then let us consider the Adlerian view.

Determinism

This position in essence says that what you are is determined by either heredity or environment, or a combination of both. Freud, for example, was essentially a hereditarian, having a biological-deterministic point of view, say-ing for example that the human being has certain innate needs or drives, such as sexual expression, and that if these needs are thwarted the individual will become neurotic. B. F. Skinner (1938), a proponent of behaviorism, is also a determinist. According to Skinner, how one experiences the consequences of one's behavior determines future behavior. Or, in short, if one is "punished" for behavior of one kind or another, one tends not to do that for which one was punished.

These points of view are compelling, and apparently logical, and many people in psychology accept the view of the determining effects of biological and social factors.

Indeterminism

An opposing point of view, found generally in the law and in religion, is that neither biological nor social factors excuse anyone from responsibility for behavior. That is to say, there is a "right" and there is a "wrong" behavior, and regardless of biological or social factors one is completely responsible for how one acts.

Soft Determinism

The Adlerian position of soft determinism is: Any human being is affected by both heredity and environment. Thus, if a person would want to run a mile in 3 minutes, he or she most probably never would be able to do so, because there are biological limits to such behavior. In other words, we all have built-in limits on our behavior, and those persons who, for example, thinks that they can fly from the top of a skyscraper by flapping their arms like a bird, or can swim the width of the Atlantic Ocean at the equator, will die in the attempt. Adlerians consequently admit the obvious: that there are limits to what any person can do. These are limitations imposed by nature.

And there are also social limits. Thus, it is not surprising that in Des Moines, Iowa, children will ordinarily speak English rather than Persian or Portuguese. They are likely to go to school and in school will be taught to use a pencil rather than an abacus for calculations. Boys will not wear skirts. Chil-dren will be induced to have particular attitudes about various religions, about various races, and various political positions. They will be told what is "right and proper" in dealing with others. In other words, they will be socialized by the environment, mostly their parents, their siblings, their friends, their rela-tives, and their teachers.

So Adlerians accept the effects of the environment and also of biology. However, here is where we depart from the others. Adlerians assume the existence of one aspect either denied or not mentioned by most other theories, *the creativity of the individual:* the possibility of an individual moving within the limits set by biology and by society, the possibility of people having creative ideas not determined by either biology or society.

In view of this position, we how have on the one side some limiting factors, and on the other side we have the responsible individual with some degree of creativity, who can "move," as it were, within the limits of social and biological possibilities. It should be evident that this position is a commonsense one, and that it gives Adlerian theorists much greater scope than presented by other theories.

Personality Theory

In the earlier section we summarized some of the elements of Adlerian personality theory, giving only names. We shall now put some flesh on these bones, and take up the theory in greater detail. Actually, to understand Adlerian group work it is most important to understand the underlying theory and philosophy, otherwise nothing will make much sense. We shall take up in greater detail the 12 propositions summarized by Ansbacher and Ansbacher (1956).

Plus to Minus

What is meant here is that the individual is seen as forever striving. Any human being at any time in his or her life evaluates his or her present position and wants to move to a better one, moving from a perceived minus to an expected plus situation.

The important part of this theory is that it is a *teleological* concept (*telos*— "goal" in Greek). (We see the person moving on, as of now, to something else.) Adler asked not *whence* (past) but *whither* (future), not from where have you come, but rather, where are you going?

This means in practice that, in studying a person, the Adlerian therapist is not so much interested in history or even present status, but rather intentions, what she or he wants to accomplish—even though, as a function of limited awareness, she or he may not be aware of what her or his intentions are.

Fictional Goal

The individual is faced immediately with all sorts of situations in life, and operates in terms of the exigencies of situations, but overall there is a final fictional goal (fictional in the sense that it is [a] a self-imposed or developed goal and [b] an ideal). If we were able to understand what that person's true goal was, we could then understand the person's behavior. For example, let us say that Jon has a fictional goal of comfort, and that he is looking for the good things of life, but without making any effort. Should this be his goal, then his whole behavior would be understood: refusing to do chores, forgetting obligations, stealing things . . . all of these signs of his real goal to have a good life without effort.

Unconscious Goal

This final, fictional goal is unknown to the individual due to a lack of self-awareness. According to Adler, the final goal is unknown to the individual. We simply do not know what we are really after, but sometimes our strange behavior gives us a clue.

Goal is Final Cause

The ultimate understanding of a person is dependent on understanding the goal. A good example might be watching a rat in a maze. Were someone not to know what the rat's goal was, the rat's behavior would be strange: the rat runs now to the right and now to the left; it then makes a right hand U-turn, and so forth, and is busy running as though it knew what it was doing. For a child, to see the rat running in this purposeful manner would be a wonder; but the experimenter who has trained the rat knows that the rat has learned a certain pattern of movement and that the rat's intention is to get to a food box. Notice how we anthromorphize the rat, in contrast to a behavioristic description. We assume that the rat has consciousness, and knows what it is after. But we assume that people really do not know their ultimate goal.

Self-Consistency

Another important theoretical element is that the individual relentlessly and consistently goes towards his or her goal, and that any deviations are only apparent. Take a horse-race bettor. One day he or she bets on Black Beauty and the next day bets on Green Fire even though Black Beauty is in the race. Is the bettor consistent? Absolutely! The goal is to win money, and on Monday he or she assumed that Black Beauty was the best horse in the race but on Tuesday he or she thought that Green Fire was a faster horse than Black Beauty. So, the bettor was only apparently inconsistent. The same with people in general: George is now in love with Helen and wants to marry her; having married her, he now falls in love with Irene. He is inconsistent in one respect, but if we know his final goal—say the pursuit of pleasure—his apparent inconsistency is quite consistent with his goal of pleasure rather than obligation.

Unified Whole

This next point relates to the person. As seen by Adler the human is always an entity and not a collection of parts: more like a tree, which came from a seed, rather than a television set, which is a collection of parts. The tree has different parts, of course—a bark, roots, branches, and so forth—but they all operate in harmony as a unified whole: nothing in conflict with other parts.

Objective Elements

We refer here to society and biology. As discussed already, they provide possibilities and set limits within which the individual can function. This explains how identical twins brought up in the same family can deviate considerably in terms of their personality. Thus, they may have the same height and weight and look alike (effects of heredity), and they may both speak the same language and wear the same clothes and eat the same foods (the effects of environment), but they may be very different in the rest of their personalities— their creativity, which they employ within the limits of the objective elements.

Apperceptive Schema

Adler's motto was: "*Omnia opinione suspensa sunt*" (Everything depends on opinions). This means in effect that people have certain predispositions to view life in particular ways, and that the reality is interpreted by people in unique ways in terms of their goals and their life-styles.

Social Conditions

An individual must be considered in terms of the environment in which he or she operates. There is no individuality apart from others. Individual Psychology is at the same time a subjective science of individuals, but they are imbedded in their society and can only be evaluated and understood in terms of others.

Social Problems

All behavior must be understood as social, in that what people actually do always relates to other people in one way or another.

Social Interest

From the Adlerian point of view the essence of normality is having a feeling of concern for others; to be interested in the interests of others. Pure selfishness, wanting power for one's self, and similar attitudes, are those of criminals. This important factor is seen as an aptitude that can be developed in people. We are not born altruistic—neither are we born as savages.

Maladjustment

The neurotic is seen as maladjusted simply because of a desire to be superior to others, to not be interested in others, to be uncooperative. Wanting to be superior to others at all costs is the prime cause of maladjustment.

Comparisons with Related Theories

In examining personality theories many forms of classification are possible. One way would be simply to discard those theories that are partial, incomplete, inchoate. This is the case with many of them. The others remaining can be examined in terms of whether they are exclusively deterministic, whether the determinism is biological, environmental or a combination of both. In effect, we find that very few personality theories are complete.

Of these we find that most of the theories that are not deterministic are really neo-Adlerian. Thus, quite definitely, both Harry Stack Sullivan's theory and Karen Horney's theory are much more in line with Adler than with Freud. The same is true with later systems: Albert Ellis's Rational–Emotive theory is a variation of Adler, as is Eric Berne's Transactional Analysis, and as is William Glasser's Reality Therapy (Roszanofsky, 1974). From my point of view all of these theories are correct—but partial. They have not as yet attained completeness, and it is my opinion that eventually they will overlap completely with Adlerian psychology as they mature.

It is my personal reaction, based on a rather detailed study of most of the current personality theories (Corsini & Marsella, 1983) that the Individual Psychology personality theory of Alfred Adler is the most complete and the most satisfying of theories; yet even though its propositions, as discussed above, are relatively simple, the system is not well known or at best imperfectly known. It is hoped that the first complete text on Individual Psychology in English (Manaster & Corsini, 1982) will help remedy this misunderstanding.

Comparisons with Other Theories

Naturally, those who accept the Adlerian point of view see those who disagree, such as the psychoanalysts with their deterministic, biologically oriented instinct system, as having essentially incorrect positions, while they also view as essentially incorrect those who take a deterministic view based on past history, such as those with a behaviorist position. Those views that accord with Adler's position—Karen Horney, Harry Stack Sullivan, Albert Ellis, Rollo May, Abraham Maslow—are seen as being neo-Adlerians, and some of them as crypto-Adlerians, taking essentially the same view as did Alfred Adler, but not giving him credit.

Adlerians regard themselves as having a commonsense point of view, and regard as plain foolishness such concepts as the Oedipus complex, or the notion that creativity is a function of one's past experiences. We consider that humans are certainly different from machines, and that any purely physical theory is inapplicable to humans; and we even consider that we are so different from the lower animals quantitatively that we are qualitatively different as well. Do animals plan? Are they aware of their mortality? Do they have a sense of humor? Are they socially concerned with one another? Will they sacrifice themselves willingly for others? We view any so-called scientific position based on either machines or on the lower animals as unscientific. Humans may have come from a common source, as have the lemurs, but we are qualitatively different from them in the important psychological variables.

THERAPY

It has already been mentioned that, from the point of view of the Adlerian, the theory/philosophy is seamless, and consequently all ameliorative treatment efforts can be seen as therapy. In "Counseling and Psychotherapy" (Corsini, 1968) it is pointed out that these two approaches differ only quantitatively. From the commonsense point of view, counseling is advice-giving for simple circumscribed problems, while psychotherapy is changing a person's view of self and others, thus changing one's life-style. In this chapter we shall label all interventions as therapy, and consider them in terms of the types of problems handled, simple and complex, surface and deep.

Theory

Adlerians believe that the main aim of individuals is to belong, to find a place in society. This strong social urge is the main goal that people have, and to achieve this aim what is called for is a sense of the group, a desire to be a working part of the society, or what we call *Social Interest*. Those who are maladjusted fall into two large groups: those who just happen to be ignorant of proper ways of operating and those who know what to do but are discouraged. The first group comes for counseling, the second for therapy.

Another basic point is that there is a tendency to health in the individual, and that if the person is given an opportunity to view self and others rationally, he or she will make good decisions. This goodwill comes out of the basic desire to belong, the existence of social interest. However, in most cases of problems, the individual tends to be discouraged, and this fundamental discouragement is the major problem to be handled.

Consequently, in the case of people who simply are ignorant, they need to be given instructions to do things differently. However, we know that people are perverse and will want to continue along unsuccessful ways if they have been operating along these ways for a long time.

Let us begin with a relatively simple example of what happened in a particular session in an Adlerian family counseling group.

The mother of six children, ages ranging from 4 to 14, stated that she had a major problem in her family of getting her children to keep their rooms neat, to make their beds, and so forth. She admitted that her techniques of complaining, nagging, punishing, and rewarding had been so far unsuccessful. After getting more data, the counselor went to the blackboard and made the following notations checking their accuracy with the mother.

Approximate number of "naggings" on this matter:

Daily	12
Weekly	84
Annually	4,000
Past 10 years	35,000
Next 10 years	50,000
Total	85,000

The counselor pointed out that so far 35,000 naggings had not succeeded and that if she continued along her ways in the same fashion until all her children were grown up and out of the house, that she would have to do some 50,000 more naggings, and did she believe that if 35,000 had not done it, would another 50,000 do it?

Now what would be the common-sense method of dealing with such a problem? Keep in mind that the counselor is not only concerned with helping that mother but also others. The counselor at this point is a teacher. How can he or she deal best with a group of people with similar problems?

The answer is to give basic information (Corsini & Rigney, 1970). And this is very important because in terms of Adlerian thinking, maladjusted people are not "sick," they are "ignorant," not knowing what to do. The Adlerian views counseling and psychotherapy as essentially a method of learning—about one's self, about others, about life.

In this particular case, the solution suggested had to do with using what Adlerians call natural consequences (Dreikurs, Gould, & Corsini, 1974), and the advice was (a) to tell the kids from now they could keep their rooms however they wished, and (b) to refuse to enter the rooms ever (except in an emergency) unless the rooms were tidy and clean.

After the usual protests on the part of the mother, she agreed to try this method, and sure enough it worked well, and she stopped her nagging and the kids began, after a delay running from several weeks to about 9 months, to take care of their own rooms, thereby learning self-confidence and responsibility.

There are two main points involved in this minor incident: first, that the counselor was not interested in learning about the history of the situation, the "why" of the mother's behavior. He was only interested in finding a workable solution. Armed with the concepts of logical and natural consequences, he could find a better solution in a short time. There was no question of sickness or maladjustment or abnormality: simply a search for a solution.

Process

The example just given illustrates by example the essential process of Adlerian group procedures: the use of logic, common sense, confrontation, explanation, direction. We have no special process: Adlerians have no special techniques that are Adlerian in the sense that the couch and free association is Freudian or pounding pillows is Gestalt or acting out is Psychodrama. We use all of these techniques if we think that they will work and if we think that they apply, but the general process is *assessment, preparation, beginning.*

Assessment

Adlerians take two positions, both quite flexible, about assessment relative to psychotherapy. The first is that in some cases no assessment is necessary, although some sensitivity as to how to deal with any specific case is called for. Thus, I have advised perhaps 100 parents about the issue of giving children their rooms, and each time that this was done there were variations depending on the clients, the size of the group (if indeed there was a group), the resistance of clients, their intelligence, and their degree of openness. But the advice is the same in the long run. However, during the process of meeting people and during the process of participation, any therapist sizes up the people. In a simple counseling-type case of this sort, no in-depth evaluation is considered necessary.

However, in the case of an individual who comes in for treatment and who is first seen in individual therapy and then later is to enter the group, some Adlerians, and I am one of them, will generally do what we call a *life-style assessment.*

The assessment is not only of the individual in terms of his or her life-style, but also the suitability of the individual for the group. This is a highly subjective matter, and on the basis of my own experience, I generally prefer groups to be more or less homogeneous, relative to three factors: (a) age, (b) social level, and (c) intelligence. That is to say, I would not want teenagers in a therapy group with mature adults; I would not want people who are wealthy with people on welfare; and I would not want persons too disparate in education, sophistication, and background. My experience is that homogeneity is called for with regard to these demographic factors, irrespective of the problems of the individuals or their personal peculiarities. So, social homogeneity and personality variability are fine. I realize that others, including Adlerians, may want personality homogeneity (such as all members suffering from depression) and social variability (mixing college professors and retarded paupers) in the same group. But, again, we run into the same situation discussed before; Adlerians have no guidelines other than their experience. Their unity lies in theory, not practice. Consequently, the material above reflects my own experience.

Preparation

Before a person enters a group, I attempt to explain the purpose of suggesting the group, and, if the group is already established, or if I know who is to be in it, then I will generally inform the person of the group's composition, saying something like this: "Well, Jim is a man of about 30, a printer, married, and has had 2 years of college; George is highly overweight, is a building manager, and is in a somewhat difficult marital situation. . . ." I would, of course, answer any questions, and if I have any belief that he or she is likely to be scared, would suggest that he try several sessions before coming to any conclusions about the suitability of the group.

Beginning

When beginning a session, it is my general practice as a group therapist (and, again, I want to insist that this has nothing to do with how Adlerians do group therapy, but rather how I as an Adlerian do it), to make some minor statements, after which I attempt to generate a hiatus, a period of embarrassment or confusion, by refusing to participate, in order to see how the group operates: who takes over, how people react to me, what they ask, how they react. I may refuse to answer questions, doing so in a pleasant manner, shaking my head with a smile, and I notice how the different people react to this treatment.

Having been infected—according to my Adlerian teacher, Rudolf Dreikurs—by my Rogerian training, my tendency is to avoid becoming the controller, which is not what I avoid when I do counseling. Adlerians see counseling and psychotherapy as related but quite different processes, and in group therapy I am much more nondirective than the typical Adlerian.

I try to give people, at least in the beginning, a lot of room in which to move around, so that I can see how they tend to operate in strange situations, and, indeed, this is a kind of evaluation which gives me greater understanding of them and also them of each other.

Mechanisms

Research (Corsini, 1957; Corsini & Rosenberg, 1955) based on 300 articles on group psychotherapy, revealed that group therapists attributed "cure" or "correction" or "change" to a total of 166 "mechanisms." Using a system of clinical cluster analysis, we found that these mechanisms fell into three groups: *cognition, emotions,* and *behavior.* Below are the names and the groupings of these mechanisms.

Cognition	Behavior	Emotions
spectator therapy	reality testing	acceptance
universalization	ventilation	altruism
intellectualization	interaction	transference

Let us now examine how these nine mechanisms are used. These mechanisms are considered universal and apply not only to groups run by Adlerians, but to all therapeutic groups.

Spectator Therapy

Essentially, this means that one client or patient in a group learns from other patients through watching and listening. In acting as a group therapist, the therapist may attempt to manipulate people to discuss problems and solutions that the therapist thinks may generate spectator therapy in a particular member or members of the group.

Universalization

Spectator therapy and other interactions in the group may lead to a kind of "ah-ha" phenomenon of universalization, the understanding that others have the same kind of problems as oneself. This can be a powerful curative force.

Intellectualization

Adlerian psychology is essentially cognitive, and we believe that true cure or improvement does not occur until there is understanding. This mechanism is facilitated by interpretation by the therapist and by a "tying-up process" such as represented by the statement: "You tell us that your fiancee gave up on you, that you have been found unsatisfactory on your job, that your parents are just angry with you, and in this particular group the various members have just complained about you. Apparently, you have the talent of turning people off. Can you find anything that you do which has generated this negative feeling on the part of practically everyone?"

Acceptance

The person who comes to therapy often has poor self-acceptance, generally is rejected by others, and feels alone and unloved. In the therapy group if a person can come to understand that there is acceptance of himself or herself despite one's having unpleasant ways, that there is a difference between disliking the behavior and liking the person, this feeling of acceptance can be a heartening experience, and gives one courage to go on. The therapist helps generate this by taking an understanding and accepting attitude which others in the group are likely to pick up.

Altruism

Whenever a person gives of self to others, spending time, showing interest, expressing concern, this is an example of altruism, and the effect of this is to help the giver and the receiver. The therapist him- or herself attempts to generate this by a loving concerned attitude, and perhaps by pointing out to resistant members how others are showing this concern.

Transference

This term as used by Adlerians is quite different from the concept as identified by Freudians. We mean by it essentially a feeling of community, an *esprit de corps,* a strong bond between members who have worked and suffered together, based on mutuality of interests and deep understanding and acceptance. The therapist generates this feeling by showing warmth and understanding, which is picked up by others in the group.

Reality Testing

Group members frequently have basic misconceptions, sometimes quite bizarre. Frequently, they have an *idée fixe* which nothing can dislodge, such as being quite unattractive. The group can be a testing ground. A therapist may say something and the client is quite likely to reject the statement as untrue, but is much more likely to accept it if the statement is made by a member of the group, or by all. So, if the entire group confronts the client on some misconception, the client is highly likely to change his or her opinion.

Ventilation

Although Adlerians do not believe too much in the curative value of a good cry, or an extreme expression of feelings as demonstrated in, for example, Scream Therapy, nevertheless, because we see it as an epiphenomenon, such emotionalism is a sign of progress, in that the person has cognitive awareness and the ventilation comes along with the new information. In view of this, a therapist may engender emotionalism to help generate a release of tension.

Interaction

The last of these mechanisms only refers to the curative factor of relationships between people, and the therapist uses this mechanism to generate openness and discussions between the members in whatever way seems best, including asking questions, telling stories, and giving personal anecdotes.

A good group therapist will understand the power of these nine mechanisms and will employ them consciously but in a natural manner.

PRACTICE

Problems

Practically any presenting problem or problem of personality can be handled by the group method as well as, and in some instances better than, by the individual method. Advantages of the group method are quite clear for delinquents, where there is a basic hostility to the therapist; or in oppressed groups such as alcoholics, drug addicts, or homosexuals, people who feel as a group inferior to others because they are likely not to relate on the basis of equality to a person whom they see outside of their group; at the same time they are not likely to accept someone within their group. If the group is indigenous, such as Alcoholics Anonymous, it can operate as a peer group.

A problem of management has to do with gaining the confidence of the group. I have run at least 100 therapy groups, and I think I found an inability on my part to establish a real group in about three or four instances. The most evident failure was with a group of passive aggressive adolescents, all referred to the group by their parents. After struggling with this group for several months, and unable to get anywhere with them, I let this be known to other therapists at the Alfred Adler Institute of Chicago, and several other therapists came in with me and later attempted on their own to establish the necessary conditions of communication for a therapy group, and everyone failed. The lesson which we all must learn over and over again is that you can lead a horse to water but you cannot make him float on his back!

That is to say, proper preparation and proper selection is important. In the case above, the group was established by fiat by someone, youths were recruited, they came in with hostility, and thereafter resisted all attempts to get them to participate in any meaningful way. It was a salutary experience for all of us. In my case, I was considered the group specialist and when I finally asked for help, I was embarrassed. Filled with confidence that they could succeed where I could not, my various colleagues came in to observe, or to participate, or even to take over, and each was as unsuccessful as I had been. The answer is that one must take a humble attitude, and should make selections carefully, or there should be preparations. Had there been several acting-out, "psychopathic" youngsters in the group, they might have mounted an attack on me, which would have been easily dealt with, but passive-aggressive people are practically impossible to handle.

Evaluation

Under this heading I will attempt to suggest how to deal with the problem of selection, and once again, I wish to say that this is not an Adlerian problem or solution, but one that any therapist has to face who works in the group process. As mentioned earlier, I try to have homogeneity with respect to age, intelligence, and social status, but try to have diversity in all other respects, including diagnostic problems. As mentioned above regarding the passive-aggressive youths, I thought that if we had had some acting-out, overtly hostile youths we would have done much better.

In discussing entering a group with any client, I attempt to explain the procedures (just talking for the most part), the size of the group (about six to eight people), the composition of the group (here I would give a thumbnail sketch of the other people discussing only demographic data, and nothing too "personal"), and any other special consideration. I might ask the person to not decide after one or two sessions but to wait for about four sessions before making up his or her mind whether to stay or to go. If there is extreme resistance or hostility to the concept of the group, I will not press the client, but suggest that we should wait until he or she is ready.

It is my custom to have constant evaluation, stopping during a session to ask: "How are we doing?" In one form of what I call *Psychodramatic Group Therapy* (Corsini, 1957), the treatment modality consisted of seven sessions, during which time psychodrama was employed, and during which time I was extremely active setting up situations, directing them, interpreting them (with Adlerian interpretations, naturally), and otherwise "running" the group. However, on the eighth session, we routinely had a relaxation session run on purely egalitarian lines, with no one in charge, with me no longer being the leader, but a participant. I strongly suggested that the major purpose of that session was to discuss me and the prior sessions and the methodology, and I endeavored to say as little as possible, avoiding taking the position of the authority in that group. After several cycles, the group members took advantage of the sessions to discuss the theory and practice of psychotherapy, to evaluate each other and me, and to prepare for a new round of seven sessions.

Treatment

There is no one method of treatment characteristic of all Adlerians. We are united in our philosophy of equality and our theory of personality development, growth, maintenance and change (see H. L. Ansbacher, 1983; G. Manaster & R. J. Corsini, 1982; H. H. Mosak, 1983) but are heterodox with respect to procedures. What I can do is describe how some Adlerians work, and even this does not help much because those who work in this way will use other methodologies as well.

Therapist A essentially interviews one client in front of the group and does the equivalent of individual therapy with that client, so that the greater part of the session (which ordinarily runs for 90 minutes) will be a back-and-forth interaction between the client and the therapist. This might be the whole session. What is going on then, if one goes back to the nine mechanisms listed on page 15, is essentially a cognitive interaction between the two. The other clients are learning through spectator therapy, and so forth. Then, at the next session, the interaction may be with another client. Essentially, the therapist comes in with a readiness to interact with any single client and will not want to be interrupted. He or she takes the position that, by operating in this manner, both the client dealt with and those listening will learn. It is the clients' responsibility to ask for the session.

Therapist B operates more or less in the same fashion, but will try to apportion time more or less equally to the various members, turning from X to Y, saying, "And now, let us see what is going on with you?" This may run for a few minutes to perhaps 30 minutes, and when the therapist believes that it is time to change, he or she will move over to another.

Therapist C seeks to interview an individual until he or she runs into an impasse, and then will turn to the group and discuss the impasse with them, attempting to get the group to unite and then to speak out, hoping that the rest of the group will see things his or her way and thus help the former interviewee to see things "properly." This person operates in a confrontive manner, more or less in the style of Albert Ellis (1962).

Therapist D likes to find some theoretical problem and likes to explain the problem, such as: "Here we have M who informs us that she has strong feelings of hostility to her parents. I don't know her parents nor whether I think she is justified in her judgments. But I wonder who can discuss the problem of the origins of hostility against parents?" And so her sessions tend to be philosophical and theoretical rather than personal.

Therapist E tends to like to upset the group, leaping from topic to topic, person to person, technique to technique, and likes to needle the group members, constantly attempting to alternately provoke and calm them, seeking emotionalism.

Therapist F is an encourager, and keeps attempting to develop feelings in the group members of self-confidence and self-worth. One technique likely used would be: "Look at each person and tell everyone in turn what you like about him or her." Therapist G, on the other hand, is more likely to say: "Look at each person and tell him or her what you dislike about him or her" or more likely to have them go over dislikes and then likes.

But surely the reader may be interested in what Adlerian therapists have in common in their procedures? Some of these features may be found in other group therapists, but some may be unique to Adlerians.

Equality

Even if the therapist takes an authoritarian position, thinking perhaps: "I am the doctor, and I know what I am doing and so I should run the show," nevertheless, an Adlerian group is always fundamentally democratic. Now this is not a function of the personality of the therapist alone. Thus, a Gestalt therapist may take on the mien of a democrat in the group or may take an authoritarian stance, depending on his or her personality and values, but an Adlerian could not shout down a person, demand something, or otherwise put down a client. We are not especially saying that other systems are autocratic, but rather Adlerians, as a function of their philosophy, are democratic.

Teaching

Adlerian therapists view themselves as teachers, because therapy is a cognitive function. We do not take a sickness point of view relative to clients, but rather an ignorance point of view, saying that people in trouble are misinformed, rather than ill. Our job is to make people see the way things are, to adjust their thinking, to see their situation in a different light.

An example is called for: A male client in a group stated that he was constantly being frustrated in his attempts to be considerate. He told the story of trying to start a parlor game at the home of some friends, but that some of the people in the group were resistant and the hosts were rude, interrupting him while he was explaining the game.

He finished and leaned back, satisfied that he had given evidence that people mistreated him.

"It seems to me," said the therapist, "that even though you are a guest in that house, you intend to run things."

This point hit home; the client could see the basic error he was making in thinking that he was helping to generate unity although in reality he was trying to dominate the others.

Openness

Adlerians do not look for confessions. They have normal interest in interesting stories that people tell, but what they really want is discussions about important things. And the important things to Adlerians are what are known as "basic mistakes" and "private logic." Take the case just discussed; the private logic of this person might be stated as: "When things are not going well, I should take charge." He saw the party was not progressing according to his views, and so took charge without permission. And his private logic might be, "If I don't take charge, someone else will, and I will not like that." And so with both of these concepts firmly imbedded in his mind, at the first opportunity he rushes forward to take charge, and if someone thwarts him, he sees this as evidence of unfairness.

Therefore, openness is not related to horror tales or confessions of "sins," but rather, the willingness to examine what is even more central, more sensitive, and potentially more hurtful: a close examination of one's viewpoints.

Courage

According to Harold Mosak (1983) the main function of an Adlerian psychotherapist is to encourage the client, who typically is discouraged, viewing life through dark glasses and seeing himself or herself in a distorted mirror. The therapist first wants to give the client better self-knowledge, but that would be an exercise in futility if the end result were only insight. Now, what is called for is action, appropriate action; but for this to be achieved, there has to be a decision to act differently, to think differently, and so forth. Just as a child who is capable of learning to swim may be afraid to go in the water in the first place, and then once in the water may be afraid to put his head under water and so forth, so too the person in Adlerian therapy, once he or she sees things differently, is led to do something about it; otherwise, all we have is insight, which means nothing much unless there is accompanying action and resulting feelings of success.

An example may be given: J believed that he was unattractive, not only in appearance, but in his style of interaction with other people. As a result of the group influence, he changed his opinion (he said) and came to the opinion that he was really a generally attractive person. Now that he had said this, he was satisfied, but not the therapist, who next encouraged him to find ways to prove this. And a new struggle started, ending with suggestions from the group as to what he could do. It turned out that he was tremendously attracted to a woman but had always felt unable even to talk to her much less ask for a date. As a result of further discussions and role playing he finally got courage to ask her for a date, and lo—she accepted happily, and during the date confessed to him that she had been attracted to him, and had wanted him to ask her for a date, but had not had the courage herself to ask him.

Consequently, the Adlerian therapist believes it is not enough to get some-one to see things differently (his or her primary task, since Adlerian psycho-therapy is primarily cognitive), but how to screw up the person's courage to actually begin to act more in line with the new understanding.

With regard to the emotions, Adlerians view them as epiphenomena, the result of but not the cause of important changes. That is, one feels good if one does good; and not the other way around. Thus, if a person gets a new and good idea about self, an insight, this is a cognitive gain, and the person tends to feel good, having learned something. If one now does something good, such as take a chance when one was previously afraid, now one feels good because one had the courage. And, of course, if things work out well, then one feels good because of the result. But these emotions are always seen as results of behavior and consequently are epiphenomena, accompanying but not really contributing to any progress.

This does not mean that Adlerians dismiss emotions as unimportant; in-deed, they are the most important thing that we strive for, to make people happy, but we see the process as first calling for new thinking, then new actions, and finally as a result, new feelings.

Adlerians see themselves as teachers more than as healers. We take the position that a person in trouble is not sick, but misguided. We try to (a) put mirrors in front of individuals so that they can see themselves correctly, and (b) put glasses on all the individuals so that they can see more clearly what is going on.

For example, at the present time in an Adlerian therapy group that I am running, there is one young man who is very bright, attractive in appearance, a pleasant person with high standards, but who has a most incorrect and dis-torted sense of self and others. I happen to know his family quite well, and can understand how he came to have these incorrect impressions of self. My prob-lem as a therapist is how to get him to trust me, and how to get him to see himself in a more correct manner. I do not want to scare him off, because he is very sensitive; and I cannot contradict his opinions, which he holds strongly. I decide, as a procedure, to see how he fitted in the group, and as I suspected he took a negative attitude toward himself and toward the other group members, arriving at the meetings with a characteristic scowl on his face. I believe that the correct thing for him to do is to make friends, but he has never had a friend. In his mid 20s, most other men of his age have girlfriends and have frequent sex. He serves himself in this area, but has conflicts about masturbation, because he is quite religious.

Consequently, as a cognitive therapist, my first task is to get him to change his attitudes about himself relative to his acceptability and relative to his sexual behavior. People tend to maintain their ideas about self, others, and about right and wrong despite contradictory evidence and despite statements of authorities. I am well aware of the stronger effect of the group. I am also aware that I must not push these matters too hard or too quickly, because I may scare him off.

The process will probably work as follows: At first he will feel intimidated by others, will retreat from contact, will be superficial. Others, bolder, will take over, and he will allow them. He will make cautious overtures, safe entries, and as time goes on and he begins to feel more comfortable through the various mechanisms discussed earlier, he will begin to have courage to speak his mind, and give us a chance to show our acceptance of him. Then will come the next phase: actual operations in the real world. Here he may need some encouragement from others in the group. One important technique is to allow the person to practice through the use of psychodrama. This will encourage him. Then, some "homework" may be prescribed, but carefully, so that he will not be discouraged by failure. But before he goes out to practice in the real world he will be informed that the only failure would be a refusal to try. If he succeeds in his endeavors, then he comes to the end of the first loop: the emotional satisfaction of success. We now start another loop: cognition—conation—affection. That is to say, first thinking, then action, and then feelings. First he has to understand and get a new view of life, then he has to act in new and more appropriate and more successful ways, and then he will have good feelings about himself. In the beginning was the thought . . . then the action . . . and then the feeling. Adlerians are concerned with the end product: greater self-acceptance, greater pleasure in life, greater happiness. But we see the process of therapy as first changing a person's thinking so that he or she will then change a behavior, and then if the behavior is correct there will be greater satisfaction.

We refer back to the earlier, simpler case of the mother with the children and her concern about their rooms. At the time of therapy, she was frustrated and angry. She knew she was a nag but did not know what else to do. In the meantime, all of her kin were upset: her husband constantly hearing her criticizing the children and the children constantly (at least twice a day according to her own account) hearing her nag at them. She was in a real bind. She wanted a neat house and she wanted happy children and a happy home. In her attempt to teach the children neatness, the only way she saw of doing it was by preaching to them, and over the many years this is precisely what she did. The fact that this did not work did not stop her. Had she stopped, she would have considered this evidence to all, including her children, that she was a bad mother. And so she was condemned, as it were, to nagging her children, failing to get them to learn the good habit of being neat, and generating a negative atmosphere in the family.

The counselor could see all this, and had a solution based on a natural consequences: let the kids alone, admit failure, let the rooms get really bad until the children eventually learn on their own to take responsibility. The natural argument that many parents give, because they do not trust their children, is that perhaps the children will never learn; perhaps they and their friends will think that the mother just doesn't care; perhaps things will get so unpleasant that others will be disturbed . . . and never will anything succeed. At this point theory and experience enter the picture: the experienced Adlerian knows that, in every single case, if the parents really follow the advice, and have the courage to do so, and will wait patiently, eventually the child will clean up by himself or herself. In terms of my own experience in advising several hundred parents on this very point, in no case did a child last longer than 9 months before finally taking charge of a particular room.

This understanding of human behavior and the comprehension of natural and logical consequences and the creative use of such functions is what makes a good counselor. Probably most people in doing psychotherapy do make use of these principles but are not aware, of this.

The courage that the therapist must call on is belief in his or her own theory and experience. Theory serves as a kind of map. If I come to a crossroads and do not know whether to turn left or right and I am fairly certain that I should turn left, and if I consult a map which indicates I turn right, then if I trust the map more than my own judgment, I turn right; if the map says at the end of Main Street when it hits State Street that Broadway is to the right, then I turn right even if a passenger assures me that left is the right direction.

Every therapist comes to some point where he or she must fly by the seat of the pants, as it were, without a guide from experience; but from these experiences comes the courage to trust one's theory.

Management

Again, Adlerians are united only in theory; they differ in almost every other respect. Some are nondirective, some are directive; some use groups and some do not; some do a lot of talking and some do very little; some do group work only after individual work, some work the other way; some like to start off with a life-style analysis, and some do not. In other words, there is diversity in all respects except in theory, and I believe that the amount of differentiation is greater among Adlerians than in any of the other well-established systems of psychotherapy.

Therefore in this section, I must simply explain how the relatively few people that I know who are Adlerians manage their groups. I shall attempt this by explaining a number of different kinds of therapy groups that Adlerians have, and how they run them.

Family Therapy

From the point of view of an Adlerian, the best method of doing family therapy is to have every one of the family in individual therapy, each with a different therapist, and periodically every person and every therapist will meet with still another therapist. Let us take the relatively simple case of a mother, a father, and an adolescent child. Let us assume that originally, the parents appeared separately to discuss their child's problems, and that the therapist came to the conclusion that at the next interview both parents and the child should be present. Let us assume that there were a lot of charges and countercharges, and that this therapist came to the conclusion that the best way to operate was to have each of the three meet with still another therapist (or, if the Adlerian therapist were a one-person practitioner, he or she would see them independently). But for the purpose of explaining the most satisfactory method of operating, let us assume that this is a group practice, and we now have Therapist 1, clients A, B, C, and therapists 2, 3, 4. And let us assume that, after the initial two sessions, therapists 2, 3, and 4 had two to three meetings with each parent and with the child. Now, all seven people are in one room.

The senior therapist (Therapist 1) now runs the session, and he or she asks each person in turn, perhaps in terms of volunteering, to report results or conclusions. I might begin with the therapists and then ask the clients; another Adlerian might begin the other way. It is a matter of style or preference or whatever may lead the senior therapist to work one way rather than another. After everyone has made a statement or given a report, the senior therapist is likely to start asking questions to get clarifications, and will interview in front of the others the various therapists and clients. They will be given a chance to comment, but always addressing the "chair" as it were, with the therapists interacting, if need be, with their own clients. Following all this, the senior therapist may come to some conclusion, ask if there is agreement and may send everyone back for more work, or may call another supergroup session if it seems indicated, and if it is approved by all.

Multiple Therapy

Still another kind of group approach used by Adlerians, pioneered by Rudolf Dreikurs (1952) is multiple therapy, which can have variations in group practice, but the usual practice is the following: The "senior" therapist[1] sees the client first, and assigns the client to another therapist to do a personality

---

[1]The term "senior" is in quotes to illustrate only that this is the title generally given to the person who plays that role. If the group practice consists of two people, each can play the role of senior at various times.

profile, called a life-style analysis (Eckstein, Baruth, & Mahrer, 1975; Manaster & Corsini, 1982). This analysis, which is a personality profile, usually gives a short description of the person, a guess as to how the person got to be as he or she is seen, the person's private logic, the person's basic mistakes, and also the person's strengths. The analysis is presented to the senior therapist in the presence of the client. The senior therapist now discusses the findings with both the primary therapist and with the client, and gives his opinions and suggestions for further study and development. The client and the primary therapist meet again for three or four sessions and come back to report to the senior therapist. One variation is when the life-style materials are presented to the senior therapist, who in turn dictates the life-style report, so that the primary therapist does not play as decisive a role in the diagnostic aspect. This variation is usually done when the primary therapist is an intern learning this form of therapy. But such "multiple" meetings occur regardless of need, that is, meetings with the senior therapist at stated intervals, usually every third or fourth visit.

Circular Discussional Groups

These are the most common type of therapy groups of any particular orientation, and the management is no different from any other form of group therapy. What is different, of course, is the type of interpretations made. Some therapists will in essence conduct an individual therapy session with one client while others look on; others will tend to shift attention from one client to another. Some will encourage group discussions between the members; some will not. However, in an Adlerian group, the general theme is to gain greater understanding, then greater courage, then on to improved behavior, which should result in better feelings.

Marriage Groups

Adlerians like to do marriage counseling in groups (Deutsch, 1967). The most usual method is to run a straight circular discussional group; however, some interesting variations have been attempted. One of them calls for the couple being discussed to sit outside the group, facing outwards, so situated that they can not see each other nor see the rest of the group. This step usually takes place after all people in the group know each other well, and the couple being discussed are volunteers. The discussion about them may well take half the usual 90 minutes of the session, and then they two can reenter the group and participate.

Another variation is to have them role-play several scenes, and then have others repeat the scene, using the so-called mirror technique. This can be quite dramatic. Adeline Starr in her *Rehearsal for Living* (1977) explicates how psychodrama can be employed for such purposes.

Family Education Centers

Still another type of Adlerian therapy group is a meeting of parents who are ostensibly there to learn about better methods of dealing with childrens' specific problems. Adlerians have concentrated on family education. Among the better known Adlerian books are *Children, the Challenge,* by Rudolf Dreikurs and Vickie Soltz (1964); *Raising a Responsible Child,* by Donald Dinkmeyer and Gary McKay (1973); and *The Practical Parent,* by Raymond Corsini and Genevieve Painter (1975). The best source for information about how such centers run is a book edited by Dreikurs, Corsini, Lowe, and Sonstegard (1959).

In this form of group counseling, children remain in a playroom during the sessions, until they are called to be interviewed in front of the group. Parents to be counseled are asked to attend at least three sessions, to learn how the group operates, before they are actually counseled. Counseling is done in front of a group, and the process usually consists of the therapist or counselor asking the parents to explain why they are there, and then, after they explain their difficulties with their child or children, they are asked to tell what they have tried to do to improve the situation. Next, the playroom worker who has observed the children for several sessions usually comes in and reports to the group what he or she has observed. Then, the child or children are brought in and are interviewed by the counselor. If anyone in the audience wishes to ask any questions, they must ask the counselor, who in turn—if he agrees that the question should be asked—asks the children. Parents usually are not in the room at the time their children are interviewed, but they may remain if they wish. Then the parents resume their seats in the front of the room, and the counselor now throws the meeting open to all present, asking them for any comments or opinions. As the final step, the counselor gives the parents very specific advice (written down by a secretary known as the *recorder*) relating to the specific problems (such as the one discussed relative to keeping one's room clean).

This kind of meeting is not as deep as the others, and is really more counseling than psychotherapy in the usual sense. However, if we assume that the two processes are essentially identical, with the differences being quantitative rather than qualitative (Corsini, 1968), this can be seen as group therapy, but certainly a group process of therapeutic value to parents, some of whom change enormously.

A by-product of this kind of group is one called a Mothers' Study Group or even a Mothers' Therapy Group. The first kind of group usually consists of mothers who meet to discuss a book (in the manner of the Great Books program); and the second kind of group usually consists of mothers who find themselves in the peculiar position of agreeing with the advice given in the Family Education Center, but being unable to follow it.

There are three other kinds of groups, Adlerian in nature, that should be mentioned. The first is the Family Council (Corsini & Rigney, 1970; Dreikurs, Gould, & Corsini, 1974), which takes place in the home. It is essentially a home project, taking place once a week for about 30 minutes, during which time the parents and the children meet as equals, with rotating chairpersons to discuss and settle family problems. The second is the Class Council (Grunwald, 1969) in which a teacher and her class stop their proceedings to discuss problems relating to the class as a whole. The third is the Marriage Conference (Corsini, 1967; Phillips & Corsini, 1982), an artificial method of communication, designed for married couples, which consists of a set of four sessions. In these, the couple meets periodically for 1 hour, one person speaking without interruption for a half hour, the other then speaking without interruption for 30 minutes, and without any discussion between the four sessions.

Primary Relationship Therapy

During the course of this chapter, I have discussed how Adlerians vary in their methodologies. I shall give one example only of a very unusual technique developed by one of my former students, Robert Postel, and which is used by among others, Genevieve Painter, my coauthor on the *Practical Parent*. In an exposition of this method which Painter coauthored with Sally Vernon (1981) these authors call it a re-parenting form of therapy for people who were, or thought they were, rejected by their parents, or who lost their parents early in life. Postel, an Adlerian, assumed that the neglected child (for whom this system is specifically designed) has a life-style not adequate for success in life. These neglected children, even as adults, feel deprived and find it difficult to make good relationships with others. Essentially, the therapist attempts to act the role of a good parent, and there may be two therapists, one playing the role of the father and one the role of the mother. The therapist-parent and the patient-child may play games, the "parent" may cuddle the "child," feed him or her, and so forth, with the intention of going through missing stages. This system usually starts with individual diagnostic sessions and then proceeds to group sessions.

APPLICATION

Group Selection and Composition

There is no Adlerian way of selecting people for groups, and composition of the groups will vary from therapist to therapist. We simply have no criteria. What I have said before applies for this section: I can only speak for myself as an Adlerian who does group therapy. Generally, I like diversity of problems and uniformity only of age, intelligence levels, and social levels, because these three permit maximum communication between the individuals. However, if one has a special notion within the field, as for example, Adlerians who do Primary Relationship Therapy, then of course the therapist would only select people who appear to need this particular form of therapy.

Group Setting

The important thing in group therapy is privacy. If one can hear extraneous noises, such as people talking, this apparent invasion of privacy can hinder interaction. The same applies for visual disturbances. If one can see others moving about, as through a window, there is a feeling of intrusion. Consequently, noise and sight pollution are to be avoided as much as possible. In doing a group, comfortable chairs are important, and also of value is a room that conveys the sense of privacy and ease. In general, the less in the way of decorations, the better. I would avoid photographs and even art on the walls, but natural objects such as plants would be desirable. The size of the room is important. I would like, everything else constant, a fairly small room, which can give a sense of intimacy. The acoustics of a room and the lighting can be important. The acoustics should be such that words carry easily and the lighting should be intermediate, neither dim nor harsh.

No special equipment is ever called for in doing Adlerian group therapy or group counseling, although some Adlerians may have the desire for soft music, or perhaps a blackboard. Generally speaking, however, all we want is privacy and comfort, nothing else is usually called for.

Individual Education

This will probably be the single most important section in this chapter, because it will tie together everything relative to the Adlerian use of groups, and will introduce a grand concept of milieu psychotherapy, as well as bringing together Adlerian theory and practice in a school situation.

In an Individual Education school (Corsini, 1977, 1979; Krebs, 1982; Pratt & Mastroianni, 1981; Whittington, 1981) run according to Adlerian principles, there exist four types of "therapeutic" groups. The reason for putting the quotation marks around the word *therapeutic* is because of the tremendous sensitivity, based on incorrect assumptions, on the part of school people about psychotherapy. However, this is no problem for Adlerians, who see psychotherapy simply as a form of learning; following the educational rather than the medical model, seeing deviations and maladjustments as mistakes in learning rather than sicknesses.

The four types of groups are:

1. *Milieu group.* The whole school runs according to the philosophy and principles of Individual Education, and all parties involved in the school, including the principal and her or his staff, the faculty, the parents and the children, operate relative to the purpose and functions of the school. Consequently, using the word properly, the whole school becomes a therapeutic environment.

2. *Homerooms.* A fairly unique aspect of Individual Education is the homeroom. In each homeroom is a faculty member known as the teacher-advisor, who plays the role of an older equal in that room. The children in the room select their teacher-advisor from all faculty members, and each member

so selected may accept the child to be in the homeroom, which occurs the first and the last period of the day. The purpose of the homeroom is to learn socialization, which, in essence, means learning how to live with oneself and with others.

Note, however, this special feature: the child selects a teacher-advisor in the same sense that adults select their doctors or lawyers; however, the teacher has the option to accept the child or not. In the homeroom the adults act as equals, and the purpose of the homeroom is to learn socialization.

The size of the membership in the homeroom will generally be equal to the student–teacher ratio, and this ordinarily means from 20 to 30 students per homeroom, depending on that school's student–teacher ratio.

3. *Small groups.* In an Individual Education school every child, over time, will tend to get the homeroom teacher that he or she prefers and will also be with other students he or she prefers to be with. The teacher-advisor informs all children that small discussion groups are to be formed which are to run in size from about four to eight children, and that the children are to self-select the children they would want to be with, but all children must be from the same homeroom. The children are given sufficient time to establish subgroups for discussion purposes. These groups meet weekly for one period a day.

The teacher-advisors do not have to run their small groups according to Adlerian principles, so it is quite possible for a teacher who, let us say, is a Gestaltist to have her or his children in the small discussion groups pound on pillows or scream to the skies. Discussion groups are thus to be run in an Adlerian educational system according to the individual desires of the teacher-advisors, but the teacher-advisors are advised to be as nondirective as possible and to participate in the group on the basis of equality.

4. *School council.* A fourth unusual element of Individual Education is a school council which consists ordinarily of about 20 to 30 people, about equally divided among three primary groups, each member of the school council being elected from their constituent groups. They are *parents, students,* and *faculty.* Thus, a school council may have one-third parents, one-third children, and one-third faculty. There must never be more than 50% of members of any group and never less than 25% of any of these three groups in the school council.

The school council is an advisory group: it elects its own officers, establishes its own agenda, elects its own chairperson, and all members representing constituent groups can bring to the school council whatever is of interest and importance to their groups. If the council comes to consensus, they write a single report which they then send to the principal, the school superintendent, or the school board. They might, for example, issue a report critical of the school's bathrooms, or critical of a particular teacher, or requesting some change in the curriculum, and so forth. If there are majority and minority views, each group can prepare its own statement on the particular issue. So, it could be that from the school council the school board might get a statement signed by some members criticizing the principal of the school while some other members might defend the principal.

The first use of the school council in one school was instructive. The council consisted of 18 people: 6 parents, 6 faculty members, and 6 children. The discussion at the first session had to do with uniform clothing that the children had to wear: all boys had to have a white shirt and blue pants, and all girls a white blouse and a tartan skirt. A resolution was brought forth by one of the children urging the abolition of these uniforms. A lively debate followed, with two of the parents strongly arguing for retention of uniforms, stating that the children looked cute in their uniforms and also that distinctions between the children on an economic basis would not occur. The vote was 16 for a change and 2 against. The two reports went to the principal, who in turn reported to the school council that she would not make up her mind on the issue until a consensus was reached. At the next meeting there was a new discussion and this time the vote to recommend the abolition of uniforms was 18 to 0. This information went to the principal who made it clear that she did not have to accept this resolution, and that she decided to abolish the school rule for uniform clothing.

It should be evident at this point that Individual Education, a school system based on Adlerian principles, represents a most complex form of therapeutic group procedures.

In addition, there are two other group procedures of the Adlerian type that accompany these schools: one of them is mandatory, the other optional. The mandatory aspect is Parent Education Sessions, and these amount to a course demanded of all parents of school-entering students on basic child psychology. They consist ordinarily of five 2-hour sessions. Usually, a book such as Dreikurs and Soltz's *Children the Challenge* (1964) is employed as a text, but other books such as Gordon's *Parent Effectiveness Training* (1970) may be used. Essentially, these groups of parents listen to lectures on parenting and are given information about the unique aspects of Individual Education, such as that children have the option to go to classes or not to go during the school day. (Incidentally, various research studies on these schools show the following advantages over traditional schools: (a) children learn more academics in much less time; (b) the schools are relatively discipline-free and orderly; (c) all adults, parents, faculty, principals strongly prefer Individual Education to traditional schools; and (d) children are better prepared for life through developing better self-concepts, gaining social capacities, improving relationships with parents, and being better prepared for social living (Manaster, 1977, 1985).

The last of the many group features of Individual Education would be a Family Education Center, which would be an optional aspect. As discussed earlier, this is a form of group counseling in which parents with problems are counseled before a group.

Probably no organization is more group-oriented or has more group features of the therapeutic type than an Individual Education School, and it appears no other school system is as completely integrated with a personality theory (Ignas & Corsini, 1979).

Group Size

There is nothing especially Adlerian about group size. I have run groups of three, myself and two clients, or myself, a student or colleague and a client, and (as an Adlerian) I have run groups of 50 or more people. It could be said that I ran a group of about 2,000, because in the city of Portland, Oregon I once demonstrated, with real cases, Adlerian family counseling and Adlerian group therapy, and if one viewed the observers as participating, then we had 2,000 participants. What would make both extremes—the group of size 3 members and the group of more than 2,000—Adlerian, had to do with the interpretation, with the discussions, with the explanations, with the attempt to make the individuals see life from an Adlerian perspective. And this means going back to our theory, our unique view of life.

Therapy Frequency, Length, and Duration

There is no Adlerian viewpoint with regard to frequency, length, or duration. Generally speaking, Adlerians, who are really eclectics, having a commonsense point of view, do precisely what most other intelligent and capable group therapists do relative to these points. The typical session runs about 90 minutes, the members meet about once a week, and the duration of the groups depends on whether the group is an open or a closed group. In an open group, new members come in from time to time and old members leave from time to time, and consequently the group can go on forever, as it were. At the start there may have been six people in the group and a year later there may still be six, but none of the original six may remain and, indeed, even the therapist may have changed. In a closed group, there is usually a start and an end point, and it may run, say, for 3 months. As an Adlerian and as a group therapist, and as an innovator and experimenter, I have tried every possible variation, including marathon groups, which have run for 36 hours.

Media Usage

If by media usage is meant, what media of communication are employed?—then any answer is appropriate. For example, I have run groups in absolute darkness, in the hope that darkness may lead some people to speak freely. I have had groups operate with their backs to the center of the room, so no one could see anyone else. I have had large groups break up into small groups. I have used touching as a medium. I have experimented with every possible variation that I can think of or have heard of. In general, I find that all gimmicks are only that, and that, in the long run, plain conversation is the important medium.

I have seen Adlerians use various techniques which are quite interesting, such as having someone stand on top of a table and act as the Supreme Boss, giving orders, with everyone obeying, but this seems to me to be artificial after a while and boring with adults, and we come back to the ever-fascinating procedure of questions and answers. Actually, if truth be told, I personally prefer, as an Adlerian, to operate as a Rogerian, and to be as nondirective and as accepting as possible. I see the nondirective method as a theory-free technique which anyone can use, and the same for the so-called couch method, hypnosis, the directed interview, role playing, and behind-the-back technique.

Leader Qualifications

I am absolutely convinced that 99% of the success of a leader depends on his or her character—personality, values, judgment, intelligence—and that training has only about 1% to do with success as a group therapist. This does not mean that a therapist should not have the best training, because that extra 1% is very important. I think that degrees or books read, including this one, are of limited value, but at the same time very important. If one starts, however, with a person who does not possess the basic qualities, no amount of training will make that person a good leader; but if one has the needed basic qualities, then training can make one a superb leader.

Now, what are these basic qualities? Essentially, I would try to define the ideal leader in terms of the by now familiar three dimensions: cognition, behavior, and emotions. The ideal leader is intelligent: this means he or she has read widely and has good understanding of people, and has a sense of timing and empathy. A second quality would be the capacity to act decisively and to seize the right moment to do the right thing. The third quality has to do with a medley of such attributes as compassion, kindness, concern and perhaps, most of all, courage.

In short, the ideal group leader is a well-balanced person. As much as I believe that some theories, such as psychoanalysis, are worthless and unscientific, I think I would rather go for therapy, individual or group, to a good person who is a psychoanalyst, than to an indifferent Adlerian. In the last analysis, it is the person, not the techniques nor the theories that count. I want my therapist, or anyone I refer to, to be someone I respect, and this is much more important than the theory or philosophy of the system one represents.

Ethics

No system of psychotherapy and no set of practitioners has a monopoly on ethics. This topic reminds me of the previous one about qualifications. An Adlerian is no more and no less ethical than anyone else, and within the field there are no Adlerians known to me who are unethical, but there may be some. An unethical practitioner will not last very long, however. The reason goes back to George A. Kelly's remark that when a psychologist sizes up another person, the other person does the same to him, so what we have are two human beings each very much aware of the other, each warily examining the other, and over time making fairly good judgments about each other. Were someone unethical, this would soon come out.

Adlerians share the same code of ethics as any other practitioners or members of professional groups. As a psychologist, I accept and try to live up to the code of ethics of the American Psychological Association. Actually, I believe that professional ethics are simply common sense, and I remember that when I first read the APA list of ethics, none of it seemed startling or unacceptable.

RESEARCH

If this section proves disappointing with respect to research in the field of Adlerian group psychotherapy, the reader should be aware that I know of absolutely no really good research at all in group therapy. As a matter of fact there is no really good research in the whole field of psychotherapy. When I use the word "research," I am taking the conventional view: the application of valid and reliable tests to measure some hypothesis—such as that people show significantly better improvement as a result of participating in group psychotherapy than with no therapy at all—by some independent and disinterested person; and coming to conclusions based on facts which would be compelling to any reasonable individual.

From *Research Abstracts of Individual Psychology: Theory and Practice* (Manaster & Corsini, 1981), I quote below a number of statements about certain published research studies:

About an Adlerian Mothers' Study Group: "Results from all three groups indicate a positive change on all measures, though not all changes are significant" (Berrett, 1975, abstract in Manaster & Corsini, 1981, p. 289).

About another Adlerian Mothers' Study Group: "Results indicated significantly less authoritarian attitudes by 'Adlerian mothers' than by the other two groups" (C. W. Freeman, "Adlerian Mother Study Groups: Effects on Attitudes and Behavior," in Manaster & Corsini, 1981, p. 292).

About Adlerian Counseling with Low-achieving Students: "Results indicated that although the group receiving Adlerian counseling had significantly better grades during the summer program, this difference began to fade as the academic year progressed" (M. O. Nelson & M. H. Haberer, "Effectiveness of Adlerian Counseling with Low-achieving Students," in Manaster & Corsini, 1981, p. 296).

All these researches are highly limited, are directed by people with an investment in proving their points, use instruments of weak or unknown validity and reliability, and generally are not in any sense crucial in proving anything.

Therefore, how do I know, or how can anyone know, whether group therapy is of any value? I suggest trusting common sense of group members and the experience of clients. In my own case, I have had perhaps two or three thousand clients. I am positive that some people got no value from attending, and some got a bit of value, and some got a great deal. I don't think anyone was harmed. In addition to my direct personal experience, I have heard from a number of people, ex-patients or ex-clients, from therapists, and all kinds of case histories which tell me, unless everyone is crazy, that group therapy works well for some people.

Now, how would I justify being an Adlerian and how would I evaluate Adlerian group therapy against any other form? The answer is simple for me: Examine its theory against any other system. If it makes more sense than others, then you, the therapist, will be more happy with it than in any other system. I personally went through two other systems of therapy before settling on the Adlerian, simply because it made more sense to me. If for example, Jung's theory or Skinner's makes more sense to you, then you should operate in these theories. However, through chance most people inherit their systems, just as some people inherit their religion and their political party. I think that this is a serious mistake, but so much time, money, and prestige may be invested in one system that one may feel quite hesitant to even examine other points of view.

In summary, it is my judgment that there is no research evidence in the usual sense supporting the superiority of the Adlerian system of thought in terms of group practice; but then there is nothing in the whole pantheon of research that supports any other system, either. We just don't know.

Group Session Illustration

From time to time in the following fictious example of an Adlerian therapy group of the usual circular discussional type, I will in parentheses make some explanatory comments. As the reader probably knows by now, these accounts are artistic endeavors attempting to show how group procedures of various types would work. And by this time, the reader well knows that what will be shown will be only what this particular Adlerian group therapist is likely to do. In this account, consequently, many things will happen in a short period of time, which ordinarily would not occur in any one session.

The therapy session takes place in an office. Chairs are arranged in a circle. At 8 p.m. the therapist enters the room. There are six people present at this time, even though ordinarily there would be eight in the group. When the others come in no one will pay any attention to them, on the basis of the therapist's instructions. His logic is that this is a work situation in which the various clients pay, not a social situation; so no one who is on time should be deprived of full time because of a latecomer. The therapist begins immediately because one of his rules is that he starts on time no matter how few are present.

THERAPIST: OK, can we start?

(The therapist waits for about a minute, looking briefly at each person. No one replies.)

THERAPIST: Well, if no one will start, perhaps I will say something. What I am now doing is called structuring the group. All groups seem to go through various stages. We have met now for about 2½ months. In my experience, about now we really start to work. How do you feel about how fast we have been moving along?

(The therapist does not want to dominate the group. He issued an invitation to all to come in, but none wanted to. He waited about 60 seconds and when he saw that there was no response, he made a comment and asked a question.)

ROBERT: I don't know about others, but I now feel less comfortable with this group than I did when I started.

(Again the therapist waits, but with body language indicates he accepts the statement, doing so by smiling and nodding his head.)

LISA: That's not the way I feel. When I first came in I was real shy and uncertain. I didn't know what would happen. I am starting to feel I belong to the group. I was scared before, but now I am not.
FRANK: Well, you know me, always sitting on the fence with my legs almost touching the ground, like the therapist said. I feel both ways.

(At a prior session, the therapist gave his impression of the various people using such illustrations as: "Sitting astride a fence with neither foot touching the ground"—for someone who cannot make up his mind; or "Keeping his ass on two chairs"—for someone who tries to have a wife and a mistress at the same time. Frank is one of these "either/or" or "On the one hand, yes, but on the other hand, no," people. The therapist prefers to indicate personality types in this manner.)

THERAPIST: So, you sometimes feel scared and you sometimes feel comfortable.

(This is, of course, a reflection, a valuable technique recommended by Carl Rogers, which this therapist often uses to make certain he does not put his foot in his mouth, as it were, and to show Frank that he understands and is sympathetic to what is said.)

DAN: I want to mention that I don't care about such things. It is just time wasting. Can't we get on with something important? Besides it pisses me off that these other two are always late.
THERAPIST: Why?

(In contrast to Rogerians, an Adlerian does not hesitate to ask questions such as this one, even though he knows that the answer may be unsatisfactory; no matter what, it can be valuable.)

DAN: Well, I feel that I have to wait for them. There is like a pressure they put on all of us. You (Dan points to the therapist) always start on time. They know it and they come in late practically every time.

ELIZABETH: What do you suggest be done?

DAN: I don't know and I don't think it should be my responsibility.

ELIZABETH: Whose should it be then? If it bothers you, then I think you should do something about it.

DAN: Well I don't have the authority.

ELIZABETH: What authority do you need?

DAN: His. (Dan again points to the therapist, who is impassive all this time.)

ELIZABETH: So, why don't you ask him for the authority?

DAN: Why the hell don't you mind your own goddamn business? If I want the authority, I will ask for it. (Dan turns to the therapist.) What do you think about this—them being late all the time?

(The therapist is now wondering what would be the best reply. Should he make a noncommittal reply; should he reflect Dan; should he do something surprising? He is not sure, so he does what he calls unburdening, and also something surprising.)

THERAPIST: Dan, like yourself I am a compulsive person, and I don't like to waste time. You can see that, can't you? I also can feel with you with your tension about the absent people (the missing two now show up, but the therapist disregards them and continues) because I feel the same way. However, there is no way I can get them to come on time if they don't want to. In a sense, I am your servant, you pay me for my services. Being late may be part of their life-style. (The therapist turns to the two who just came in, Mary and Lisa.) Dan was mentioning that your being late is tension-producing for him. Seems he finds your absence annoying or something like that.

MARY: I am sorry about that Dan.

LISA: Screw you, Dan. Mind your own business. I don't control you and don't you try to control me.

DAN: I would think that if you want to get the maximum benefits of the group you would come on time. And if you had consideration of others you would come on time.

LISA: Did you ever think, that if I could do that I wouldn't need group?

DAN: That's a copout. Anyone can be late once in a while, but you two make a big production out of it. You flaunt it.

THERAPIST: (The therapist realizes that this situation needs some unraveling.) Well, let me come in. I see things as follows: Dan is upset by Mary and Lisa coming in late; Mary is somewhat apologetic about this and Lisa is aggressive about it. And everyone involved is making a big deal of this. Now you all know the applicable Adlerian statement about problems do you not? What is it?

SANDY: A problem is an opportunity.

THERAPIST: Right. But what does it mean in this case? Just take the three participants: Dan who is angry because Mary and Lisa are frequently late; Mary who is apologetic about this; and Lisa, who is angry with Dan, sees him as trying to control her. What can we make out of all this action?

SANDY: I don't know.

ROBERT: I think it tells something about their life-style?

THERAPIST: Right! (The therapist, a cognitive therapist, wants the group members to get a better understanding of themselves and each other.) What conclusions can we come to about Dan, Mary and Lisa just from this little scene?

DAN: I suppose you are going to say I am hostile. (There is a long silence, and then Dan begins again.) Maybe I am hostile, but aren't there times when one should be hostile? Remember in the New Testament when Jesus got angry and took a cord and scourged the moneychangers out of the temple? After all, it bothers me and isn't that what group therapy is all about? I just express my hostility; maybe others feel just as angry and don't want to show their feelings? I don't know if I am more hostile than others.

FRANK: If it walks like a duck, and if it quacks like a duck, then it is a duck.

DAN: You are *so* smart! (Dan remarks sarcastically.)

THERAPIST: (The therapist wants to keep feelings under control.) OK, all this is very good and I think rather complicated. Just because Dan expresses himself strongly does not mean that he is more hostile than others; Frank is saying that hostility is behavior. Is Dan saying that hostility is an internal matter? And is Frank saying it is an external matter? (The therapist is trying to defuse the situation, so that instead of people just getting angry, they can try to make sense out of the situation. He realizes that just plain emotionalism will be of no value, so he decides that it is time for him to lecture a bit.)

You see we run first into a semantic problem: What is hostility? Imagine someone so hostile to you that he is planning to kill you and yet you may think he likes you. So, in this case, we can say one is subjectively hostile. Now, if someone deliberately steps on your toes, he or she is objectively hostile. But of greater importance, I think, is this: Is Dan usually more inwardly and outwardly hostile, and if so, what is the reason for it? I believe I know what the reason is, but first I would like to turn to Dan: is it OK to talk to you and try to explain something about you to the group, as I see it?

DAN: Sure, be my guest.

THERAPIST: It appears to me that in terms of overt behavior that you are one of the angriest persons in the group. Would you agree to that?

DAN: Sure, but how about her? (Dan points to Lisa.)

THERAPIST: She is a close second to you. Would you agree to that Lisa?

LISA: I don't want to be too close to him. (The group laughs.)

THERAPIST: OK, now, it also seems to me that you both are love-starved, angry with your parents, feel alone, and have no friends to speak of. Would you both agree? (They nod.) OK, now, what connection could there possibly be between a person who feels friendless and, say, coming late or getting angry if someone comes in late? Where, if anywhere, is the dynamic connection?

What's the link? Feelings and thinking. I assume that there is something inside, which Dan and Lisa are not aware of perhaps, which results in their outside behavior, which is very aggressive, and which pushes people away. You see, behavior is a function of thought. For example, I had a client who went to a movie with his pregnant wife and when they came out it was raining heavily. He went to call a cab but the cab companies said they were too busy. He waited outside the movie house for maybe 15 minutes. The wife wanted to walk in the rain. He would not let her. So he went around the block, found an unattended car with its keys in the dashboard, got in the car, picked up his wife and drove her home, dropped her off and brought back the car where he found it, and then walked home in the rain.

Now, why do I tell you this story; what's the meaning; what's it got to do with Dan and Lisa?

MARY: You are saying that your thinking is different from this man's.

DAN: Are you saying this man is more hostile than you?

FRANK: I think he is saying that he would not do that under those conditions, but this other fellow did, and the difference is in their thinking: the other guy thought it was the right thing to do but our therapist would not do that.

THERAPIST: Exactly. All voluntary behavior, such as coming in late, or bawling out people—what Lisa and Mary did and what Dan did—is directed by thoughts, by what we may call private logic—meaning that we think it is right to do what we did. As I see it, both of them are unusually aggressive; both of them state that they have no real friends; both of them have had a rather unhappy childhood; and it appears to me to be logical that there must be some connection between their thinking and their behavior.

ELIZABETH: Are you saying that because they were treated brutally that they are now aggressive? _

THERAPIST: Not at all. But it may be that they thought they were treated brutally, and consequently their reality for them is their belief.

DAN: I know damn well how I was treated. I was there. I still have scars on my body that my father inflicted on me.

THERAPIST: I am not denying that. You and Lisa both say that you were treated brutally. This is your opinion and it is your conclusion. I believe in reality you were so treated. I am not so sure about Lisa. But she believes it was true, and that makes it true for her.

LISA: How could I prove it to be so?

THERAPIST: No way, and it is not important; the fact that this is your conclusion is enough. It is your reality; it is true for you. If we could bring your father from the grave; if we could have all your brothers and sisters swear that there was no brutality, you would still believe it. So, we deal with your reality; what you believe is true for you and you operate on the basis of your conclusions and convictions. Is that clear? (Everyone nods.) Now comes something important. Both Dan and Lisa have given some of their early recollections, which all of you know are important for understanding a person's view of life. I already have permission from all of you to state these. (The therapist takes out a notebook and starts to read.)

"I remember once when I was about 7 years old I wanted to wrap a kite line around a stick the way I had seen older boys do, and I had a big ball of cord and I began to spread it all over the room, and then I heard my father come in the house, and I was scared because he might get angry at what I did, and when he came in he asked me what I was doing and I told him, and he called me a fool and he hit me so hard that he knocked me out."

Now, what do any of you make of the meaning of this early recollection? I will argue that if you understand it, you understand a good deal about Dan; and if Dan understands it, he will understand a good deal about himself. Who would like to interpret it, and explain what it means?

ROBERT: I think it is self-evident. Dan remembers this because his father was in reality so brutal.

THERAPIST: I beg to differ. I have found clients who gave me early recollections when we started, and then at the end of the sessions when the therapy was completed, they had forgotten them. No, an early recollection tells one's view of life; and if therapy is successful, we have another view of life, and so we have different memories.

SANDY: I think the memory states that he expects people to be hostile to him.

THERAPIST: That's exactly as I see it. He tends to expect people to be hostile. Now, it is not experience necessarily that leads to expectations, but rather interpretations. This is why even so-called Siamese twins can come to different conclusions about life: they have exactly the same heredity and the same environment, but each can construe life differently.

DAN: You are saying then that my conclusion is an invention and not a necessary one from the facts?

THERAPIST: Not quite. It may be a necessary conclusion, maybe not; but whether the conclusion is based on facts or not is not important: what is important is that you expect hostile behavior and are prepared for it. Therefore you act in a hostile manner since you expect hostility.

LISA: I understand that, and it applies to my case too, but what can be done about it?

THERAPIST: Can you see what Lisa means, Dan?

DAN: Could you run that by me again?

LISA: You have a hostile attitude. You take everything personally. And the reason you have this attitude is that you expect everyone to be your enemy. This is a conclusion you came to. And it doesn't matter whether the conclusion is based on valid facts or not. Unless you change your thinking, you won't change your behavior.

DAN: OK, I'll buy that. It makes sense. But how can I change my attitude? Now, that we know that, where do we go from here?

THERAPIST: Now, you must change your behavior if you realize that when you are hostile, others react in a hostile manner to you, and, that as a result, your relations with others are negatively affected.

DAN: But that is not enough.

THERAPIST: OK. I agree. Would you like to role-play the same situations we had a few minutes ago when both Mary and Lisa came in? Do you remember what you said when they came in?

DAN: Somewhat. . . .

THERAPIST: How about redoing the scene in two ways. . . . First more or less in the way you did it and then in a new way. Meantime, we can watch you in both situations and give you our opinions.

Comments

I hope that this scene indicates the therapist's thinking. He views behavior, that is to say overt behavior, as intermediate to two other types of behavior: *cognitive*, which comes first, and *affective*, which follows overt behavior. People are usually aware of their feelings and not of their thinking. Dan got angry with Lisa and Mary, and so he was aware of his feelings and responded to them in an angry manner. His feelings are something like this: "You are unfair to me." And so he responds in a hostile manner when they appear. Now, the therapist knows that this person has a generally hostile manner and knows from his theory that inside Dan's head is a view that people are not good, they are not fair, they don't do what is right, and they act in ways to harm him. Coming late, which bothers nobody else, is seen by Dan as a hostile act. The therapist did not feel this way nor did anyone else, but it was a real matter for Dan. Consequently, the therapist attempted by discussions and lectures to show Dan that his individual unique response was based on certain conclusions that Dan had about others; and when Dan caught the idea and asked for help, this therapist thought that role-playing the prior situation and a new way of responding might be advisable. Another Adlerian, at this point, might ask for further discussions, or might just drop the matter, hoping that the client would get to understand his particular reaction.

STRENGTHS AND LIMITATIONS

At the risk of sounding somewhat arrogant, I believe that the Adlerian approach to life, its philosophy and its theory, is the most correct of all systems of personality. A consequence of this is that if a therapist follows the theory and the philosophy, better results will accrue relative to any other system. Now, this statement calls for a lot of qualifications. It does not mean by any means that an Adlerian therapist is better than, say, a Jungian therapist. What I mean to say is this: keeping therapists constant, I think Adlerian therapists would achieve better results in a shorter time than other kinds of therapists.

The reason is simple: Adlerian psychology is nothing but common sense. We have no crazy ideas, such as that boys want to have sex with their mothers, or that they carry in them the memories of past ancestors. We don't have complicated schemes such as dividing the individual into parts: the parent part, the child part, and the adult part. We don't have single dimensional ideas, such as everything depends on feelings. We are not limited in our methods of treatment, such as never giving advice or asking questions.

The important thing about being an Adlerian is something that few people realize: it is really the equivalent of a religion, a secular religion, and this point of view stresses respect and equality. It is also a hard-headed personality theory, accepting nothing that offends logic. It is also an open system, and Adlerians are eager to accept anything new in theory or in practice that makes sense and works.

In view of this position, Adlerian psychology is as good as the people in it, and it does not limit them in the way other systems do. For example, as has been stated over and over in this chapter, when it comes to treatment we have all kinds of ways of operating, and indeed you will find some Adlerians using the therapeutic couch, some, and I am one of them, using Moreno's psychodrama, Rogers's reflection theory, and Ellis's disputational *ABC* system, finding them all consonant with my particular view of how to operate.

Adlerian therapists do tend to use early recollections as a projective tool, and I personally have used the Rorschach and the Thematic Apperception Test (TAT), but I believe that this early-recollection method, developed by Adler, the first of all the projective techniques (Munroe, 1955), is the best way to find out unobtrusively peoples' thinking—to isolate their hidden private logic—and, consequently, it gives the Adlerian therapist an enormous advantage over those who do not use this procedure (Olson, 1979).

I hope this is clear: the most important element in psychotherapy is neither the theory nor the technique—it is the therapist. But keeping therapists and training constant, the best of all theories I see as the Adlerian. It can do what any other theory can do: it has the utmost flexibility; it is really the only truly eclectic theory; and many other theories and systems, such as Glasser's, Berne's, and Ellis's, are essentially derivations of Adlerian theory (Rozsnafszky, 1974).

In short, I see it as the most nearly complete and, consequently, the most satisfactory of all therapies known to me. This does not mean that new and better ones may not emerge, but what will probably emerge is this: Adlerians will probably accept any new ideas or new practices as part of their already comprehensive philosophy and theory. However, all this does not necessarily mean that Adlerian theory or therapy is the best for all practitioners; there is a subtle relationship between these practices and one's own personality (Corsini, 1956). So, if you happen to be an authoritarian, then this would not be the system for you; if you like cognitive complexity and find Adlerian ideas simplistic, then this is not the system for you; if you want to impress others and use fancy language, this is not the system for you.

It must always be kept in mind that the most important elements in Adlerian thinking are the concept of *Gemeinschaftsgefühl*—which can be translated as good will to all persons—and *Common Sense*. Whoever has common sense and good will to others is an Adlerian, no matter how that person may label himself. This is something that Adlerians have been saying for a long time: a lot of people are Adlerians and don't know it. They are in the same position of Molière's *bourgeois gentilhomme,* who had been speaking prose all his life and only recently found out.

Summary

In this chapter I have attempted to explain that Adlerian Group Psychotherapy is quite different from any other sort of group psychotherapy in that it is not restricted in any way by procedures, and, given 1,000 Adlerians doing therapy in groups, there would be very little similarity in how they operated. Were one to attend a variety of groups run by followers of the six therapeutic systems here included, I daresay that there would be quick identifications of the encounter groups, the Gestalt groups, the Transactional Analysis (TA) groups, the Rational-Emotive Therapy (RET) groups, and the Behavior Therapy groups, but I believe that misidentifications would be likely relative to the Adlerians running groups, simply because at times they could be operating like any of these other five groups.

Also I have tried to explain that, quite differently from any other system I know of, Adler's psychology stresses a philosophy of values, known in English as *Social Interest* and in German as *Gemeinschaftsgefühl* (best defined by Heinz Ansbacher, 1983, as interest in the interests of others). Essentially, this is a humanistic, egalitarian philosophy which stresses the importance of mutual respect.

Relative to group methods, I have attempted to show that in addition to the usual circular discussional group which characterizes most other group methods, Adlerians use not only such variant techniques as Behind-the-Back and Psychodrama, but all the techniques employed by others, if they think these techniques will achieve good results. In short, we are truly eclectic. In addition, since Individual Psychology is a social psychology, we employ groups in a variety of ways intended to help people. To illustrate this, I have described in some detail a complete educational system based on Adlerian psychology, which uses group procedures in at least a half dozen ways, much more than any other known educational institution or any other formal group or organization.

Still another difference has to do with language. Certainly, in comparison with the "big three" (Freud, Adler, and Jung), we use simple language and simple concepts. Probably even within this book our language usage appears relatively simple. Compare our language with, for example, that of Transactional Analysis.

The most important argument is that Adlerian psychology is a total system of living: a philosophy of life, equivalent to a religion, and that its theoretical principles are of the commonsense type. Everything follows from these two points. Consequently, group therapy for any participant is a process intended to give that person better values, increased self-confidence and courage, and a more wholesome view of life.

REFERENCES

Adler, A. *Study of organ inferiority and its psychical compensation*. New York: Nervous and Mental Disease Publishing, 1917.

Adler, A. *The neurotic constitution*. New York: Dodd Mead, 1926.

Adler, A. *The practice and theory of Individual Psychology*. New York: Greenberg, 1927.

Adler, A. *What life should mean to you*. London: George Allen & Unwin, 1962.

Ansbacher, H. L. Individual Psychology. In R. J. Corsini & A. J. Marsella (Eds.), *Personality theories, research and assessment*. Itasca, Ill.: Peacock, 1983.

Ansbacher, H. L., & Ansbacher, R. R. (Eds.). *The Individual Psychology of Alfred Adler*. New York: Basic Books, 1956.

Berrett, R. D. Adlerian mother study groups: An evaluation. In G. Manaster & R. J. Corsini (Eds.), *Individual Psychology: Theory and practice*. Itasca, Ill.: F. E. Peacock, 1982.

Corsini, R. J. Freud, Rogers, and Moreno. *Group Psychotherapy*, 1956, *9*, 274–281.

Corsini, R. J. *Methods of group psychotherapy*. New York: McGraw-Hill, 1957.

Corsini, R. J. Immediate therapy in groups. In G. M. Gazda (Ed.), *Innovations to group psychotherapy*. Springfield, Ill.: Charles C Thomas, 1967.

Corsini, R. J. Counseling and psychotherapy. In E. Borgatta & W. Lambert (Eds.), *Handbook of personality theory*. Chicago: Rand-McNally, 1968.

Corsini, R. J. Individual education. *Journal of Individual Psychology*, 1977, *33* (2a), 295–349.

Corsini, R. J. Individual education. In E. Ignas & R. J. Corsini (Eds.), *Alternative educational systems*. Itasca, Ill.: F. E. Peacock, 1979.

Corsini, R. J., & Marsella, A. J. *Personality theories, research and assessment*. Itasca, Ill.: F. E. Peacock, 1983.

Corsini, R. J., & Painter, G. *The practical parent*. New York: Harper & Row, 1975.

Corsini, R. J., & Rigney, K. *The family council*. Chicago: Rudolf Dreikurs Unit of the Family Education Association, 1970.

Corsini, R. J., & Rosenberg, B. Mechanisms of group psychotherapy. *Journal of Abnormal and Social Psychology*, 1955, *51*, 406–411.

Deutsch, D. Group therapy with married couples. *Individual Psychologist*, 1967, *4*, 56–62.

Dinkmeyer, D., & McKay, G. *Raising a responsible child*. New York: Simon & Schuster, 1973.

Dreikurs, R. Patient–therapist relationship in multiple therapy. *Psychiatric Quarterly*, 1952, *26*, 590–596.

Dreikurs, R. *Group psychotherapy and group approaches: Collected papers*. Chicago: Alfred Adler Institute, 1960.

Dreikurs, R., & Soltz, V. *Children: The challenge*. New York: Duell, Sloan & Pearce, 1964.

Dreikurs, R., Corsini, R. J., Lowe, R., & Sonstegard, M. (Eds.), *Adlerian family counseling*. Eugene: Oregon University Press, 1959.

Dreikurs, R., Gould, S., & Corsini, R. J. *The family council*. Chicago: Henry Regnery, 1974.

Eckstein, D., Baruth, L., & Mahrer, D. *Life-style: What it is and how to do it*. Hendersonville, N.C.: Mother Earth News, 1975.

Ellis, A. *Reason and emotion in psychotherapy*. New York: Lyle Stuart, 1962.

Freeman, C. W. Adlerian mother study groups: Effects on attitudes and behavior. In G. Manaster & R. J. Corsini (Eds.), *Individual Psychology: Theory and practice*. Itasca, Ill.: F. E. Peacock, 1982.

Gordon, T. *Parent effectiveness training*. New York: Peter Wyden, 1970.

Grunwald, B. Roleplaying as a classroom group procedure. *Individual Psychologist*, 1969, *6*, 34–38.

Ignas, E., & Corsini, R. J. *Alternative Educational Systems*. Itasca, Ill.: F. E. Peacock, 1979.

Krebs, L. Summary of research on an Individual Education school. *Journal of Individual Psychology*, 1982, *38*, 245–252.

Manaster, G. (Ed.). (Whole issues). *Journal of Individual Psychology* 1977, *33*; 1985, *41*.

Manaster, G., & Corsini, R. J. (Eds.). *Individual Psychology: Theory and practice*. Itasca, Ill.: F. E. Peacock, 1982.

Mosak, H. H. Adlerian psychotherapy. In R. J. Corsini (Ed.), *Current psychotherapies*. Itasca, Ill.: F. E. Peacock, 1983.

Munroe, R. *Schools of psychoanalytic thought*. New York: Dryden Press, 1955.

Nelson, M. D., & Haberer, M. H. Effectiveness of Adlerian counseling with low-achieving students. In G. Manaster & R. J. Corsini (Eds.), *Individual Psychology: Theory and practice*. Itasca, Ill.: F. E. Peacock, 1982.

Olson, H. O. (Eds.). *Early recollections: Their use in diagnosis and psychotherapy*. Springfield, Ill.: Charles C Thomas, 1979.

Painter, G., & Vernon, S. Primary relationship therapy. In R. J. Corsini (Ed.), *Handbook of innovative psychotherapies*. New York: John Wiley, 1981.

Phillips, C., & Corsini, R. J. *Give in or give up*. Chicago: Nelson-Hall, 1982.

Pratt, A., & Mastroianni, M. Summary of research on Individual Education. *Journal of Individual Psychology*, 1981, *37*, 232–246.

Rogers, C. R. *Client-centered therapy*. Boston: Houghton-Mifflin, 1951.

Rosznafsky, J. Three free-will therapies of the sixties. *Journal of Individual Psychology*, 1974, *30*, 234–241.

Silverman, N. S., & Corsini, R. J. Is it true what they say about Adler? *Teaching of Psychology*, 1984, *11*, 188–189.

Starr, A. *Rehearsal for living*. Chicago: Nelson-Hall, 1977.

Whittington, E. Critical incidents: Traditional and Individual Education. *Journal of Individual Psychology*, 1981, *37*, 247–271.

Glossary

Basic Mistakes. As we grow up we tend to develop certain concepts about ourselves, life, others, which are incorrect. These ideas, central to our personality, are practically always unknown to us, even though we live by them. It is these ideas, such as: "I really cannot trust anyone" or "People should give me special treatment" which generate problems for individuals. In Adlerian therapy we attempt to locate such mistakes and make the person aware of them, so that they will be clear, so that the client will now be able to operate in a more intelligent and commonsense manner.

Counseling. The Adlerian view of counseling is simple: first, learn the problem; second, find out what was done in the past to solve it; third, decide whether you (the counselor) know the right thing to do; fourth, inform the client how to handle the problem; fifth, try to convince the client to do what is necessary to solve the problem; sixth, do not go ahead with any new solutions until the first problem is solved.

Early Recollections. An early recollection is a specific memory that could start with "Once" rather than "We used to . . ." which occurred before memories started to be continuous. They are of special significance in that they give the clinician clues relative to the client's misperceptions of reality and help to indicate the client's life-style and basic mistakes.

Emotions. Adlerians view the emotions as "handmaidens" to cognition: means of getting the person to do what the intellect has already decided to do. Emotions are movers or motivators, and are at the "service" of the intellect. So, it is the intellect and not the emotions that generate behavior. The intellect steers the wagon and the emotions push it.

Encouragement. Adlerian counseling and psychotherapy depend strongly on two things: cognition (which we call common sense) and emotions (which in terms of change is called encouragement). In other words, we need the courage to do what will work, to behave properly and sensibly.

Family Constellation. It is generalized by Adlerians that being in certain family positions, such as first child, is likely to generate particular patterns of behavior. Research evidence is equivocal about such relationships.

Horizontal–Vertical View. Adlerians see most psychological problems as due to people's having a vertical view of themselves and others: feeling inferior to those whom they see as superior to them, and feeling superior to those they see as inferior to them. The attempt by Adlerian therapists is to have clients "be on the level" and see all people as different and yet equal—to have a horizontal view.

Inferiority. There are two distinctly different elements involved here. "Inferiority feelings" are common and normal and have the effect of motivating the person to greater superiority—that is, to make compensatory efforts to improve. "Inferiority complex" has just the opposite effect—to discourage one and leads one to give up. The first is normal and useful, the second is abnormal and useless.

Life-Style. This term is roughly equivalent to the word *Personality*. It is the way one operates in life, the approach one takes to problems, the view one has of others; the totality of the person in thought and action.

Logical Consequences. This concept is used a good deal in Adlerian family counseling. It relates to the behavior of a parent who reacts to the behavior of a child. Instead of the parent rewarding or punishing the child (seen as opposite sides of the same authoritarian view) the parent will respond for the purpose of training in a logical manner. Thus, if the child comes home late for dinner, he may find that everything has been eaten, and plates put away. The latecomer now has to take care of his own dinner and clean up after himself.

Natural Consequences. This is an important concept in child training. Essentially, it means that the parent should not intervene, allowing the child to receive the natural consequences of his behavior. Usually, a parent will inform a child of a certain consequence, and if the child persists in wanting to do a particular thing, the parent will permit it (if not potentially dangerous), such as allowing a child to go out of the house improperly dressed, in the expectation that the weather, or other children, and so forth, will react in such a manner as to make the child learn.

Private Logic. The disturbed person tends to develop a viewpoint about life which departs from *sententia communis* or "common sense." The private logic is a unit concept within Basic Mistakes. "I am really special" is an example of a private logic, and could also be a basic mistake.

Psychotherapy. From an Adlerian point of view, the therapy consists of having a mirror put in front of a client showing him or her what the reality of the person is. In this way one sees one's mistakes. The therapist now attempts to encourage the client to act in ways to remove or reduce conflicts and tensions and to operate in a more healthful manner.

Punishment. Adlerians see no place for rewards or punishment in human relationships, because these are elements relating to superiority–inferiority. Instead Natural and Logical Consequences are substituted.

Rewards. Adlerians see rewards as the analog of punishment, the other side of the same coin: only a superior can give rewards—or punishment.

Social Interest. This is probably the single most important Adlerian concept. The term *Social Interest* does not really do justice to Adler's German term *Gemeinschaftsgefühl*. The term means literally, "Feeling for community" and relates to the concept of a person belonging to a community, feeling part of it, and having its interests in mind. Perhaps a better single term might be "Belongingness." The uniqueness of this term is that it is value-laden and so Adlerian Psychology differs from all other personality theories in this respect.

Soft Determinism. Instead of taking the view of determinism as held by behavior modifiers and Freudians, or the opposing view of indeterminism held by courts and some churches, Adlerians view the person as limited by circumstances beyond his control (biological and social limits) but that within these limits individuals have considerable potentialities for creative decisions. In short, we are responsible even though our responsibility is affected by outside factors.

Unconscious. Adlerians are holistic. They view the person as an entity, indivisible. There is no separate unconscious but rather any individual at any time has a limited amount of awareness. There are some elements that one is unaware of (a fish may be unaware that he is swimming in water). An example would be one's private logic.

2

Transactional Analysis in Group Work

JOHN GRIMES

Introduction

I have been adventuring with Transactional Analysis (TA) for more than a dozen years. I originally met TA in Tom Harris's book, *I'm OK—You're OK* (1967). And it was there I learned my first lesson about TA. It was *understandable*. It talked of "ego states" and helped me lay hold of the way things were within myself.

A second characteristic of TA was its ability to reach toward both ends of the healing continuum (Figure 1). It gave a new *wholeness* to the therapy I was doing.

In those days I was learning to work in the "here and now," clarifying with clients the middle ground of "where are you now?" TA added to this by showing me the nature of *early decision* ("Where did you come from?") and the nature of *re-decision* ("Where are you going?").

A third characteristic of TA was its concern for the client and its willingness to incorporate the techniques of other disciplines whenever they would add to the effectiveness of a healing strategy. TA is, in a word, *eclectic*. If it works, use it—as long as it is moral and appropriate to the moment!

A final, fourth characteristic, seemingly inherent in the approach of TA, is its *ability to create* new tools when the known tools are not getting the job done. An illustration of this is seen in the question: "How does it help?" When the client, the group, and I are stuck, then it becomes a question of "How does it help to stay stuck?" And because what we do within ourselves and among ourselves is always reasonable, at some level, the question has an answer. Our answer then becomes a stepping stone on the way out.

TA is an exciting teacher—understandable, whole, eclectic, and creative. Within the light of this approach, both therapists and clients know themselves to be traveling together in an adventure of learning and healing.

John Grimes • 3480 Dixiana Drive, Lexington, Kentucky 40502.

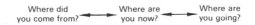

FIGURE 1.   The healing continuum.

DEFINITION

TA is three things: a philosophy, a theory, and a system of techniques. All three are thoroughly interconnected (Woollams & Brown, 1978, p. 1).

As a *philosophy*, the basic assumption of TA is *OKness:* I'm OK, You're OK, We're OK, They're OK, and It's OK. On this base, the client and the therapist stand as equals, adult to adult. As such, we can negotiate contracts which satisfy our needs. The rightness of positive strokes for each of us is accepted. Based on our adult-to-adult relationship, it is agreed that we will speak a common language using terms that are clear. It is also understood that the aim of our work is success—and that this success for new life decision is in the hands of each of us.

As *theory*, TA explains the development of the individual personality, the internal transactions of the individual, and the transactions of individual with individual. TA theory is used to account for the way we are and act in the present, to understand how the feelings and behavior of the past relate to the present, and to clarify the options for change in this moment and in the future.

As a system of *techniques*, TA offers a wide variety of therapeutic approaches. TA encourages freedom in both the selection and creation of techniques, according to the specific context of a client's contract for change. TA also acts as an umbrella of guidelines for the choice of techniques consistent with its own theory and philosophy.

At this point in its history, TA is a developing field enjoying great creativity and much cross-fertilization between itself and other therapeutic disciplines, and among the various schools of TA (Barnes, 1977, pp. 3–31; Dusay, 1977b).

HISTORY

TA history begins with Eric Berne, M.D. (1910–1970). He is the originator and primary developer of TA and is referred to almost with the mystery of sainthood in TA circles (Woollams & Brown, 1978, p. 2).

The genius of Berne lay in his willingness and eagerness to cut through the accepted formulas of therapy. He seemingly did not believe that anyone is incurable. He only believed that, where there was failure, there was still ignorance, that we, as therapists, did not yet know how to do our job well enough. He saw the therapist's job to be that of healing the client as quickly as possible. "Making progress" was not the goal, and any goal less than *cure* was either dishonest or immoral (Berne, 1971).

Berne was trained as a psychiatrist and a psychoanalyst, but was never fully accepted by the psychoanalytic community. He was impressed with the insight and depth of psychoanalysis and was highly influenced by it in his thinking and writing. However, Berne was impatient with the slowness and rigidity of psychoanalysis.

In 1957, Berne wrote "Ego States in Psychotherapy" (Berne, 1957). It was here that he first mentioned the three ego states (Parent, Adult, Child) and used three circles in a diagram (Figure 2).

The story is told that in the early 1950s, Berne came to the genesis of his theory in a series of therapy sessions with a young lawyer (Dusay, 1977b). The man was a habitual gambler, and, when in Reno, would employ several kinds of personal magic in an effort to win. He made sure he did not step on any cracks in the sidewalk on his way to the casino. He took careful baths after winning. He performed mental gymnastics to convince himself he was ahead when he was actually behind. Berne and the young man realized, as they talked, they were looking at two separate kinds of thinking. One belonged to the successful, everyday professional life of the man and was logical and realistic. The other belonged to the superstitious gambler part of his life and was illogical and unrealistic.

In further work, Berne's client began to share his memory of a vacation with his parents, on a dude ranch, when he was 8 years old. He remembered wearing his cowboy clothes, helping one of the workhands unsaddle a horse. As he did so, the workhand turned and said, "Why, thanks, cowpoke." The client remembered himself answering, "I'm not really a cowpoke, I'm just a little boy." At that point the lawyer looked at Berne and said, "That's the way I feel now, like I'm not really a lawyer; I'm just a little boy."

Berne began to see that the two thinking patterns could be behaviorally identified by voice tone, facial expression, memory, and feeling. These patterns he called ego states. The logical rational system he called the "Adult" ego state. The magical, nonrational and creative system he called the "Child" ego state. In diagramming them he drew a circle around each of the two showing them as separate, complete and total (Figure 2a). At a later date, Berne deline-

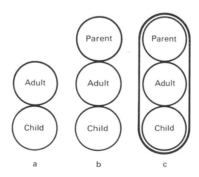

FIGURE 2. The basic TA diagram of human personality.

ated the "Parent" ego state, adding a third circle (Figure 2b), and drew a second line around all three to indicate wholeness (Figure 2c) thus completing the basic TA diagram of the human personality (1972, p. 12).[1]

In 1958, Berne named this new approach "Transactional Analysis" and, in the same article, mentioned "games" and "scripts" (Berne, 1958). Also, in 1958, Berne began the first TA seminars—called the San Francisco Social Psychiatry Seminar (*Transactional Analysis*, 1985). The seminar grew, membership increased, and TA began to be used and discussed around the country (Woollams & Brown, 1978, p. 3). In 1962, the "Transactional Analysis Bulletin" was created and later (1971) expanded into the *Transactional Analysis Journal*. In 1964, with members in most of the 50 states as well as Canada, Costa Rica, and England, the name of the organization was changed to the International Transactional Analysis Association (ITAA).

Presently the ITAA publishes the *Journal* and a newsletter (*Script*), has established a publishing house (Transactional Publications),[2] holds two national conferences per year, promotes TA as an area of specialization, and is very active in the training and certification of its members. World membership totals 6,000 persons.

High standards and demonstrated competence are expected of ITAA members who offer counseling, treatment, consultation or teaching in Transactional Analysis. Those who have attained certified membership are authorized to call themselves transactional analysts (*Transactional Analysis Journal*, 1982). These categories of membership are: Special Fields Member (SFM), Clinical Member (CM), Special Fields Teaching Member (SFTM), and Clinical Teaching Member (CTM).[3]

GOALS

The goal of TA, as it is used in a group setting as well as in other situations, is to open doors of power, of insight, and of healing to the participants. In the accomplishment of this goal, the transactions within the group itself are understood to be basic to both diagnosis and cure. Verbal interactions, behavioral reactions, and feeling responses are all grist for the therapeutic mill.

A further expansion of this goal is the intentional creation of a group environment which supports for each member the underlying TA philosophy of OKness. In this context there is freedom to feel, opportunity to try new behavior, encouragement for positive stroking, learning to accept responsibility for self and to account for thinking and feeling, and finally clarification and redecision around earlier messages within the self (Goulding, 1972, pp. 105–

[1]For the sake of convenience, the more informal diagram of Figure 2b is ordinarily used.
[2]Trans Pubs, P.O. Box 3932, Rincon Annex, San Francisco, CA 94119.
[3]For further information about the ITAA, membership, or training standards, contact: The International Transactional Analysis Association, Inc., 1772 Vallejo Street, San Francisco, CA 94123.

134). It is an environment designed to facilitate the client's successful completion of her[4] contract for change and the client's development of personal autonomy.

Basic Concepts

TA Theory can be divided under the two headings: *diagnosis* and *cure*. The first has to do with the active process of discovering the inner-outer, relational dynamics of a personality. The second has to do with the revising of these dynamics, both intellectual and emotional, so that the objectives of the client for personal life change are achieved.

The assumption is that both diagnosis and cure can be accomplished. No matter what the present state of affairs within an individual or the reasons, either ancient or recent, for the creation of that situation, it is possible to understand it and it is possible to put together new plans for new behavior that is satisfying within the context of what, in effect, becomes a new life.

Diagnosis

There are four areas of analysis within the scheme of TA from which diagnosis is made. These are: *structural analysis, transactional analysis, game* and *racket analysis,* and *script analysis.*

Structural Analysis. Structural analysis is used to understand what is taking place within the individual personality (Woollams & Brown, 1978, pp. 8–12). Each person is understood to have three "functional" parts called *ego states.* Berne defined an ego state as "a system of feelings accompanied by a related set of behavior patterns" (Berne, 1964b, p. 23). As we have already seen, he identified these three as Parent (P), Adult (A), and Child (C).[5]

Within structural analysis, ego states are examined *functionally* and *structurally.* A functional diagram of a personality is drawn with the Parent and the Child ego states divided vertically (Figure 3). The two sides of the Parent point to the double function of the Parent in both controlling and nurturing. The left side is ordinarily labeled the Controlling or Critical Parent (CP). The right side is labeled the Nurturing Parent (NP). The function of the Critical Parent is to store and dispense the rules and protection for living. The function of the Nurturing Parent is to care for, to nurture.

The function of the Adult is to compute the probabilities and make appropriate decisions in terms of data drawn from the Parent, the Child, and the environment.

The two sides of the Child, like the Parent, indicate the double function of

[4]The gender of pronouns is alternated throughout the text.
[5]Words denoting ego states are capitalized.

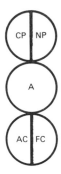

FIGURE 3.   A second-order functional diagram.

this ego state. The Adapted Child (AC), on the left, adapts to the rules, patterns of behavior, and wishes of the Parent ego state within the self or others. The adapting may take two forms: either "adapted compliant" (following the rule) or "adapted rebellious" (rebelling against the rule). These two forms of the Adapted Child may appear quite different, but in fact, are flip sides of the same coin, because both depend upon the existence of the explicit, implicit, or imagined rule in order to act. The Free Child (FC) on the right, sometimes called the Natural Child, reacts only to itself and according to its own needs without regard for the rules or wishes of Parent(s).

There are four ways to identify the ego state a person is in at a particular moment: behavioral, social, historical, and phenomenological (Woollams, Brown, & Huige, 1977).

Behavioral clues embrace an individual's choice of words, voice tone or level(s), dress, posture, facial expression, movement of hands or feet, and other visible, auditory or even olfactory indicators. *Social* clues to the identification of an ego state are drawn from the reactions of others to the individual. As an illustration, a person coming from Critical Parent may pick up either the Compliant or Rebellious form of the Adapted Child in another person. *Historical* data is gathered by looking into the past for a similar situation with similar feelings to those that are being experienced in this moment. A person may suddenly realize that her father, for instance, stood just this way and sounded this way. The *phenomenological* clues are given when the individual looks within himself. He then decides, according to the experience of the moment, as it ties into the experience of the past, which ego state, Parent, Adult, or Child, is in executive control.

The structural examination of ego states is accomplished by way of implication. The basic PAC diagram (Figure 2b) is understood to be a first-order structural diagram. For a more complete understanding of the nature and development of personality, it is helpful to draw what is termed a second-order structural diagram (Figure 4) (Woollams, Brown, & Huige, 1977). In this diagram the ego states are divided horizontally with the vertical also being used in the Parent to indicate the different sources of input.

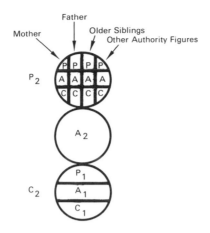

FIGURE 4.   A second-order structural diagram.

The Parent (P_2) is formed as the individual, as a child, records what she perceives as the behavior and the messages of mother, father, and others in authority. These recordings of collected knowledge direct the person how to live, survive, and manage in the world. They become rules for living that tell how "grown up" people act and, therefore, how the individual "ought" to act. However, the doors of learning are never completely closed and further information can be added to the Parent at any time throughout life.

The Adult ego state gradually forms its logical, computerlike abilities and appears to complete its development at about the age of 12 (Woollams, 1977).

As the Parent is created to record what significant others are doing, so the Child is created to record what is felt (C_1), thought (A_1), and decided (P_1) about what is happening. These recordings in the Child form the basic dynamic from which all behavior of the personality flows. The Life Script is written by A_1 (the "Little Professor"), the intuitive part of a person, and is stored in P_1 (the "Electrode").

In the use of structural analysis to diagnose psychopathology, two types of malady come to light: *contamination* and *exclusion* (Woollams & Brown, 1978, pp. 36–39). When ego-state boundaries break down and the Adult ego state becomes contaminated by the Parent, the Child, or both, contamination is said to have occurred.

Contamination results in the Adult computing Parent or Child recordings as though the material were factual data. Prejudice is the result of a Parent contamination of the Adult (Figure 5a). The Adult really believes that "Men are animals" or "Women can't think." Phobias and delusions spring from a Child contamination of the Adult (Figure 5b). In this case, the Adult believes it to be an objective fact that "mice are scary." When both the Parent and the Child are part of the contamination of the Adult, (Figure 5c), the individual is hearing the Parent message and reacting in a feeling way from the Child with both inputs

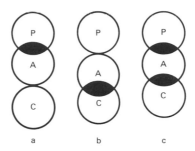

FIGURE 5.   Contamination of the Adult ego state.

feeding through the Adult. An example of this would be: "Women can't be trusted" (Parent), "I don't deserve to be happy" (Child), and "I am afraid my wife is unfaithful, therefore, I am suing for divorce!" (Adult contaminated).

The second form of psychopathology, exclusion, is seen when a single ego state habitually dominates a person's behavior.

The constant Parent is diagrammed in Figure 6a. This is the person who has a rule for everything and is preachy and authoritarian about it. Examples of the constant Parent might include some ministers, teachers, or military figures. The constant Adult in Figure 6b is a person who seems to function like a computer, without feeling. Examples might include some mathematicians, engineers, or scientists. The constant Child in Figure 6c is the individual who, always in the here and now, seems to lack the ability to see the broader picture, that is, either the context or the outcome of his behavior. Examples might include some comedians, a social butterfly, or the practical joker.

Exclusion is also seen when a person habitually uses only two ego states out of the possible three (Figure 7).

In the case of the excluded Parent (Figure 7a), the person may have recorded either very heavy or contradictory messages in the Parent which, rather than being structurally helpful or protective, result in pain to the Child. Therefore, in an act of desperation, the Parent is excluded from an active part in the

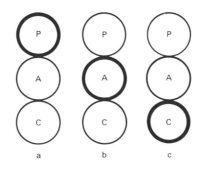

FIGURE 6.   Constant ego states.

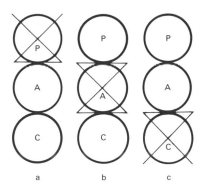

FIGURE 7. Excluded ego states.

personality. The person may then appear to act irresponsibly or without conscience. The individual with an excluded Adult (Figure 7b) may switch from
Parent to Child without regard for external reality. An extreme example is the
manic-depressive adaptation. When a person excludes the Child (Figure 7c), it
is likely a defensive move to protect the personality from pain that was, at
some point, repeatedly brought to bear whenever feelings, desires, creativity,
or other evidence of Child activity was displayed. Examples of this particular
internal strategy might be found in victims of a concentration camp experience
or those who have undergone electroshock treatment. More familiar is the
individual who seems to have little fun, does not allow himself to get close to
others, and expresses few feelings.

A further approach to understanding ego states is the *egogram* (Figure 8)
developed by John Dusay (1977a, pp. 3, 4). Though the genesis for individual
behavior seems always, upon close examination, to spring from the Child, very
different levels of energy may be invested in the various ego states.

A basic assumption in the egogram is that the amount of energy is constant. Therefore, when there is an energy level change in one ego state, there
will be a change in one or more other ego states. In Figure 8, the individual
may want to increase the energy in her Free Child. A likely approach would be

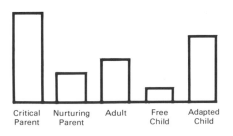

FIGURE 8. An egogram.

to work toward moving Critical Parent energy into the Nurturing Parent and Adapted Child energy into the Free Child. In practice, this involves teaching a client ways of nurturing both herself and others and opening avenues for Free-Child activity. One use of egograms as a therapeutic technique in groups is explained under "Media Usage" (p. 84).

Transactional Analysis. The second diagnostic tool of TA is transactional analysis (Woollams & Brown, 1978, pp. 23–80). It is based on the understanding that, in order to communicate, people use *transactions.* A transaction can be seen as an exchange of energy or strokes between two people, involving a *stimulus* and a *response.* The analysis of the transaction will reveal the specific ego states utilized in the transaction.

There are three kinds of transactions: *complementary, crossed,* and *ulterior.* With each of these there is a corresponding rule of communication (Berne, 1972, pp. 14–21).

A complementary transaction is one in which a stimulus is sent from an ego state of one person and is received by a single ego state in another person, followed by a response from the receiving ego state and received then by the stimulus-originating ego state (Figure 9).

In the complementary transaction the stimulus–response vectors are parallel. The *first rule of communication* in TA is that, as long as the vectors remain parallel, the dialogue can continue indefinitely.

A crossed transaction is one in which a stimulus is sent from an ego state of one person and is received by a single ego state in another person, followed by a response from an ego state other than the receiving ego state (Figure 10).

In the crossed transaction, the stimulus–response vectors are *not* parallel as they are in the complementary transaction, and are diagrammed to intersect or cross. The response crosses the stimulus, and the *second rule of communication* in TA is brought into play—when the vectors are not parallel, the dialogue ceases. The breakdown may be only temporary; nevertheless, something different is likely to follow.

A crossed transaction can also be experienced even when the vectors, at

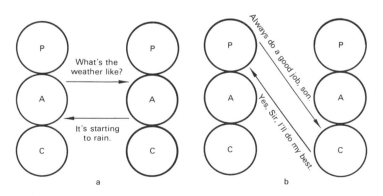

FIGURE 9.   Complementary transactions.

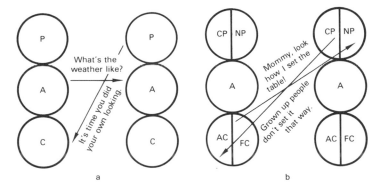

FIGURE 10.   Crossed transactions.

first glance, seem parallel. In Figure 10b the stimulus moves from the Child ego state to the Parent, which in turn sends a response back to the Child. However, because the vectors are from different sides or functions of the ego states, it is a crossed transaction.

An ulterior transaction can be either "duplex" or "angular." In either case there is a *social* and a *psychological message*. The social message is the message that is heard intellectually. It is diagrammed as a sold line. The psychological message is heard at the emotional level, that is, it is felt. This message is diagrammed as a dotted line (Figure 11).

The *third rule of communication* in TA is that the outcome of a transaction will be determined by the psychological vector. This is illustrated in the duplex form of an ulterior transaction in Figure 11a. Here four ego states are involved, two in each person. As the duplex transaction is experienced by the participants, a single conversation will seem to be occurring. This is the social level. However, at the psychological level there is a second, hidden conversation.

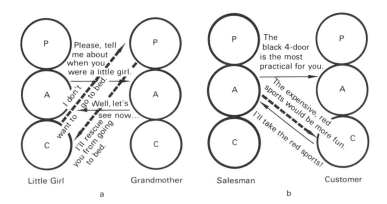

FIGURE 11.   Ulterior transactions.

The same rule of communication is also illustrated in Figure 11b. Here the angular form of an ulterior transaction is diagrammed, and three ego states are involved. The salesman appears to be coming from an information-giving, Adult position when, in fact, he is also including a psychological message to the Child of his customer in the hope of hooking that ego state.

In the angular transaction, the salesman is aware of the hidden message he is attempting to put across. The customer is cognitively unaware of that message, and yet reacts in accordance with it. In the duplex transaction, neither participant is cognitively aware of the hidden, psychological message. Still, in both transactions, it is the psychological vector that is felt, reacted to, and, in effect, determines the outcome.

Game and Racket Analysis. Game and racket analysis clarifies the nature of transactions that lead to bad feeling payoffs. It is the third diagnostic tool of TA. Games and rackets are actually separate tools of understanding but are looked at together here because they are similar in many ways (Woollams & Brown, 1978, pp. 127–149).

Both games and rackets are substitute ways for living (Woollams, Brown, & Huige, 1977), both are learned systems for structuring time and acquiring strokes, both call for a discount of self and/or the other person, both are used to confirm not-OK life script and not-OK life positions, and both provide predictable strokes and bad feeling payoffs. In both there is a quality of manipulation of events and of others.

The difference in the two lies in the tendency of rackets to be an internal process, while games involve an external process. Rackets can include others in their operation, but essentially they are private, inside procedures designed to produce the desired bad feeling. Games always include two or more persons from beginning to end.

Rackets and games are often intertwined. Rackets can be used to lay the groundwork for a game, and games can open doors for the further running of a racket.

RACKETS. A *racket* is Berne's term for behavior that pretends to be one thing while actually it is quite another (Berne, 1972, pp. 137–139) as in "racketeering" (English, 1976) in which one, apparently legitimate business is used as a cover for the real, illegitimate business that is kept hidden. With TA rackets, the issue is feelings. A racket can be defined as an inappropriate interpretation of events and transactions used to support a main bad feeling as a substitute for other, less acceptable feelings.

Rackets come in all the shapes and forms of all the feelings that people are capable of feeling. There is the person with the mad racket who is afraid to get close to others and so will manage, whenever things begin to get intimate, to turn fun or honest sharing into an imagined slight. This person is often afraid of losing control, becoming vulnerable, and, therefore, uses her anger both to cover her fear and as a manipulative tool to keep herself in control. On the other hand, an individual may use the feelings of sadness to hide his anger. It can be assumed as quite likely that he grew up in a home where sadness was an acceptable feeling and anger was unacceptable. Or another may escalate her feelings of fear and fantasies of disaster in order to keep from celebrating success and her reasons for happiness. There is, it seems, even the use of glad feelings in a racket form—marshaled to the defense of all that is positive against even the hint of a negative—in the facade of the Pollyanna, the glad-hander, and the eternal optimist. There are also guilt rackets and confusion rackets among the more usually chosen forms of this substitute behavior.

The key to grasping the nature of rackets is their quality of unrealness and their tendency never to be finished. On first encounter a rackety expression of feeling may appear to be real, but as the experience is extended, the reality of its underpinnings becomes suspect. The first two or three times an individual picks up on a flaw in transactions with a new friend and uses that flaw as a reason for anger, he will likely be given the benefit of the doubt by his friend. But by the fifth or sixth instance of such behavior, a judgment may have been made by the friend that this person is "always angry." The "always" quality points toward racket. Racket feelings may be delivered from a base of much reality, little reality, or almost total fantasy, but ultimately the base itself will be felt as inadequate for the feeling that is expressed.

Racket feelings go on and on and come up again and again. In contrast, straight, nonracket feelings are felt, learned from, dealt with and let go of, and the person moves to the next experience and the next feeling (Woollams, Brown, & Huige, 1977).

GAMES. By *game* Berne means a psychological game and defines it as "an ongoing series of complementary ulterior transactions progressing to a well-defined, predictable outcome" (Berne, 1964b, p. 48). A game comes about when people use duplex transactions to communicate, saying one thing at the beginning and then switching to a "surprise" ending which ordinarily results in bad feelings for all participants.

The first game recognized by Berne and those he worked with was "Why Don't You, Yes But" (Berne, 1964b, p. 116). In this game the initiator seems to be saying that she wants to be helped, but as she and those who try to help transact together, she is able to state a "good" reason why each of the suggestions will *not* work. At the conclusion everyone gets to leave with bad feelings—the initiator because no one was able to help her and the helpers because they weren't able to help!

There are five ways used in TA to analyze games (Woollams & Brown, 1978, p. 135): (a) *formal game analysis* focuses on the specific "advantages" of a game; (b) the *drama triangle* clarifies game roles and role exchange; (c) *transactional diagrams* show ego states, the movement from one to another, and the duplexes; (d) the *symbiosis diagram* identifies the preferred ego states of each participant; and (e) *formula G* delineates the steps of a game in its flow from the initial moves to payoff.

These five are used to focus on the different facets of games. However, in the analysis of a specific game, they are often woven together.

Learning to recognize games usually begins, after a game is completed, with a new look at the bad feeling payoff. Of course, as long as the bad feeling is accepted and feels comfortable the game continues to accomplish the purpose of its original design and there is no motivation for change. But when the old, familiar, bad feeling payoff no longer feels fully comfortable, then the learning can begin.

At this point, the question can be asked: *What do you get out of playing this game?* Formal game analysis points to six kinds of *payoff* or *"advantages"* (Berne, 1964b, pp. 70, 71): (a) internal psychological, (b) external psychological, (c) internal social, (d) external social, (e) biological, and (f) existential. An illustration of these payoffs can be seen in the game of "I'm Only Trying to Help You" (ITHY), which opens with the therapist offering advice to a client. The client seems to agree and says he will "try it out," but later returns to report that the suggestion would not work. The therapist feels let down but may go ahead and offer further advice with the same cycle being repeated. His "let down" feeling then becomes frustration and, if he and the client continue to play a few more rounds, the frustration becomes a feeling of inadequacy and finally bewilderment (Berne, 1964b, p. 144).

The advantages of this game to the therapist are (a) internal psychological: the therapist gets to feel like a martyr; (b) external psychological: he doesn't have to face his inadequacies; (c) internal social: he gets to think about the ingratitude of others; (d) external social: he gets to talk to other therapists about the deep-seated quality of this patient's problems; (e) biological: he gets sympathetic stroking from his wife or other therapists who have had similar clients; and (f) existential: the therapist gets to prove again that he is not as good as he thought.

Once the payoff of a game has begun to be identified, the game player who wants to quit can move a step back into the process and begin to spot the *switch* and the *cross* (p. 27) which occur just before the payoff blossoms. The switch can be demonstrated using the Drama Triangle (Figures 12 and 13) with its three roles of *Persecutor* (P), *Rescuer* (R), and *Victim* (V) (Karpman, 1968). Looking at the same game (ITHY), we see first of all the therapist in the role of Rescuer and the client in the role of Victim (Figure 12a).

The Drama Triangle postulates the theory that all drama is based on these three roles and the excitement of the dramatic situation derives from the exchanges that occur among the roles. In this case the client as Victim exchanges this role for that of Persecutor and the therapist exchanges his role of Rescuer for that of Victim (Figure 12b).

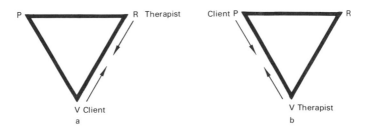

FIGURE 12.   The drama triangle.

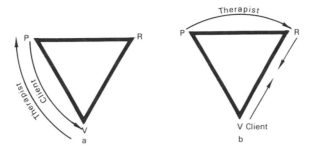

FIGURE 13. Role switches in the drama triangle.

Games can be played within games or fuse into other games. Here our Client-Victim might well be playing a game of "Wooden Leg" (Berne, 1964b, pp. 159–162) in which he presents himself as unable to follow through with the therapist's suggestions because he is alcoholic or had some difficult childhood experience. And the Therapist-Rescuer (now Victim) might, once he has gotten enough of frustration and bewilderment, set up a game of "Now I've Got You, You Son of a Bitch" (Berne, 1964b, pp. 85–87) in which he makes some "final statement to the client that puts him down mightily. He would then switch from Victim to Persecutor and the client as Persecutor would exchange places with him as the new Victim (Figure 13a). Finally, if the victim were properly apologetic, the therapist could with good conscience return to his original role of Rescuer (Figure 13b) and they would be ready for the next round.

Transactional Diagrams show what is happening within the duplex transactions and among ego states as various game responses are made by the participants (Berne, 1964b, p. 55). The transactions at both social and psychological levels are illustrated in Figure 14.

Notice in these Transactional Diagrams that the switch is seen as a change in ego states at the psychological level. It will feel to the therapist that he has been crossed up and if Transaction 1 is placed over Transaction 2, the psychological "cross" is clearly seen.

The Symbiosis Diagram (Schiff & Schiff, 1971; Woollams & Brown, 1978, pp. 130–141) is used to focus on the preferred ego states of the participants (Figure 15). In ITHY the therapist prefers to be both Parent and Adult, and so take care of the seemingly inadequate, helpless client who is in his Child. In order to do this the therapist and the client must discount the Parent and the Adult of the client (who can't be trusted to handle the difficulties of life) and the Child of the therapist (who isn't allowed to openly feel his frustration). In the symbiotic relationship neither participant can allow himself to be seen as a complete person. When the switch in the game comes, the client flips from the Compliant to the Rebellious form of his Adapted Child and temporarily comes on from his Parent as was seen in the Transactional Diagram. He manages to prove the "know-it-all" Parent-therapist wrong in that moment, but the symbiosis remains the same.

The fifth approach to game analysis is Berne's "Formula G"—diagram-

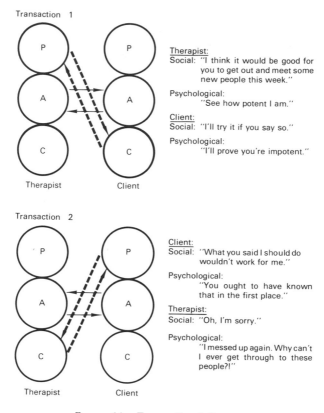

Transaction 1

Therapist   Client

Therapist:
Social: "I think it would be good for you to get out and meet some new people this week."

Psychological:
"See how potent I am."

Client:
Social: "I'll try it if you say so."

Psychological:
"I'll prove you're impotent."

Transaction 2

Therapist   Client

Client:
Social: "What you said I should do wouldn't work for me."

Psychological:
"You ought to have known that in the first place."

Therapist:
Social: "Oh, I'm sorry."

Psychological:
"I messed up again. Why can't I ever get through to these people?!"

FIGURE 14.   Transactional diagrams.

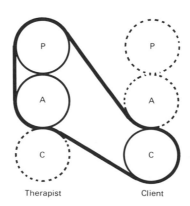

Therapist   Client

FIGURE 15.   A symbiosis diagram.

CON + GIMMICK = RESPONSES ➡ SWITCH ➡ CROSS ➡ PAYOFF

FIGURE 16. Formula G.

med in the form of an equation (Figure 16). Illustrations of the *con* and the *gimmick* are seen in the Transactional Diagrams (Figure 14, Transaction 1) in which the "social" statements of the client and the therapist mask the "psychological," ulterior messages. The therapist pretends he is doing one thing, that is, helping the client, while in reality he is doing something else, that is, setting himself up for frustration and bewilderment. This is a con. It only works because there is a weakness it can hook into, that is, a handle or gimmick (Berne, 1972, p. 23). Here the gimmick is the client's desire to prove authority figures wrong.

The *switch*, as has already been pointed out, occurs with the switch in ego states at the psychological level. The *cross* is the momentary feeling of confusion, and of being "crossed up," felt by the therapist. The *payoff* is all of the "advantages" gained from participating in the game (p. 23).

Games can be played at first, second, and third degree levels of intensity. A first degree level is merely uncomfortable; second degree is socially embarrassing; and third degree involves tragedy and/or tissue damage (Berne, 1964b, p. 64). In the therapist's game of ITHY, first-degree game playing might result in only a vague feeling of frustration, second degree a 2-week depression, and third degree could go all the way to suicide.

Games can be ended at any point in their development: as an individual becomes sensitive to the moves of his game, he can learn to spot an invitation to play in the opening duplex. Adult, cognitive awareness of the steps within a game, the feelings that go with each step, and the various advantages of the payoff can go a long way in helping the individual stop a game. But, in the final analysis, game playing does not cease until the reason behind it is dealt with. The connection here is with script and the life decisions which are reinforced as strokes are gained from each play of the game.

Stamps. In TA, *stamps* is the term used to represent incomplete transactions at the feeling level. Stamps are saved-up fellings or strokes used to support rackets and games, and to justify game and script playoffs (Berne, 1964a, p. 127; Woollams & Brown, 1978, p. 146).

Time Structuring. Games are one of six categories worked out by Berne in his list of human *time-structuring* activities (Berne, 1972, pp. 21–26; Woollams & Brown, 1978, pp. 81–92). These six categories include: (a) withdrawal, (b) ritual, (c) pastimes, (d) work, (e) games, and (f) intimacy. Each is designed as a structure for time in which the desired strokes will most likely be produced.

Withdrawal describes activities that involve only one person who mentally separates himself from others for a long or short period of time. Examples are daydreams, fantasy, and meditation.

Ritual involves two or more people who, through stated or implied agreement, speak or act in a prescribed and predictable fashion. We see ritual in religious services, graduation exercises, and the daily greeting of two people in the hall.

Pastimes are less regimented than rituals but also tend to be fairly predictable. They are organized around common interests which are "talked about" when no goal of "doing anything" is contemplated. Common subjects for pastiming include automobiles, sports, children, places to eat, food, and dieting.

Work is goal directed toward some objective product. Examples include the job a person holds to earn her living, the chores given to a teenage son, and the hobby of gardening.

Games begin with and are played using ulterior transactions—ordinarily out of Adult awareness. They follow a well-defined course and end in a predictable outcome. The payoff will be in terms of each player's favorite (usually bad) feeling.

Intimacy is understood to be the most rewarding of the six ways to structure time. It can be defined as a relationship of sharing and trust, that is honest, game-free, lacking ulterior motives, and with the straight, spontaneous giving and receiving of strokes. It occurs in times of courage when people decide to level with each other, or when persons, in love, share the joy of being themselves with each other.

Any of the six forms of time structuring can be used to gain either positive or negative strokes (see pp. 73–75), good or bad feelings. As an illustration, it is possible either to withdraw into depression or to use withdrawal for spiritual renewal. The same is true for the other five forms—though games in large part are employed to fill time with negative feelings and intimacy must ultimately move toward the positive or dissolve itself in the process.

Script Analysis. The word "script" is used in TA to denote the life plan created by an individual at an early age to ensure survival within the world (Woollams & Brown, 1978, pp. 151–189), as the young child perceives that world, and which is then used as the basic ground plan for the living of the rest of his or her life (Berne, 1972, pp. 25, 26). A very large part of the child's environment is the grown-ups around her and any older brothers and sisters who may exist. From these people she receives the food, shelter, and caring that she needs to survive. The young child is able to process an enormous amount of data and from this computes the safest and shortest ways to the satisfaction of her needs. As these ways to satisfaction, whether by crying, screaming, or cooing, become generalized into some sort of rules for living, the script has begun to be written.

In terms of the influence of parents and others on the child, the script is input with strokes. What mother comes running for and smiles at, become important foundation stones for the script. Even negative attention can be an important stroke if the small child computes that that is the only attention he is going to get. This then is the person who may become a behavioral problem for his teachers in school.

A life script is similar to the script of a dramatic stage play (Berne, 1972, pp. 35–39). There is a general theme which can be stated in a few words. This is called the *injunction*. Certain roles are called for. These will be filled as the individual selects particular persons as friends, employers, or married partner(s). There will even be certain lines to be spoken and times to laugh, to look sad, or to be angry. Finally, as in the stage play, there is a climax and conclusion in the life script; there are climactic scenes and–or statements and the individual proceeds to her preprogrammed life-script payoff.

Ordinarily a script is in operation for a lifetime. A person will modify the external forms to accommodate the particular situation he finds himself in, but the original thrust of the script will remain. However, scripts can be changed either under extreme duress of danger, tragedy, or faith in which a person "converts" to another point of view, or in the conscious redecision process of a therapeutic setting.

Scripts can be similar, but, like fingerprints, no two are exactly alike. In general, scripts can be categorized as *loser, nonwinner,* or *winner* (Berne, 1972, pp. 203–205; Capers, 1975). In the loser script there is more negative experience, negative thinking, and negative feeling than positive. Loser scripts with tragic endings are sometimes called *hamartic.* This term is drawn from Greek drama, in which the hero blindly commits a tragic error and destroys his life. In the nonwinner or *banal* script the negative and the positive just about balance each other out. In the winner script the positive far outweighs the negative. Losers are the problem people whom judges and jailers frequently see. Nonwinners are those who almost make it but never do. Winners accomplish what they set out to do.

Berne observed that scripts structure time in the following ways (Berne, 1972, pp. 205–207): (a) *Never* scripts never get to do or have what they want the most; (b) *Always* scripts must always follow a particular line of living such as always working; (c) *Until* scripts rule that the individual must wait until something happens or until a certain time before doing the wanted thing; (d) *After* scripts point toward trouble after marriage, after success, or after age 50; (e) *Over-and-Over* scripts program the person to almost succeed but never quite; and (f) *Open-Ended* scripts make no plans for what the individual will do when the script program is completed, that is, when the children leave home, the fortune is made, or retirement is achieved.

Another way to look at scripts is in terms of the fundamental stance chosen by the individual as he faces his world. This stance is summed up in the various forms of OK and not-OK. The four usually pointed to in TA are: I'M NOT-OK—YOU'RE OK; I'M OK—YOU'RE NOT-OK; I'M NOT-OK—YOU'RE NOT-OK; and I'M OK—YOU'RE OK (Harris, 1967, pp. 43–50). It appears that most people, in the process of early training, decide on the I'M NOT-OK—YOU'RE OK stance. It makes sense in a world in which the little person finds himself smaller than all the others and dependent upon others for almost everything. The I'M OK—YOU'RE NOT-OK stance is chosen under extreme duress and may end in some form of sociopathy. The I'M NOT-OK—YOU'RE NOT-OK stance results from an environment of heavy double messages and can end in a schizophrenic orientation. The I-M OK—YOU'RE OK stance is usually decided in the Adult ego state later in life, while the other three are decisions of the Child at an early stage.

In order to clarify the way in which a script is created from the various

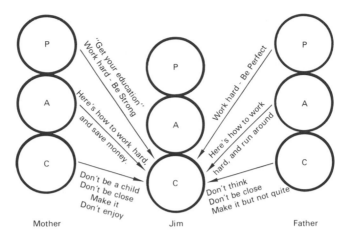

FIGURE 17.   Jim's script matrix.

inputs impinging upon the personality, it is helpful to draw a *script matrix* (Fig. 17) (Steiner, 1966).

Jim is a workaholic, a perfectionist, and sometimes steps out on his wife. He has done well in business. He is quite sure that he loves his wife. What he does not understand is why he periodically jeopardizes everything they have built together, his reputation, and his business, in order to start seeing someone outside his marriage. It begins to make sense as the elements of the puzzle come together in a life-script matrix.

The material for the matrix is gathered, in large part, from the original intake and the life-script questionnaire. Various questions are asked about what the individual was told concerning his birth, how he feels about his name, his favorite story as a child, his favorite game, his heroes, his favorite bad feeling, and what his mother, his father and others were like when he was a child.

In Figure 17 Jim received strong Parent messages from both his mother and his father to work hard. They modeled work-hard behavior and gave Jim positive strokes for work that he did. From his mother Jim received an unequivocal message to "make it"; the message from his father tended to be "make it but not quite." Jim's mother regularly told her 10 children to "get an education." She was careful with the money she got from selling eggs and garden produce. His father was a sharecropper and, off and on, managed to get close to owning his own farm but then would get "taken" in a land deal, drink up his money, or spend it on affairs with other women.

In his life Jim has, for the most part, lived in his *drivers* (see p. 70): Be Strong and Be Perfect. His work is a model of perfection. But though the rewards of financial success and community standing have come to Jim, his script prevents him from ever relaxing. He cannot feel the childlike parts of himself, enjoy his achievements, or be close to his wife, because he must always be strong. With his drivers he sets himself up for the script injunctions of Don't Be A Child, Don't Enjoy, and Don't Be Close.

Jim took a Don't-Be-Close injunction from the behavior of both his parents, in that neither showed much open affection with each other or with their children. From his father he also gets the injunction, Don't Think, and it is this life decision that allows Jim to escape the constant heaviness of working hard and being strong. This injunction operates as a "release" from pressure. The periodic affairs which have been a complete mystery to Jim's usual, careful-thinking self begin to make sense as the bones of the script matrix are laid bare.

The life script can be divided into *script* and *subscript*. Script injunctions are drawn by the Child of the individual from messages coming from the Child of parents, parent figures, and others held in authority. The primary script is formed around these script injunctions. Some 15 of these have been identified: Don't Be Close, Don't Belong, Don't Make It, Don't Be Well, Don't Trust, Don't Feel, Don't Be You, Don't Grow Up, Don't Be Sane, Don't Think, Don't Enjoy, Don't Be Important, Don't Be A Child, Don't Be, and Don't (Goulding, 1972, p. 107). There are also, of course, many positive script injunctions, but it is the negative ones that give us trouble and therefore are the ones we work with. Script injunctions are pre-Oedipal, nonverbal, preconscious, and visceral. They usually are not stated in so many words by a parent to the developing child, but are intuited by the child from the parents' words, voice tone, expressions, and behavior.

The subscript injunctions are drawn from the Parent of the parents and others. They are less potent than the script injunctions and give rise in the developing personality to a secondary script, the subscript. This secondary script was originally termed the "counterscript" in that the injunctions were so often experienced as opposite to the script injunctions (Steiner, 1966). In Jim's script (Figure 17) the Be-Perfect driver expectations of the subscript are experienced in opposition to Jim's Don't-Think script injunction with its periodic "mess up" behavior.

Taibi Kahler, in his work with the *not-OK miniscript* (Kahler & Capers, 1974), has identified five general forms of subscript injunctions: Be Strong, Be Perfect, Please Me, Hurry Up, and Try Harder. These five are called "drivers," and he sees them as primary in the individual's setting herself up for activity in her script. The sense is that the person is "driven" by herself to do what she does.

THE NOT-OK MINISCRIPT. The miniscript is designed to clarify the playing out of a script in the bit-by-bit, momentary living of life. It is diagrammed with four positions: Driver, Stopper, Payoff, and Provocation. The makeup of each position is described using four categories: Injunctions ($\lfloor$), Feeling ($\gtrless$), Thinking ($\mathfrak{y}$), and Behavior ($\longrightarrow$).

In Figure 18 the individual plays her script out in less than an hour as she begins again and again to copy her letter, trying hard to make it perfect so that she can please whoever asked her to write it or the one who will receive it. It could be played out in even less time if, for instance, in trying to properly introduce a guest at a party she mispronounces the name. She can then go quickly through her awareness of having messed up, feeling confused, feeling depressed and down, withdrawing for a while, and then somehow putting the blame on her husband who should have done the introduction in the first place!

Cure

Following diagnosis, there appear to be four areas of special focus within the TA treatment approach. These are *contract, stimulation, structure,* and *decision.*

Contract. Contracts are used by TA therapists to clearly set down the conditions and goals of treatment. Contracts afford a clearly defined structure which is safe, satisfying, and profitable for both client and therapist. There are three types of contracts used (Woollams & Brown, 1978, p. 250): the business contract, the treatment contract, and the working agreement. Contracts are part of the original intake session. They are taken seriously and are understood to be the underlying key to ongoing and final success in treatment.

The *business contract* clarifies the nature of the professional relationship which the therapist and the client are entering. Steiner states that there are four important considerations to focus on: mutual consent, valid consideration, competency, and lawful object (Steiner, 1971, pp. 101, 102). *Mutual consent* says that the agreement to work together is voluntary on the part of both therapist and client. *Valid consideration* calls for each person to put something of value into the relationship. For the therapist this usually means his time, his skills, and an appropriate place to meet. For the client, it usually means the payment of fees, though in some instances there can be an exchange of services. *Competency* implies that the client and the therapist are both competent to enter the therapeutic relationship. *Legal object* calls for the use of both legal and ethical means in bringing about legal and ethical ends.

Invitations to game are often given and sometimes accepted at the point of the business contract. An illustration is the husband who comes for counseling under the threat of divorce if he does not. The therapist who treats this situation as fully voluntary is letting himself in for a game and is likely to be disappointed in terms of final results. Valid consideration, too, can be a problem for therapists. The therapist who feels she is being paid too little for her time may have begun as a Rescuer; if so, she will soon begin to feel Victimized and may end up as an angry Persecutor. However it goes, the client will feel what is happening, that is, both the therapist's anger and, ultimately, his own anger at being Rescued. Therefore, the business contract, no less than the treatment contract, is part of the therapeutic process both in terms of diagnosis (as the therapist becomes aware of the kinds of game he and the client seem most likely to play) and in terms of cure (as the therapist carefully sets up a straightforward, game-free structure).

The *treatment contract* is also called the "Change Contract." As "threatment" the emphasis is on the therapist who is offering her ability, training, skills and concern in the service of the client and, as such, will "treat" the client. This is in line with the medical model and continues to have validity (Dusay, 1977b). As "change" the emphasis is on the client who has something he wants to change about himself and must furnish the energy to effect that change. The notion of "contract" tends to keep these two emphases in balance.

The treatment contract sets up specific goals for work between therapist and client. The creation of this contract for change is seldom an easy process as therapist and client struggle with each other and within themselves toward a bedrock of clarity, in terms of motivation and behavior, that both are willing to accept.

In my own practice I use a printed contract sheet. On that sheet are three questions, equally spaced down the page: (a) *What is it you want to change about yourself?*; (b) *What is the significant behavior?*; and (c) *What will success look like?* Toward the middle of our first session, I give this sheet to the client and we begin to work through it.

It is vital in the creating of a viable contract of this kind that the power for change in the individual be contacted either subtly or openly. This means, in TA language, that her Child be invited to speak. Contracts can be made from the Parent, the Adult, or the Child (and all three ego states will, and need to be involved in the final edition of a strong, workable contract) but if the Child is left out, cure will not take place. This calls for moving toward the wants and feelings that are underneath the long, good sounding words that often come out first, for example, "relationship," "communication," and "self-image."

But even if the client is using small, Anglo-Saxon words, it is important for the therapist to check out the underpinnings. With the client who says she wants to "feel her feelings," the therapist may well ask what her feelings are. The answers to this question will be written in the second part of the contract having to do with behavior. The therapist will continue questioning as the line of reasoning and sharing progresses until he and the client are satisfied that they have made the best sense of the client's desire for change, at that point. As the client does her work, in the weeks that follow, the therapist knows that she will gain greater clarity about what it is she is doing, and if the first attempt at contracting is less than solid, the client or the therapist, will recognize it and suggest a change that is more on target.

The treatment contract is used in this manner to clarify the wants of the client and the thinking of both the client and the therapist about what they are willing to attempt together. During the process all ego states of both participants are checked[6]: (a) the Child (of client): Is this what I want and do I feel comfortable with it? (of therapist): Do I feel good about working with this person on this matter in this way?; (b) the Parent (of both): Is this right and moral?; and (c) the Adult (of both): Does it make sense the way we have set it up?

The treatment contract, as noted above, includes data on the client's be-

---

[6]Ego-state names (Parent, Adult, and Child) may be but are not necessarily used at this early stage.

havior surrounding the issues the client is focusing on for change. In sharing her behavior the client gives the therapist a sense of where she has been and often clues as to how she got there. In the telling there is also the opportunity to begin clearing out unhappy pieces from the past with their tragic endings, stamps, and racket feelings.

Finally, the treatment contract includes a picture of success. This third part is a verbalization of the client's inside picture of herself *successfully* living out the changes she has accomplished. It is written in the present tense. In allowing herself to see herself where she wants to be, in new health and new freedom, she is setting herself up to do just that. For example, an individual with a contract stating, "I want to learn how to be close to others," might create for herself a success picture which reads: "I am in a room of new people; I am feeling relaxed; we are enjoying each other's company; I am making new friends."

Once drawn, the treatment contract becomes the guide for what is done in both individual and group sessions. What has happened since the last session is reported in terms of contract goals. What the client wants to work on in this session can be checked out in terms of its connection with the contract. The contract is sometimes referred to in the middle of work when it is helpful to make contact with the work's direction. Again, as the work as a whole progresses and clarity is gained, the client may find himself uncomfortable with the way he originally put the issue. Contracts may be added to as new levels of insight are broached and contracts may be subtracted from as goals are achieved. Finally, the contract is the checkpoint against which cure or success is tested when the client announces termination from the group. If his treatment contract was originally solid and has been kept up to date, then termination becomes a time of celebration for both the client and for his group.

The *working agreement* is a specific task the client will agree with her group to accomplish. These are working contracts or subcontracts which are sometimes referred to simply as "contracts." They are created by way of requests from the therapist and/or group members, and sometimes are suggested by the client herself. A client may, for instance, "contract" to be the "Martian" in the group and give feeling (versus thinking or judgment) feedback throughout the session no matter what else is happening. When there is an agreement for behavior or performing a specific task outside the group, this is called "homework." Working agreements are designed to give the client permission and protection as she moves in her life to accomplish her stated goals for change.

Contracts are nearly always the beginning point for therapists working in the TA model. One of the few times a contract is temporarily bypassed is when the person who has come for help is so emotionally torn by her situation that the requirement then is for the therapist to: (a) listen carefully to the client—letting her know she has been heard, (b) encourage her to feel her feelings and get them out, and (c) give her permission to give herself peace. When the main force of the trauma has abated somewhat, the therapist and the client can begin to move toward goals and contract. In almost all other therapeutic situations, contracts are the order of the day (Groder, 1976), and, in the way they are put together, they, in large part, determine the success or failure of the work.

Stimulation. All needs and wants finally come down to either stimulation or structure. We need stimulation in order to survive and we create the structure we need in order to produce that stimulation in the most efficient manner possible.

A form of stimulation that is vital to human life and development is the "stroke." A stroke is a unit of social intercourse and social attention (Berne, 1972, pp. 23, 24). A stroke can be physical, verbal, or nonverbal. Research has shown that infants require physical stimulation or strokes in order to develop properly and even to survive (Spitz, 1945). And, in fact, strokes are so important that if positive strokes are not available, negative ones will be invited. It is better to be spanked than ignored, and a negative stroke is better than none.

There are many forms of stroking. Physical strokes go all the way from being held in a mother's arms to arm wrestling and sexual intercourse. Verbal strokes include words of encouragement, arguments, the daily exchange of greetings, and the close words of intimacy. Nonverbal strokes include smiles, birthday gifts, a name in lights, and election to public office.

Strokes can be categorized as *Positive Conditional, Positive Unconditional, Negative Conditional,* and *Negative Unconditional* (Woollams & Brown, 1978, pp. 50, 51). The positive conditional stroke is a positive stroke which carries a condition: "I like the way you look in that dress." The positive unconditional stroke is positive without condition: "I love you." The negative conditional stroke is a negative stroke that carries a condition: "I don't like you when you smoke." The negative unconditional stroke is negative without condition: "I hate you." Conditional strokes tend to be the ones most easily accepted, whether positive or negative. The positive unconditional is usually the most difficult of the four to accept. The negative unconditional can, of course, be devastating.

Positive strokes, conditional or unconditional, allow interaction, dialogue, and negotiation to move smoothly. Positive strokes, when they are accepted and absorbed, build up the courage of the Child, that is, the courage to take the risk of change. Positive strokes are vital, therefore, to the healing process. Depression, for example, cannot exist in the midst of a matrix of positive stroking. Depression depends upon a supply of negative strokes, and as positive strokes are accepted the depression begins to evaporate. With further positive stroking, clarity and courage come forward to deal with the anger seemingly always beneath depression.

Clients of TA therapists are taught to aggessively listen for strokes and to seek them out. They are taught five ways in which to get all the strokes they want: (a) *Ask* for the strokes you want, (b) *Give* the strokes you want to give, (c) *Accept* the strokes you want to accept, (d) *Refuse* the strokes you do not want (or that aren't good for you), and (e) *Self-stroke* yourself. Each of these tends to contradict old training and scripting (Steiner, 1974, pp. 114–117), because to ask was considered conceited, giving was based in "ought to" rather than "want to," accepting was discouraged in favor of self-discounting, refusing was impolite, and self-stroking was the twin of pride.

People who enter therapy are often stroke-starved. The old rackets, games, and scripts are not producing acceptable strokes any longer, and a stroke void has been created. Also, as these same rackets, games, and scripts are brought to light, they become even less palatable as a stroke source. However, unless the stroke hunger is met and the void filled, the individual, out of desperation, will return to old behavior belonging to the old script. So the retraining of group members in terms of their need of strokes, recognition of strokes, and acceptance of strokes is vital to successful therapy.

The concept of *discounting* (Holloway, 1977; Woolams & Brown, 1978, pp. 112–115) is a part of this retraining. Discounting means simply the making of less value that which is of greater value. It is possible to discount the value of things, accomplishments, behavior, and persons. The continuation of bad feeling rackets depends on an inner program of discounting of self and/or others. All games begin with a discount. Scripts can be looked upon as discount screens through which only certain portions of the surrounding reality are allowed to pass in order that original script decisions can once again be "proven" by the incoming "data."

As an illustration of the many ways it is possible to discount, the statement: "I love you," might be answered by: (a) *denying:* "No you don't"; (b) *distrusting:* "What do you mean?"; (c) *ignoring:* "I'm afraid it's going to rain"; (d) *inflating:* "If you really knew me, you'd love me more!"; (e) *exchanging:* "I love you too"; and (f) *explaining:* "We were meant for each other."

In the group experience, certain words and phrases come to be recognized as discounts and will be brought to the attention of the one who is discounting (Berne, 1972, pp. 325–334). When a client uses the phrase "you know," it often is a discount of his own knowledge. Though it may seem to be simply a conversational "filler," it is likely he has moved into the Child ego state and is inviting the other person to move into Parent. The word "try" can signal an intent to "try and fail." When a client reports a piece of new behavior and that she "finally" did it, it is well to ask her to say the same sentence again without the "finally." It is a word which detracts from full celebration of accomplishment. TA therapists will, in a similar way, ask a client to substitute "won't" for "can't" since the "can't" is usually a discount of the client's own power to change.

Stopping the discounts and increasing the positive strokes are two sides of the same therapeutic coin as the client learns to supply himself with new, positive stimulation for living. As a part of this same OK stimulation, clients are taught to feel their feelings, to give feedback and to receive it, to celebrate accomplishment, and to care for each other. The teaching is done through word, through example, through acceptance, and perhaps through the vibrations themselves within the group.

Structure. As the stimulation of a person's life is renewed and replaced so also must the structure that sets the scene for that stimulation be renewed and replaced. This is accomplished by taking the TA tools of diagnosis, as discussed above, and using them now for cure. As they were used previously to clarify the specifics of the not-OK position, with its bad feeling payoffs and its tragic endings, so now structural analysis, transactional analysis, racket and game analysis, and script analysis are used to facilitate the move to an OK stance and process.

Utilizing the insights of structural analysis, the TA therapist will endeavor to offer the Child of her client: (a) *protection,* (b) *permission,* and (c) *potency* (Woollams, 1977). Protection has to do with the therapist's willingness and ability to set up a protective environment, both physically and psychologically, in which the client can safely try out new behaviors, search out the emotional roots of her script, make a redecision, and then begin the reordering of habits to support that decision.

In the safety of this protection, a client can be offered permission to succeed, to exist, to think, to feel, to be close, to trust, to belong, or to be important. In effect, it is a permission to temporarily use the Parent of the therapist and/or group members in place of the client's own Parent. *Space* is, in this way, given to the Free Child to grow and *time* is allowed in which the client can update her Parent.

In order for the therapist to offer believable protection and permission, there must also be potency. The script is powerful and was created in the midst of parental pressure and life and death alternatives. The potency of the therapist must be of this same power quality. It is achieved in the therapist's own OK acceptance of herself and in her careful use of all three of her ego states: (a) her Parent cares about her client and has life promoting values at her fingertips; (b) her Adult is able to present pertinent data according to the needs of the client; and (c) her own OK Child allows her full use of her power, creativity, and intuition.

Transactional analysis is used to gain insight into what is happening within the transactions of clients inside and outside the group. The familiar PAC diagrams are drawn with vectors to indicate the direction of the transactions. This insight and understanding is part of the healing endeavor. However, once this is done, the next step is taken and the client is offered the opportunity to restructure the diagram, to look for new options, and to decide on a course of action in line with both insights and options. Various communication techniques may also be taught by the therapist and time will be given for the practice of these when appropriate.

An awareness of rackets and games is utilized in the group as a guide to understanding the behavior and interaction that are finally self-defeating. Rackets and games exhibited by an individual can be ignored for a while and even allowed to run their course, confronted immediately if previously seen several times, or missed completely when played so expertly that neither the therapist nor the group members "catch on" until the bad feelings of the payoff begin to surface. But at some point, the racket or game will be recognized, confronted, and dissected.

Rackets and games are an early adaptation designed to produce the necessary strokes for survival. In terms of that adaptation at the Child level, a person's rackets and games always make sense though, to his Adult, they may appear quite illogical. Still, it is helpful to congratulate the Child on the care with which those early survival adaptations were worked out. And in dismantling a racket or game the client is encouraged to replace each part with something better and to move no faster than his Child is willing to part with the old designs.

The script itself is similarly used for insight and then for the building of a satisfying guide to living. A script matrix (Figure 17) may be drawn on the board. Data are elicited from the client as the drawing proceeds and this is augmented with material from the life-script questionnaire, transactions remembered by the group from earlier sessions, and insights that are gained in the midst of the exercise itself as pieces come together. This work brings to the client's Adult awareness the heretofore mysterious sources of early, life-script decision.

At other times, the miniscript form of the script is diagrammed. The not-OK miniscript, as explained earlier, is used to focus on injunctions, feelings, thoughts, and behavior which accompany the movement of the script in its everyday circuitous route (Figure 18). Once clarity on this has been achieved, an *OK miniscript* (Kahler & Capers, 1974) can be drawn utilizing the same situation with OK injunctions, feelings, thoughts, and behavior (Figure 19).

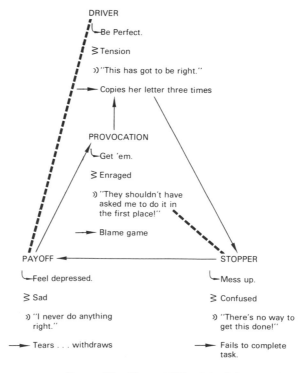

FIGURE 18.   The not-OK miniscript.

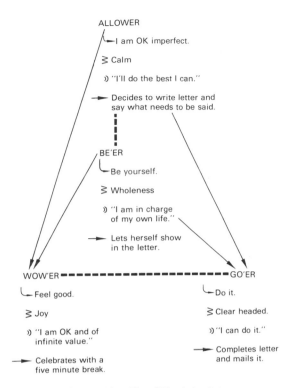

ALLOWER
⤺ I am OK imperfect.

⪼ Calm

⟩ "I'll do the best I can."

→ Decides to write letter and
say what needs to be said.

BE'ER
⤺ Be yourself.

⪼ Wholeness

⟩ "I am in charge
of my own life."

→ Lets herself show
in the letter.

WOW'ER ▬▬▬▬▬▬▬▬▬▬▬▬▬▬▬▬▬▬▬▬▬▬▬ GO'ER

⤺ Feel good.

⪼ Joy

⟩ "I am OK and of
infinite value."

→ Celebrates with a
five minute break.

⤺ Do it.

⪼ Clear headed.

⟩ "I can do it."

→ Completes letter
and mails it.

FIGURE 19.   The OK miniscript.

Decision. The script, and the rackets and games supporting that script, in turn fed by the negative feelings derived from them, all began with decisions. A person's life plan, or script, is not laid on her willy-nilly. There can be, of course, enormous pressure from the early living situation and the people belonging to that situation so that the options for survival are quite limited. However, it is the person herself who decides what the script shall be (Goulding & Goulding, 1978, pp. 10, 11). Beneath this decision is the basic decision to live. As an illustration, an early decision to "don't be close" is made in the midst of an environment where trying to get close to the grownups brought pain and/or danger to the child. So, the decision to survive, by way of a Don't-Be-Close injunction, though originally made by the individual to protect herself, later becomes the cause of other pain when she wants to get close to someone and finds herself again and again unable to do so.

What is important here is that old decisions be seen for what they are: adaptations chosen and decided upon for the purpose of survival. A feeling of guilt or despair at earlier decisions made within the child's limited environment is inappropriate. This is said clearly to the client who is beginning to be in touch with her roots of early decision. She is encouraged to see the decision in terms of survival, and to understand that that same power of decision is available to her in the present moment.

It is also useful to understand that the same level of decision must be part of any new script decision if the new decision is to have the same power in the client's life. Adult awareness and insight are the first step toward redecision. The next step is the emotional "getting in touch" with that part of the Child which made the original decisions. Gestalt techniques, psychodrama, or guided meditation may be used to gain this kind of contact. With the accomplishment of insight and deep emotional contact, a viable and lasting redecision becomes possible.

A redecision is not a promise made by the client to the therapist, to the group (Woollams & Brown, 1978, p. 205), or to some figure in authority either living or dead. It is not even a promise made by the client to himself. Rather, it is an intention of direction decided by the client, in full view of his wants and needs, that is viable from the point of view of all three ego states—moral to the Parent, logical to the Adult, and comfortable to the Child.

As intention, the redecision can be trusted. It has been made and that particular piece of it does not need to be made again. Further steps involve the client focusing on specific behavioral changes she sees belonging to the redecision. She will, during the next weeks and months, increase the strength of her new scripting as she, step by step, assimilates it into behavior and feelings, weaving it into her belief system.

Under physical or emotional stress, bits of old script which still have not been worked through will sometimes surface. It is important that both therapist and client be aware that this can occur. And when it does, the experience can be used for further insight and further growth. The tendency of these later episodes of script activity is to become less intense and shorter in duration.

Summary

The basic concepts of TA theory can be divided under: (a) diagnosis and (b) cure. Diagnosis includes four techniques of TA analysis: structural analysis, transactional analysis, game and racket analysis, and script analysis. Cure includes four areas of approach in TA therapy: contract, stimulation, structure, and decision.

Assumptions about Human Nature

We are born OK. I'm OK, You're OK, We're OK, They're OK, It's OK. This is the way we were born to live (Wollams & Brown, 1978, p. 1). Whether a person accepts his own basic OK or not, whether he or I act in an OK manner, or whether we even feel OK, still we are OK (Grimes, 1975). Within TA, this is the basic philosophical stance on the nature of persons. For the individual, the OK becomes a decision made about himself and others. It can be made either consciously or out-of-consciousness, though for most people it is a conscious decision.

We are in charge of our own mental and physical health. If we are sick, it is because, in some basic part of our system as a human being, it makes sense to be sick. If we play a bad feeling game or have a headache, we have good reason for what we are doing. It may not make sense in view of our present environment, but it makes sense. It is, therefore, necessary to uncover that "sense" if we are going to make the changes we want in ourselves.

We are also the product of our decisions in terms of relationship to others. What others do to us began with our decision to transact with them and continues in our various decisions along the way to accept or refuse what is offered. In this sense, whatever is done is only seemingly done to us. And, in that we are the ones who made the original decision, we can redecide when and how we will change it.

Finally, we carry within us much of the necessary data for redecision. A particular decision may have been made out-of-consciousness at an early age and is therefore "preconscious," but it is never "unconscious." If we decide we need to, we can go to the roots of that decision and search out the data we need.

Personality Theory

Personality is developed in response to the young individual's own stimulus and structure hunger and in response to the stimulus and forms of structure received from her parents and/or other significant persons. It is a milieu of the growing person's wants and feelings shaped by her experiences within an expanding context of decisions.

Decisions make sense out of the incoming mass of data. The stimulation experienced as satisfying becomes the stimulation that is preferred and sought. The structures that facilitate the arrival of the wanted stimulation are the structures that are chosen. It is a process of action and reactions. If the child cries, someone will come. If she cries quietly, perhaps she will be cuddled. If she cries in the middle of the night, she may cry louder and will continue to cry until she is taken care of. If she is startled, she cries loudest of all so that "they" come quickly. Crying *in various ways* is her structure. Being taken care of is stimulation.

During this phase, the parents are also applying *their* structure. They do not like to hear the crying, so they respond quickly. After a time, however, they may come to feel they have let the baby take over. Then, the old structures within themselves begin to whisper that they are "spoiling" this child. So they rethink their structure and perhaps decide to put the baby "on a schedule" and suffer through the first few times of her crying rage.

During the process of action, reaction, and struggle between those who are already here and the babe who just arrived, the development of personality takes place. The new individual again and again decides what she wants and how she can get it. Decision is added to decision, decisions are made about decisions, and personality is formed.

There are as many subtle variations on this theme as there are human beings. It is here that the life script is written. This script is the "owner's manual" created by the individual word-by-word, feeling-by-feeling, and decision-by-decision, as the just born baby, then the growing toddler, and again the little child battles for life and selfhood.

Obviously, in such a prodigious project there is room for error when that life-script plan is applied to later living. The plan is *always* correct in terms of the needs and perceptions of the young child. However, it can be most unsatisfying in terms of later awareness of self, mature forms of need, and a broadened perception of the environment.

In this awareness, an individual will sometimes recognize the need for change within herself. This is often a scary proposition. It can be experienced as the personality operating against itself, even at war with itself, as one side attempts to force on the other side an "obviously necessary" change and then meets unyielding resistance. This resistance may not be noticed at first and the action for change may be thought to have been accomplished, but it will not have been so, for early decisions at the deeper level will prevail (Woollams, 1977).

This internal struggle is the same old battle originally played out between the parents and their little child. The little one learned long ago how to win this kind of battle, and just because the new regime of grown-up Parent and Adult sees itself as logical, this does not mean it is felt in the Child as logical.

The battle can continue with one side even calling the other evil: "I know that nothing good dwells within me, that is, in my flesh. I can will what is right, but I cannot do it" (Romans 7:18, Revised Standard Version of the Holy Bible, 1952). In fact, the battle will go on until the logical, grown-up side of the personality begins to treat the primitive, early decision maker and script writer with dignity. At this point, the listening of each to the other and the negotiation of internal differences can begin. Old, seemingly weird decisions can be honored for their service in keeping us alive, but rethought, now, in terms of present needs and expanded awareness. Accordingly, the personality updates itself and brings about desired change.

Comparison with Related Theories

According to the thinking of Milton Erickson (Haley, 1967, p. 535; 1973, pp. 17, 18) and the recent work of Bandler and Grinder (1975, pp. xiii, 2), at a deep level, similar things occur in all successful therapy. Whether the work is done in consciousness or out-of-consciousness, the client's perception of the structure of reality is opened to a reexamination of her original experience of reality. In the process, previously unseen options appear and a base for redecision is created.

It appears that what we are seeing when we look at the various theories of therapy dedicated to the healing of persons is, in actuality, *points of entry*. Each approach tends to have a favorite door by which it enters the healing relationship.

In orienting clients as to their position within the healing continuum, I sometimes use what I call the *Life Change Circle* (LCC) (Figure 20). This diagram is helpful in quickly pointing the client to other areas of awareness which need emphasis in the completion of the healing process.

It appears that all four ways of knowing, *belief, image, feeling,* and *behavior,* are part of fully knowing. They are necessary to both the conservation of old life patterns and the integration of new patterns. Each of the four is enhanced by the other three, for example, new *belief* is strengthened as the individual *images* in his mind the way it might be, then allows himself to sense how this would *feel,* and, finally, plans changes of *behavior* and carries them through. The belief base, then, is broadened, as the new behavior affirms the new belief. The image comes more easily, the feelings are felt, and the process continues.

On the other hand, when parts of the LCC are left out, the desired life change either will not result or will be only partially inaugurated. This happens when there is new insight and new thinking (perhaps about early childhood influences and decisions) but the person has no image of herself actually living out her new understanding. Or, new behavior is begun (quit smoking, go on a diet, get a job), but the client continues to believe "it won't work," and truly it will not.

The same LCC diagram can be utilized to illustrate therapeutic points of entry. Freudianism, Rational Emotive therapy, and TA tend to enter at the point of *belief.* Their concern is first of all with the client's thinking, insight, and belief about herself. Therapies which begin with art, music, fantasy, and meditation are entering at the point of *image.* Illustrations of these are: art therapy, psychodrama, prayer groups, and meditation for cancer control (Simonton, Matthews-Simonton, & Creighton, 1978). Therapies belonging to the *feeling* point of entry are Gestalt and Encounter Therapy. Therapies beginning with *behavior* are Reality Therapy and Behavior Modification.

Therapists of one persuasion or another may argue with my placement of their approach at a particular point on the LCC. However, it is important to understand that whatever the point of entry into the healing continuum, all

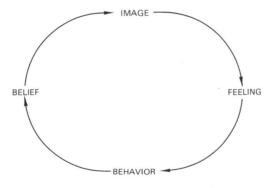

FIGURE 20.   The life change circle.

four ways of knowing must, in the final analysis, be adequately integrated by the client. TA theory, for example, with its grasp of ego states and life script, would be of limited usefulness if used alone. It is interesting to understand transactions and this, in itself, can be healing to those who are already standing on fairly solid psychological ground. But in order to be well-rounded and successful as a therapeutic approach, TA must either borrow or create theory and method to enter the other aspects of human change. In the same way, it appears that Gestalt therapy, which begins with feeling, must reach out for pegs of thinking and belief on which to hang the uncovered feelings and awareness. The behavior therapies must do similarly—for as long as a person thinks poor, sees herself poor, and feels poor, she will ultimately create the conditions of poverty even though, in the moment, she is rich. And, in the area of image, a program of meditation on wellness without a parallel change in belief may even be a setup for further stress and sickness.

Therefore, to the extent that the practitioner of a particular modality is willing to do what is necessary to fulfill the conditions for healing in the wholeness of human personality, the theory used, whichever it is, will produce successful results. My impression is that this is true even though some theories may actually be clearer, better integrated, or generally more successful than the one being used.

THERAPY

Theory

We, each of us, created our life script in relationship with others. This usually means a family environment, but may be true of other kinds of groupings. The script is written in the group environment as a roadmap for getting from point A (the need) to point B (the satisfaction).

If the needs of the infant are responded to quickly, appropriately, and with a minimum of fuss, the script will tend to be written as a winner script. If the early environment is otherwise, for example, the hungry infant is slapped when he cries instead of being fed, then substitute behaviors will be developed. Loser and nonwinner behaviors will be worked out in order to win whatever can be won in the situation. Passivity and manipulative techniques will be instituted by the young child instead of assertive, nonmanipulative behavior.

The point of therapy is to teach the client how to meet her needs appropriately and effectively in a straightforward fashion. It means the dismantling of the old script, with its unsatisfying substitutions, and the creation of a new script. In this process discounts of self and others are confronted and the client is encouraged to account for her feelings, thoughts, and needs.

In the therapeutic group milieu an individual has the opportunity to rethink the original base of the old script. To a greater or lesser extent, various members of the group will be experienced as mother, father, or other family members. Old feelings, incompletely dealt with in the past, can be brought to the surface and examined in the light of day.

In addition to this, the openness to being heard and the permission to make himself heard is both a model for new behavior and also an environment in which new techniques for living can be worked out and inaugurated by the client.

Process

The process of therapy (Woollams & Brown, 1978, pp. 261–265) can be divided into seven steps: (a) trust in the other, (b) trust in self, (c) moving into group, (d) work, (e) redecision, (f) integration, and (g) termination. These seven steps intertwine with each other and seldom are clearly separate.

Trust in the other may never be openly stated between therapist and client, but must be built if success is to be achieved. This trust begins with the first telephone call requesting an appointment. The process continues during the first session, with the gathering of data: why the client has come, name, address, referral source, state of physical health and other background information. During the same session, the working out of a treatment change contract is begun; questions are asked to determine whether there is active third degree behavior; and a business contract is negotiated.

Beneath this surface activity is the underlying trust building process either being accomplished or not depending on how it is done. For the client, trust in the other means confidence in the therapist as a capable professional who is willing to work with him, accept him as he is, and who uses a therapeutic modality that works. For the therapist, trust in the other means confidence that the client has enough motivation to work in order for the therapist to invest his time and himself in this person.

Trust in self tends to follow the building of trust in the other and is dependent upon it. The meaning here for the client is that change, real and lasting, is possible both in the abstract and specifically for him. The meaning for the therapist is that the abilities and skills he has to offer can be appropriately helpful to this client.

Moving into group begins during the first session when the client is advised by the therapist that group work is ordinarily part of the counseling process in his practice. Feelings and reactions to this news are dealt with in a relaxed manner. Later, after five or more sessions, when he feels the client is ready, the therapist will invite him into a group. At this point the therapist has decided that (a) there is a good level of trust between himself and the client; (b) the client has begun to trust himself and the process; (c) the client is regularly and successfully working in session and between sessions; and (d) the client will profit from the group experience. In my experience, it is important to success to exercise this kind of care in moving persons from individual work to group work. However, others may use far fewer individual sessions or perhaps none, placing the client immediately in group and even completing the intake during a group session (Berne, 1966b, p. 10).

Work, of course, is going on from the time of my first question to the client, "What brings you here to see me?" to the time of my last words, "Have a good life." Work means doing what is necessary to accomplish the changes called for in the treatment contract. Work includes the deconfusing of the client's Child, the updating of the Parent, the clarifying and strengthening of the Adult, and the rewriting of the script.

Redecision is central to successful therapeutic work. It begins with a growing awareness on the part of the client and the therapist of the nature of the original decisions and script. This awareness is deepened both intellectually and emotionally as the client works. A lasting redecision on his life plan calls for the participation of all three ego states, as explained under "Basic Concepts" (pp. 77, 78).

Integration may be overlooked or slighted in the excitement and celebration of redecision. However, as the old script took time and effort to achieve its standing in all the facets of life, so the new options for living, as new script, take both time and effort. This means that the client may continue in group for some weeks or even months following his basic redecision as he integrates the redecision and its effects upon the various relationships and parts of his life.

Termination from active therapy comes about when the dividends no longer warrant the expense in time, money and effort. A ground rule, in our practice, is that the client give a three session termination notice in group. This allows time to go over the treatment contract during this first session when termination is announced. During the second session, the ego states of the client are looked at separately to determine the thinking and feeling of each regarding termination. The final session is used for words of love, well-wishing, and goodbye. The time and focus utilized for termination also allow the client the opportunity to feel comfortable with his decision to terminate or to realize otherwise and to contract for further work.

Mechanism

There are five parts to the mechanism of therapy as it is used in our groups: (a) the contract review, (b) the work of the client, (c) the participation of the group, (d) the contribution of the therapists, and (e) the establishment of the environment.

The *contract review* is done at the beginning of the session with each group member, in turn, stating her change contract, what she has done about it since the last session, and what she wants from this session. This is done in a few sentences taking from 30 seconds to 2 minutes. It is immediately followed by a single word of feedback from each of the other persons in the group. After everyone has completed the contract review, an opportunity is given for clarification on any feedback received.

The *work of the client* is the responsibility of the client. She must initiate the work, that is, ask to work and state what it is she wants to work on. She may be asked for further clarity, where she wants to end up with this work, or how it relates to her contract.

The *participation of the group* adds a quality of reality and broadness to the work that is unavailable in individual therapy. There develops in the group a group memory which operates both generally, in support of the group milieu, and specifically in terms of remembered data given by the client at an earlier date. The feeling response of the group to the person and work of a fellow member is often a turning point in that client's work. The affirmation of each other within the group operates as a continuing and trusted base.

The *contribution of the therapists* includes the general modeling of relaxed OK behavior which forms the base for the group environment and the specific use of various therapeutic techniques, diagrams, and theory.

The *establishment of the environment* is originally begun by the therapists and continued by the group—though it may be added to by the therapists from time to time. The nature of this environment is based on an unqualified acceptance of self and others as OK. This is followed by the encouragement to "feel your feelings," to "make sure" you get the amount of positive strokes you need, to "account for yourself," and to know you are "in charge" of your life.

PRACTICE

Problems

When Clients Are Afraid to Work

When a client has only recently entered the group, she may be reluctant to work. It is usually best to let the client handle this herself. Otherwise, it is easy to get into games of Rescue that end in frustration for both therapist and group. However, when four to six sessions have passed and the client has not yet begun to work, the suggestion may be made that it is probably time to begin. If there is a problem of trust, then this needs to be dealt with before other work can be done.

The issue here is that, though the therapist and the group can make statements, ask questions, encourage, and confront, the initiative is best left in the hands of the client. If the client is inviting the group to Rescue her and the group does so by beginning to do her work for her, then, of course we are into game. The recognized game can, at this point, become the work. But here too it is important to ask the client if the game, now brought into Adult awareness, is what she wants to work on. In this way the initiative is again returned to her.

When Clients Terminate Inappropriately

Inappropriate termination means the client is terminating from the group (a) before he has completed his change contract, (b) before the first 3 months are up that he originally agreed to, or (c) without giving three sessions notice of termination.

Occasionally, a client will simply drop out, and at other times the client will write a letter saying "I'm sorry . . . but." However it is done, it is probably a bit of script showing and may be an invitation to game. To try to draw the client back with a letter or telephone call is a continuation of the game. It is better for the therapist to recognize in such a situation that he had his chance with this person and did not succeed, to feel the loss, to learn from the failure (his and the client's), and then to forgive himself.

When Age, Illness, or Tragedy Tempt Us to Rescue

Older people, like others, may enter a group hoping for some magical cure to their discomfort in life. Then when the awareness begins to come through that therapy takes work, they may feel "at their age" that the effort is not worth it. So they spend their group time sitting and waiting, discounting the seriousness of their problems, giving out Parental platitudes, and perhaps mentioning their age and how they know they aren't "with it."

Sometimes I find myself being overly protective of the older person in group. I am aware of the amount of energy it took to secure the positions they hold in life, how life has not been easy, and how devastating the knowledge of missed opportunities can be. But when I, in my misplaced kindness, Rescue that person, I am setting myself up to feel Victimized when she doesn't get her work done or terminates inappropriately. Instead, it is better to be real with the older person—asking her to do what she came to do.

The same applies to the client who has six children and an alcoholic husband, or the client who is terminally ill, or the client whose wife has left him. Empathize, at times be tender, understand, but do not Rescue. Rescue invites the other person to give up being in charge and to be less human than he or she is.

When Clients Are Late and Other Useful Data

When a member of the group is late, he usually apologizes and I thank him for the apology. I also let myself be aware of it. If there is a second time, I am aware of this. It is data. That is all. If there is a third time, I will ask what is going on or perhaps a member of the group will do so. There is always a good reason at the Child level. It may be fear of the opening contract review or he may be out to get negative strokes from the group because he really does not trust the positive ones. So the "late behavior" becomes an avenue to new understanding for the client and the group.

When Clients Want to Smoke in the Office or the Group Room

I ask people not to do this. They accept the restriction.

When Clients Bring Coffee, Pop, and Other Distractions to the Group Session

Things in a client's hands get between him and doing his work and between him and his relationship with the group. For the most part, our clients do not bring food or drink to a group session. However, if a person does, I ask him to stop.

In the same vein, people will sometimes twist keys in their hands while in group. At some point, maybe even after a session or two, I or one of the group members will mention it. This can then lead to further work. Sometimes a female client will hold a purse or sack of knitting on her lap. I am reluctant to say anything about this and almost never do. After a while, the person will usually put the article down. Sometimes a client will want to take notes. This can be a good thing, but if it appears to get between the person and the group, I will say so.

The point is to get the offending item out of the way without violating the part of the person for which the item has protective value.

When It's Time to Talk about Money

All subjects are acceptable for discussion and/or work in the group. This includes money as well as sex and other sensitive issues. Berne recommended that money matters be worked through in the group (Berne, 1966b, pp. 7, 8). We have found it to be good advice. Negotiating openly in the group helps prevent the development of a game around a client's fee. If a sliding-fee scale is used, it is clarifying to have the arrangements carefully thought through and in printed form, plus a sheet of figures showing the fee amounts for each level of income. This added structure permits a feeling of increased security in that the client knows what is required and that the requirements are the same for everyone.

Evaluation

There is much that is tragic in the things clients tell their therapists day after day. Without guides to evaluate the work being done, the therapist can soon "burn out." Good evaluation furnishes the data both for celebration of work completed and improvement in the therapeutic approach.

Five avenues of evaluation come to mind: (a) the contract review, (b) reaction in the group, (c) reports of improvement, (d) termination, and (e) later feedback.

The *contract review*, discussed earlier (p. 85) under *Mechanism*, gives the therapist a once-a-week, bird's-eye view of where things are with the client.

Reaction in the group includes the therapist's observations of the transactions between the client and others, the behavior of others toward the client, and the therapist's own feelings and images concerning the client. Sometimes evaluation is as simple and as subtle as feeling more comfortable than before in the same room with this person.

Reports of improvement range from reports of psychological and physical improvement to evidence of improved communication at home or at work. One client may tell of her amazement at being able to stop her recurring fantasies of disaster. Another may report that her blood pressure is down, or still another that his migraines are no more, sleep comes regularly now, there's better sex, she talked straight with her mother for the first time, he and his wife had a good week together, her symptoms of arthritis have greatly lessened, and he went for his first job interview.

Termination, discussed earlier (p. 85) under *Process,* is a time of focused evalution. The client is asked to read through the items for change in his contract and, using specific behavioral evidence, say how each has been completed. He is then asked to read his "picture of success" (the third item on the contract) which was written early in the therapeutic process. He is asked if this has taken place. Further evaluation of the client's work and achievement is arrived at using the ego-state squares, as explained under "Media Usage" (p. 93).

Later feedback comes in the form of letters, Christmas cards, the referral of friends, and calls and visits from former clients telling of their continuing success in the ordering and living of their lives.

Treatment

In practice, treatment includes anything that holds promise of success for the client. TA appears, by nature, to be eclectic, and transactional analysts use many forms of treatment in the groups they lead.

Included among these forms are: the usual explanations of TA theory, experiential devices to make clear the meaning of the theories, diagrams to further facilitate understanding, the use of transactions within the immediate group situation as well as reported material from outside the group, the use of Gestalt techniques and psychodrama to help the client separate self from parents and ego state from ego state, the use of meditation, techniques from art therapy, various suggestions for reading, and the use of homework for specific action during the week.

These and other therapeutic strategies are used by the therapist as she listens to the client's words and behavior, to the transactions taking place between the client and the group, and particularly to the feeling tone in the room as she perceives it and checks it out with others from time to time. She will look for feeling under feeling, for belief behind the feeling, and for images and memories the client is carrying. The group is invited into this mix of work, awareness, feeling, and understanding for whatever reaction, thinking, advice, or experience is immediately available. At times the group is allowed to take over the work with the client while the therapist listens for and supports the kinds of transactions and advice that seem to help. Any particular intensity between the client and another group member may be drawn upon in that moment to give the client a track to run on—utilizing in the process the group's memory, support, insight, and power of confrontation.

In the sense of the above creative convolutions, successful treatment seems, in effect, to call for an individualized therapeutic approach contoured for each client and even for each piece of the client's work (Groder, 1977).

Management

Management in a therapeutic practice begins with the *referral* of clients. In a private practice, referrals come from various sources including other professionals, workshops given, present and former clients, and self-referrals of the clients themselves. Other professionals are generally lawyers, ministers, psychotherapists, and physicians. Self-referrals are made on the basis of hearing about our work from another, hearing one of us give a talk, or finding our names in the "yellow pages" of the telephone directory. The large majority of our referrals come from our own clients and are usually the best referrals. The least hopeful referrals are self-referrals made from the yellow pages with no other support.

Appointments are made in a relaxed manner with a minimum of talk. Day and hour are agreed upon. Referral source and the client's telephone number are requested, and directions to our office are given. Information on fee structure is also given if requested by the prospective client. Our experience is that volunteering further information than this tends to invite the client into game.

An *intake* is begun and perhaps completed during the first session. The intake we use is designed to get down both basic background information and some indicators of where the client is in terms of here and now feelings and script matrix.

The negotiation and building of a *treatment or change contract* is also begun during the first session. The nature of this contract is discussed on page 71 under *Basic Concepts*. As this contract is developed, (a) the thinking of the client begins to clear, (b) the nature of the client–therapist relationship begins to form, (c) the seriousness of the client's willingness to work is tested, and (d) a structure for the work ahead is begun.

At the end of the 1st hour printed *guidelines* for individual, marriage, and group therapy are gone over with the client.

The client is also given a printed *fee schedule*, including information on the "sliding-fee scale," and an income–fee table. From this material the therapist and the client quickly come to an agreed upon amount for each session. If the client's income allows the use of the sliding-fee scale, then it is also agreed that as his income changes, he will advise the therapist and a proper adjustment will be made.

A printed sheet of *ground rules* is shared with the client before entering group. These cover a variety of areas, including: the confidentiality of the group experience, the use of the treatment contract, a minimum 3 month time-contract, a three session notice before termination, announcement of planned absences, the necessity of asking for what you want, and requests for individual sessions.

Successful management requires that careful records be kept. A write-up is done on each individual session, read over to the client at the next session, and included in the client's file along with the intake, treatment contract, and life-script questionnaire.

A write-up is also done on all group sessions. Each group member who has "formally worked" during a particular session writes on the group sheet a summary of her work and what she is taking from the session. The therapists later add to this their grasp of the work.

A client's individual records are available to the client whenever requested. The group notes are kept in a notebook and can be reviewed before or after the group session by group members.

Careful records are also kept of fees received, of when the client entered therapy and when she terminated, whether the termination was appropriate or not, and whether the work contracted for was completed.

APPLICATION

Group Selection and Composition

We presently work in our practice with three weekly, ongoing groups. The members are drawn from among clients we are seeing individually.

Many people come to us expecting to enter a group. For others it is a completely novel and scary idea, and for these persons entering a group can be a major decision.

Group selection is made at random (Berne, 1966b, pp. 4–6) according to which client is ready for group, the client's schedule, and which group or groups have openings. We make it a practice, before the client enters a group, to share with the client the names of the group members and to share the client's name with the group. The point here is to eliminate the surprise of an acquaintance suddenly appearing in group and to deal openly with the matter ahead of time.

The composition of the groups tends to average out in terms of age, sex, and type of client problem. The age range is from late teens to early 60s with a bulge in the late 20s.

Group Setting

The setting for our group sessions is a room measuring 16′ × 25′. At one end are double glass doors opening to the outside. Facing in from the doors is a bookcase on the right containing an assortment of books that clients can check out.

Most of the wall space is covered with subdued paintings. The exception is the wall at the far end of the room which we use as our "blackboard." With masking tape we stretch sheets of butcher's paper across the length of the wall. This provides space for diagrams, noting comments that seem important, or working out a script matrix.

The group is arranged in a circle using canvas director's chairs.

Group Size

The size of our groups is ordinarily from five to seven, with eight being the maximum number we will place in a single group (Berne, 1966b, p. 3).

The optimum number for doing group work is achieved through balancing (a) the need for adequate interaction among group members, (b) the therapist's need to be aware of what is going on, and (c) the client's need to have the time and space to do his work. Too few or too many persons in a group tends to slow down the work. Too few persons lowers the number and variety of transactions and makes it too easy for the client to work—because little effort is required to push in. Too many in a group also slows the transacting because there is little time for each person to get in his or her say.

Therapy Frequency, Length, and Duration

Our groups meet once a week for 90-minute sessions. These are ongoing, open-ended groups. A person enters the group with a contract for change and with the agreement to be in the group a minimum of 3 months. When the person completes her work she announces termination. As there are openings in the group, others are invited into the group.

Nine months to a year seems to be the length of time needed by most people to complete their work. There are, of course, those who feel complete in fewer sessions and there are a few who take far longer. With those persons who take a short time, the original contract is the amount of work that is usually completed. With those who take longer, there is a completing of the first contract, then an adding to it and, for some, a writing of several complete contracts in the process of moving from one level of awareness and new behavior to other levels.

Media Usage

I will consider here media as: (a) the spoken word, (b) the written word, (c) the group members, (d) the group room furniture, (e) paper and pencil, and (f) other media. Beyond any of these, of course, is the personality of the therapist—teaching, leading, and patterning through the multiple avenues of her gestures, voice tones, pauses, choice of words, eye movements, and other avenues both recognized and unrecognized.

The *spoken word* is taken quite seriously in TA. The awareness is that the words we speak are behavior, reinforcing beliefs about ourselves. Reference to the way words can, on the one hand, be detrimental and, on the other, changed for cure is found on page 75 under *Basic Concepts*.

Often in working out a treatment contract, we will ask the client to use "9-year-old words." Our purpose is to get around Parent and Adult words in order to let the Child speak. For when we know what the Child is feeling and wanting, we then have a base on which to facilitate change.

Also, most of the stroking we do and the expression of feeling is done in words. Words are the train we ride on as we shuttle back and forth among our transactions, giving and accepting stimuli, affirming and updating our structures.

The *written word* as media is seen in our use of the blackboard, described on page 91 under *Group Setting*.

In writing or drawing diagrams, it is helpful to use different colors in order to separate thoughts from feelings, one feeling from another, Parent from Child words, and to show movement in the work. As an illustration, brown might be used for statements of depressive self-talk, blue for new options, and green for redecision.

For the most part, the therapists use the board, but it can be helpful at times to have the group member, who has just completed a piece of work, strike out or add a word or sentence in affirming the new decision being made.

We use the *group members* as media in setting up psychodrama. The client may be asked to choose his "family" from the group. The client is then instructed to move these people around until she feels they are in a proper spatial relationship to each other. Lines can be given to the participants by the client or they can say what comes to mind in the role as mother, grandfather, and so forth. The variations are infinite.

The *group room furniture,* in this case the chairs, become the media in the use of the Gestalt technique of the "empty chair." An empty chair (sometimes several are used) is set in front of the client and, according to the work being done, she is asked to place a particular person, thing or part of herself in the chair. A dialogue is then begun by the client with whomever or whatever is fantasized in the chair. As feelings are gotten out from one side, the client is asked to become the other side and respond. In the process the client has an opportunity to clearly delineate between the sides of herself and to reintegrate the energy she has been using to stay at war with herself.

In using *paper and pencil* as media we have what we call, "ego-state squares." These are simply 8" × 11" sheets of paper (or cardboard) with large letters drawn on each to represent an ego state. We use six sheets to stand for Critical Parent, Nurturing Parent, Adult, Adapted Compliant Child, Adapted Rebellious Child, and Free Child. The ego-state squares are introduced at the time of a client's termination and at any other time when there is a need for clarification among ego states. In the process the client is asked to place the ego-state squares in the center of the group and then to stand on each, one at a time, saying what that ego state says about termination or whatever else is being worked on.

The medium of paper and pencil can, of course, be used in many ways. One that yields excellent results for us is the drawing of egograms (Figure 8). Each group member and leader is given paper and pencil and asked to do an egogram for each person in the group, including herself. The drawing of the egograms is done quickly, in perhaps 8–10 minutes. Then, focusing on each person in turn, the egograms are read aloud. After this feedback has been completed for the whole group, time is given for clarification. The exercise is often illuminating in terms of how a person sees herself coming across to others and can open new avenues of awareness.

Other media which I have found useful are: collage, colored chalk, clay, and paint used on large sheets of paper. These media, however, are time consuming, both in using them and in gleaning insights from them. They are, therefore, more appropriate to the 6-hour minithons we set up, from time to time, for the groups.

Leader Qualifications

I am a Clinical Member (CM) of the ITAA. The training that goes into becoming a CM takes from 2 to 4 years and is meant to prepare the therapist for a high level of competence (Woollams & Brown, 1978, p. 4). It involves (a) a training contract with a Teaching Member, (b) at least a year of involvement in a TA training program, (c) a year of supervised clinical work, (d) the setting up of a group, (e) a comprehensive written examination, and (f) an oral examination.

Among TA therapists there is a wide variety of professionals represented: psychiatrists, psychologists, physicians, social workers, nurses, teachers, ministers, and others.

Ethics

Ethical issues in a therapy group revolve around: (a) confidentiality, (b) power, (c) role, and (d) truth.

Confidentiality is vital to working close with people who want to make basic life changes. The agreement with the client before she enters a group is that the names of group members and the specifics of others' work stay in the group. Confidentiality of this kind is necessary to the building of trust so that each member does his work with the confident assurance that privileged information remains just that.

Power is part and parcel of the potency of both the therapist and the structure set up to produce a healing environment. However, it is necessary that the therapist be sensitive to his own or others' misuse of the power available in a group. Manipulation is a form of misuse and can sometimes appear in a therapist's or group's overeagerness for decision on the part of the one who is working. Anger, as power, can also be misused, and, though it is necessary for the therapist to be aware of, and straight in accounting for, his anger, he should also be aware that his position as therapist tends, in the eyes of his clients, to magnify his expressions of anger. Finally, there is the power of permission. As permission is given to a client for new thinking and new behavior, equal energy needs to be put into consideration of the requirements of protection for that person.

The *role* of the therapist, it appears to me, should be kept clear. The therapist is the therapist; she is not a group member. She is not less (or more) of a human being for being a therapist, but in the therapeutic situation that is who she is. She can receive strokes in the group as well as give them, her feelings are real, and she can enjoy the group. But she needs to sensitize herself to the difference between this and using the group for self-gratification, her own therapy, or her own basic stroke source. For this she needs to look elsewhere. I also believe it is difficult to mix therapeutic and social roles. Friends and acquaintances come to us for counseling, but during the contract period we ordinarily do not socialize. To do otherwise appears to lessen the force of the work and is probably confusing to the client's Child.

Truth is vital to the clarification of past and present. There are often unpleasant truths that have to be faced by the client and often enough broached by the therapist. But the therapist needs to be aware that truth expressed without love (a feeling and caring approach based in an underlying concern) is only more weight added to the burden the client already carries. In effect, "truth without love" becomes a destructive confrontation. The reverse of this, "love without truth" is also destructive and will ultimately be seen for the insipid falsehood that it is (Bonhoeffer, 1963).

RESEARCH

Eric Berne urged that TA be tested and refined and then retested. Since his death in 1970, serious efforts have been made in this direction.

A minimum of 25 studies have researched the effects of TA group workshop training—plus additional studies which evaluated the effects of TA therapy in juvenile rehabilitation institutions, public school settings, political science, and business (McClenaghan, 1978, p. 3).

During the years 1963–1980, 124 doctoral dissertations related to TA have appeared in the *Dissertation Abstracts International*. The four most frequent research topics were "effectiveness," "theory," "test development," and "education" (Wilson, 1981).

Recent research (1977–1982) published in the *Transactional Analysis Journal* has included a variety of subjects and projects. In one study of the effectiveness of an introductory course in TA (77 participants), the author concluded that the group, as a whole, had applied TA to everyday life, improved job productivity, and improved interpersonal relationships (Spencer, 1977). In another study of attitude changes during a 4-week TA workshop, it was concluded that all measured attitudes of the group changed in a positive direction (Bloom, 1978). In a comparison study of a 12-session ongoing weekly therapy group and an 188-hour marathon group, it was found, as hypothesized, that the marathon group showed greater positive change initially and the weekly group evidenced greater positive change in the latter two-thirds of the treatment period. Interestingly enough, however, the marathon participants did not show a loss of their initial strong change toward health, as was originally hypothesized. Seemingly, both approaches are capable of producing lasting change (Steere, Tucker, & Worth, 1981).

Two particularly interesting studies have been published on ego states. The first has to do with a psychophysiological approach to the existence of ego states. Eighteen graduate students were asked to respond to a questionnaire (designed to evoke Parent, Adult or Child ego states) while measurements of changes in skin temperature, respiration rate, heart rate, and skin conductance were recorded. The conclusion was that the physiological changes which accompany shifts in ego states provide empirical evidence of the existence of ego states (Gilmour, 1981). The second study utilized photographs and videotape records to analyze basic human posture and its correspondence to specific ego states. Two of many conclusions were (a) shifts in the spinal cord (trunk shifts) are the key to changes from one ego state to another and (b) changes in ego state may be elicited by encouraging clients to alter their posture and realign their spinal cord (Steere, 1981).

Two recent studies in the area of family life are of interest. The first describes and discusses outcomes observed in five families who participated in a 7-day residential family workshop. Five similar families (nonparticipants) served as controls. The Family Environment Scale, the California Psychological Inventory, and Shostrom's Personal Orientation Inventory were administered prior to the workshop, at its completion, and 8 weeks after. The evidence indicated clearly that the families in the study changed significantly. The results also suggest that a 1-week multiple family therapy workshop is an effective format for promoting change (Bader, 1982). The second study was of nine physically abusive (PA) and nine seriously neglectful (SN) mothers who participated in a 12-week TA/Redecision group psychotherapy program to evaluate short-term effectiveness of this therapy model with such patients. Criteria considered in the evaluation of the program included the Minnesota Multiphasic Personality Inventory (MMPI) change scores, therapists' and social workers' evaluations of behavioral change, and so forth. Significant changes were identified for each of the criteria. The TA/Redecision model, with its emphasis on locating the power to change in the patient rather than in the therapist, appears to be effective in the treatment of PA/SN mothers (Sinclair-Brown, 1982).

Three other interesting research projects concerned with the use and effectiveness of TA centered on (a) TA and problem drivers, a highly successful teaching program in Florida for problem drivers who had lost their licenses (Prothero, 1978); (b) TA and customer relations department employees, a productive training program resulting in both an increase in employee perceptions of customer satisfaction and customer reports of satisfaction (Martinko & Luthans, 1981); and (c) TA used in the field of education to examine the charac-

teristics of more helpful and less helpful consultative experiences as viewed by
the consultee (Fine, Franz, & Maitland, 1982).

Finally, two research studies on stroking are of particular importance. The
first has to do with the stroking treatment effects on depressed males. The
treatment consisted of four weekly 2-hour group sessions focused on positive
stroking—utilizing lecture, exercises, discussion and homework. The main
finding was that depression levels of the eight reactively depressed adult males
were decreased from a group mean score of 19.00 on the Beck Depression
Inventory pretest to a group mean score of 11.63 (Fetsch & Sprinkle, 1982). The
second study looks at the relationship between positive stroking and self-
perceived symptoms of distress. The findings of the study strongly supported
the hypotheses that as positive stroke acquisition frequency increases, self-
reported symptom distress decreases (Horwitz, 1982).

GROUP SESSION ILLUSTRATION

This is a Monday evening group.[7] The session runs from 6:00 P.M. to 7:30
P.M. There are eight members in the group. The group assembles on the hour
or slightly before and has a few minutes for pastiming with each other before
the two therapists come in at 6:05 P.M.

The group sits in a circle of chairs, already set up. The seating arrangement
of the participants varies somewhat from session to session, but the members

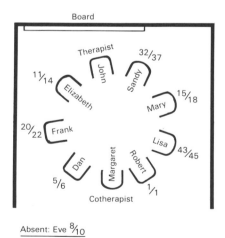

FIGURE 21.   Group seating diagram.

---

[7]A fictional group derived from experience with many groups.

tend to choose approximately the same seat each time. Figure 21 diagrams the seating arrangement for this session.[8]

The therapist and the cotherapist verbally greet everyone and the session begins.

COTHERAPIST: Eve called and said her son was down with a cold so she's staying home with him and won't be here tonight. She said to tell the group her work last week really helped. (The group responds.)

THERAPIST: Robert, it's good to have you in the group.

ROBERT: It's good to be here.

THERAPIST: As I said to you in our last individual session, we do a Contract Review at the beginning of each group session. This means you say basically in three sentences: what your contract is, what you did about it this past week, and what you want from this session. Then you will receive a word of feedback from each member. OK?

ROBERT: I remember; I just hope I can remember all of my contract.

THERAPIST: All right, let's begin. Lisa, you start and we'll go counterclockwise and end up with Robert.

LISA: My contract is to stop confusing myself and to allow myself to enjoy my life. This week I got into a lot of confusion . . . heh, heh. I know you all will think I do it on purpose, but I don't think I do. And, I did do one good thing and that was starting to take walks each evening in our neighborhood and that felt good . . . mostly . . . but I still don't see how that's going to solve my problem. Anyway, tonight I think I ought to work on my feelings for my mother.

GROUP RESPONSE: Clearer. . . . Gallows (cf. Berne, 1972, pp. 334–337). . . . Discounting. . . . Child. . . . Confusing. . . . Ought. . . . Beginning. . . . Game.

MARY: My contract is to quit smoking, to feel my feelings, and to say what I want to say. I have been meaning to tell the group that I quit smoking 4 weeks ago . . . and I am holding to it. I think I am feeling my feelings. . . . I sure got angry this week at Sam . . . and I told him just how I felt . . . so I guess I am doing pretty good. Tonight I need to take a little time and look at why I got *so* angry.

GROUP RESPONSE: Making it. . . . Celebration. . . . Wow. . . . Disbelieving. . . . Hopeful. . . . Great. . . . Good. . . . Help!

SANDY: My contract is to keep my job, to stop going round and round in my head and to be good to myself. I have a new job now and I think I like it but I may not. It mostly depends on my boss. I went to dinner twice this week and to a movie . . . so I was good to myself . . . but now I'm out of money. Tonight I just want to listen and I might work if there is time.

GROUP RESPONSE: Good Grief. . . . Another? . . . Better. . . . Moving. . . . Work! . . . Getting it. . . . Might. . . . My boss.

---

[8]The numbers by each name denote the individual ratio of total sessions attended to total sessions possible. The total group ratio here is: 135/153 or 88% attendance (Berne, 1966b, p. 11).

ELIZABETH: The contract I have with the group is to listen to my feelings, to quit making things feel bigger than they are, and to plan to give myself some fun. I am so mad today I can't think. Everything seems to be going wrong for me. My boss is looking at me like he wants to fire me. I called three friends to try to get them to go out with me Friday night and none of them would. And then today I had a flat right there on Main Street and that's money I couldn't afford. I know I ought to work but I don't want to.

GROUP RESPONSE: Heavy. . . . Hurting. . . . Angry. . . . Escalating. . . . Trying. . . . Mad. . . . In touch. . . . Angry.

FRANK: My contract is to make it in school, to talk straight, to quit judging others, and to work through my anger for my stepfather. Well, I had one exam this week and two coming up next week . . . and I think I did OK on the one this week . . . oh, heck, I know I did OK . . . I had that material down pat. And my stepfather called this week . . . and I could see how the work I did here two sessions ago was right on. He is inviting me into a game with him . . . and I'm supposed to try hard and fail . . . so, thanks everybody. And tonight I just want to be a part of the group.

GROUP RESPONSE: Terrific. . . . Excellent. . . . Good going. . . . Making it. . . . Yeah. . . . Good. . . . Successful. . . . Learning.

DAN: My contract is to quit using alcohol to relax, to work out my marriage, to get my work in on time, to stop overspending, and to learn to listen. I don't know whether I have done any of that this week. But maybe I did; I don't know. I started on the surveys and got three of them almost done, but Mr. Barlow laid me out this morning because I said I might not finish them by tomorrow. Oh, well. (Dan sighs.) And Doris and I got into it over something really nice I bought for the house and she thought we could have done without it, but it was such a good bargain. Tonight, I want to work on why I procrastinate and set myself up for making such a mess.

GROUP RESPONSE: Coming along. . . . Good. . . . Negative. . . . Daddy. . . . Mother. . . . Sigh. . . . Bargain. . . . Good.

ROBERT: My contract is to stop being afraid when it's not necessary, to like myself, and to learn how to make friends with people. Well, I'm scared right now. This is the first time I have ever been in a group. I guess I must have liked myself some or I wouldn't be here right now! Oh, yes, and what do I want tonight? . . . I just want to kind of see how you do it and begin to get acquainted a little.

GROUP RESPONSE: Courage. . . . Straight. . . . Afraid. . . . Scared. . . . Good. . . . Welcome. . . . Trying. . . . Beginning.

THERAPIST: Does anyone want clarification on any feedback you got?

DAN: Elizabeth, what did you mean by "Daddy"?

ELIZABETH: It was the way you said "Mr. Barlow" . . . I got the notion that he might be like your daddy.

DAN: Thank you. You may be right.

SANDY: John, what did you mean by what you said?

THERAPIST: What did I say?

SANDY: You don't know? . . . Oh, well . . . no, wait a minute . . . you said "work" . . . what did you mean by that?

THERAPIST: It sounded to me like it was time for you to *work*.

SANDY: Oh . . . OK.

MARY: Lisa, what did you mean by "disbelieving"?

LISA: I thought you were having trouble believing your success.

MARY: I hadn't thought of that. Hmmm . . . maybe so.

THERAPIST: Anybody else? . . . All right, let's work.

MARY: I want to work on what I said in the Contract Review . . . about why I got so mad at Sam.

THERAPIST: OK . . . go ahead.

MARY: I was kind of glad I said what I said, or a lot of it . . . but I didn't like the way I said it. It was like I was beside myself. I don't know if I was ever like that with him before.

DAN: What was it you said to Sam? Seems like to me it couldn't have been all that bad. Maybe you only thought it was so bad. Sometimes I do that to myself. (Mary is looking down.)

THERAPIST: What are you feeling, Mary?

MARY: I am feeling covered up by what Dan is saying . . . like it's too much. It's all good, but like it's too much.

THERAPIST: So, maybe you better tell him.

MARY: Okay . . . Dan, I'm feeling covered up with your words. Would you ask your question again?

DAN: I've forgotten what it was . . . I'm sorry . . . no, I remember . . . I said, what did you say to Sam? I just couldn't believe it could have been that bad. And, even if it was, I don't think you would have meant it.

FRANK: Dan, you're doing it again . . . covering Mary up with words.

DAN: I am?! I just can't seem to say anything in a few words. I don't know what's wrong with me. I have diarrhea of the mouth! I just go on and on. And this is what Doris says about me! Just yesterday, we were sitting at the table and I.

THERAPIST: Stop! Please ask Mary your question in one sentence.

DAN: You mean again? (The therapist nods.) OK, . . . in one sentence. Mary, what did you say to Sam?

THERAPIST: Good.

MARY: I called him a goddamn sonofabitch and told him he never listens to me and I am really angry. I knew I did it wrong . . . not at the time . . . at the time I felt good about it . . . but later it didn't seem right. You know?

THERAPIST: And what do you want to do with it tonight?

MARY: I want to figure out why I went so high.

THERAPIST: Okay. Pick someone in the room . . . call them by name and in 4 or 5 . . . maybe 10 sentences, tell what happened.

MARY: All right. Lisa. Three years ago Sam met this couple on his bowling team . . . or, at least, the man and then later his wife. Matt and Vickie are their names . . . and he wanted to have them over and for us to get acquainted. I wasn't too thrilled about it, but you know, so we had them to supper and Sam thought it was grand but I couldn't stand either of them. He's a chauvinist pig if there ever was one and she likes it that way. I'm not a woman's libber but they are too much and I said so to Sam. But he said I just needed to get to know them. One night we were out with them for supper and Matt started acting sexy with me . . . coming on strong . . . and I told Sam about it, but he said that's the way Matt is and don't worry. Boy, that hurt! . . . And so we've kept on seeing them. Sometimes we go to some fun places, but so what, you know,[9] and then Sam came home on Friday and said he and Matt had signed up for some sort of boat trip going down a river in West Virginia, camping out at night and I blew my top. That's when I called him all those names. But he doesn't listen. And even then he said wait till *I* see the brochures.

LISA: I can see why you got so angry.

MARY: Thank you. That helps.

FRANK: I don't know why you stay married to him . . . if he never listens. I'm mad at him myself and I think you ought to be!

MARY: Oh, I'm not mad at him now. I was when I said those things to him but not now. He's really good to me. Sometimes I think he worships me almost and I feel guilty for not wanting to go on this trip he's so excited about.

FRANK: Now it feels like you're trying to protect him. What's going on?

MARY: I'm not protecting him. I am just saying, well, that he's good to me in a lot of ways.

THERAPIST: What are you feeling, Frank?

FRANK: I didn't know it till you asked but . . . frustrated . . . angry. Yeah, *angry!*

THERAPIST: Have you ever had this reaction before, Mary?

MARY: Sometimes Sam feels that way. I think.

THERAPIST: Think?

MARY: He doesn't exactly say it, but he'll slam doors or maybe mope around for a day or two . . . and that's part of why I don't want to hurt him about the trip. Just can't do it, you know.

THERAPIST: Mary, what's your favorite fairy tale?

MARY: Oh . . . Sleeping Beauty [cf. Berne, 1972, pp. 50, 51]. I guess.

THERAPIST: Will you tell us the story, please?

MARY: It's been a long time since I heard it. . .

THERAPIST: Tell us what you remember.

MARY: Well, once upon a time (many giggles), there was a king and a queen and they had a baby girl . . . a princess . . . and they sent out invitations to a big ball to celebrate the birth of the princess and everybody came except one old witch who they forgot to send an invitation to. But she came anyway and was so mad at not being invited, she pronounced a curse on the princess

---

[9]Mary's self-discounting expression, "you know," is allowed to pass, but at some future point it will be gently confronted.

that would happen when she was 18. And that's what happened . . . when the princess was exploring the attic one day . . . and there was the old witch . . . only the princess didn't know who she was, and the witch was spinning and the princess wanted to learn how . . . and the witch said "Oh, I'll teach you how," and that's when the princess pricked her finger on a poisoned needle and fell asleep for a hundred years. That's all I remember . . . though there's something else about a prince coming to take care of her. . . .

THERAPIST: Thank you. Are you open to feedback?

MARY: Yes . . . (quietly).

THERAPIST: Anybody.

SANDY: I think it's a beautiful story and you are a lot like a princess.

MARY: Why do you say that?

SANDY: It's like you're very sensitive and very quiet at the same time. Like you don't quite belong in the world. I'm not saying it very well but do you see what I mean?

MARY: I think so.

DAN: I don't know . . . but the wandering around and getting hurt in the attic . . . isn't that kind of like what you told us about the way you started smoking. You were at the beach and met some people and they offered you a cigarette and you said you didn't *think* about . . . you just kept on smoking after that. It's the not thinking, in the wandering around, not knowing exactly where you are that I am hearing. I could say more (Dan grins) but I won't.

THERAPIST AND GROUP: Way to go Dan . . . yeah (etc.).

MARY: Wow. That sure sounds like me, Dan.

COTHERAPIST: Who are you in the story, Mary?

MARY: I'm the princess.

COTHERAPIST: Okay. Good. And who is the old witch?

MARY: She's just the witch in the story.

COTHERAPIST: Let yourself visualize her there in the middle of the room. Will you? (Mary nods.) Do you see her?

MARY: Yes. . . .

COTHERAPIST: Describe her.

MARY: She's dressed all in black, black shoes . . . and she's got on a blue hat with a little blue feather on it.

COTHERAPIST: Nice . . . Now, look at her face.

MARY: OK.

COTHERAPIST: Who do you see?

MARY: (With a start) My mother.

COTHERAPIST: Good . . . and what else?

MARY: She's frowning.

COTHERAPIST: Ask her what the frown means.

MARY: You mean out loud?

COTHERAPIST: Yes.

MARY: All right. Mother, why are you frowning? (She waits a moment.) She says she is angry because I've been bad. (Mary starts to cry.) She always was saying that I'm bad . . . one way or the other.

COTHERAPIST: Feel your tears, Mary.

MARY: I am.

COTHERAPIST: What are they saying to you?

MARY: That I'm sad. I'm sorry I don't ever seem to please her.

COTHERAPIST: Good. Anything else?

MARY: Yes . . . no . . . yes. . . . I'm feeling hurt.

COTHERAPIST: Good. Go ahead and say that to your mother.

MARY: Now?

COTHERAPIST: Yes . . . see her there . . . and say how you feel to her.

MARY: Mother . . . I am feeling sad that I never seem to please you. Even now and I'm married and hardly ever see you. Nothing is ever right in anything I do!

COTHERAPIST: Keep telling her how you feel.

MARY: And I'm hurt . . . that you don't like me as a daughter. I try hard and I want you to love me but I'm never good enough. (Mary sheds more tears . . . then sobs.)

COTHERAPIST: You're doing good work, Mary. Let the tears come out. (*More tears . . . then they begin to let up.*) What else are your tears saying?

MARY: That I am really, really hurt. She never has accepted me . . . and I have tried like everything.

COTHERAPIST: Say that to your mother. (Mary does so.) Now, tell your mother the feeling underneath what you've just said.

MARY: (Mary looks toward a fantasized mother.) I am frustrated.

COTHERAPIST: Good. And the feeling under that feeling. Tell her.

MARY: I am upset, Mother.

COTHERAPIST: Anything else?

MARY: Mad . . . (with a quick uptake of breath) . . . I hadn't seen that at all.

COTHERAPIST: Tell your mother.

MARY: Mother, I am mad. I am so mad. I am *so* mad at you (*tears*). . . . You have been frowning at me *all* my life and I have been trying to be good and nothing I ever do works with you. And nothing Daddy ever does works with you. But I keep on trying and trying. And being stupid . . . just like Daddy did and still does. God, I've been stupid . . . when I think of all the times. And I am mad. . . .

COTHERAPIST: Mary, stand up and be your mother.

MARY: Oh, wow! . . . (The group laughs. . . . Mary stands . . . puts her hands on her hips . . . then puts them down . . . and frowns.) I just don't understand you Mary. The time and effort I've put into you. I did it all for you. (Mary's no longer frowning.) And now you say these things to *me*. You've hurt me more than you know. And I'm very disappointed in you. (Mary turns to the cotherapist.) That's all she says.

COTHERAPIST: OK. Good . . . come back and be yourself. And this time, stay standing. (The dialogue continues, back and forth, with Mary getting her anger out and Mary, as her mother, beginning to see Mary's point but still insisting she did the best she could.)

COTHERAPIST: Good, Mary. Now, go ahead and in a few sentences, finish the dialogue with your mother.

MARY: Mother, I have been angry with you for a long, long time . . . I see that now . . . and I have gotten a lot of it out today . . . I may want to say some of this to you, really . . . but I haven't decided that yet . . . I can see I really do love you and I might even be able to kiss you the next time you all come over . . . but I am through (she beats one hand in the other) . . . I am through with trying to please you and always feeling guilty sleeping through my life so I never have to grow up. (Her voice *softens*.) . . . Hear me, Mother, I am deciding to be grown up now. (Mary speaks to the group.). . . Whew . . . that's it . . . and thank you.

LISA: That was really good work, Mary. I can see a lot in that for *me* and I think you did my work for me tonight. Thank you.

MARY: You're welcome (smiling) and thank you.

DAN: Good work, Mary.

MARY: Thanks, Dan.

ELIZABETH: You got the anger out!

MARY: Yes. Thank you.

THERAPIST: Good, Mary. (Mary smiles.) Quickly tie what you've done tonight in with Sam.

MARY: It's all the same thing, I think. I've been sleeping . . . staying a child . . . and expecting Sam to treat me like a princess. It's been a game. And so he does all that.

ROBERT: You said he almost worships you.

MARY: Thank you, Robert, I had forgotten that. And then when he does worship me and goes ahead and plans everything, then I get mad and call him names. But he doesn't listen because he sees me as a child. I can't believe it . . . I've done it to myself.

COTHERAPIST: You can believe it.

MARY: Yes . . . yes, I can.

THERAPIST: This week, Mary, be aware of the game, and maybe write it down when you see yourself inviting Sam to treat you as a little girl . . . or a sleeping princess. And we can talk more next week about the payoff you're getting out of playing the game. OK?

MARY: Yes.

THERAPIST: Good. Who else wants to work?

ELIZABETH: Mary's work reminded me I need to work on *my* anger.

THERAPIST: Good . . . go ahead.

ELIZABETH: Well, I know you're always saying we're in charge of our own feelings, but I just don't think we are.

THERAPIST: Oh?

ELIZABETH: No, like Mary . . . her mother has a big piece of that . . . it's *not* just Mary's fault. And, no matter what you say, my boss is looking at me like he wants to fire me . . . I know he is . . . and he's already fired two others . . . he has the reputation.

THERAPIST: Elizabeth, are you angry with me?

ELIZABETH: No, I'm not angry with you! You said that the last session! And I was then but I'm not now!

THERAPIST: It feels like you are.

FRANK: I think you're angry. I can feel the vibrations.

ELIZABETH: Well, I am now because you all are saying I am.

THERAPIST: And what will you do with it?

ELIZABETH: Feel it, I guess.

THERAPIST: And then what?

ELIZABETH: Save it. (She laughs.)

THERAPIST: For what?

ELIZABETH: I don't know, but I know I do.

SANDY: I think you save it to get us later. You're always mad. Oh . . . I don't think I should say that! But you are. And it never seems to go away. Just stays . . . like a dark, polluted cloud over your head . . . and you try to get other people in your cloud with you. I am sorry . . . but I *think* I'm right. Do you see what I mean?

ELIZABETH: I'm taken aback . . . but I see what you mean . . . and it doesn't feel very good.

SANDY: Well, just look at all the people and things you're mad at this week . . . your boss, and your three friends, your flat tire . . . your money, I guess, and John . . . I agree with Frank!

ELIZABETH: Oh . . . I see.

SANDY: Do you really? What do you hear me saying?

ELIZABETH: That I am angry all the time. You may be saying more, but that's what I am hearing . . . loud and clear.

SANDY: That's right. Thank you for hearing me. (She smiles.)

ELIZABETH: You're welcome. (She smiles for the first time this session.)

THERAPIST: Your smile seemed to say something special.

ELIZABETH: I was suddenly seeing myself angry all over everything like the time I vomited all over everything and my grandmother's good blue rug just as we were about to leave and I didn't want to go . . . and then we *had* to stay another 2 days till everyone was sure I was well enough to travel. Oh, I was a real mess. (Elizabeth laughs.)

THERAPIST: Sounds like it! Interpret what you've just said in terms of now.

ELIZABETH: Well, I used the getting sick so we couldn't go home and I could stay at Grandma's a while longer and everybody would *have* to be nice to me and serve me meals in bed and ask how I was . . . because I was sick . . . though I wasn't all that sick. I know now. . . .

THERAPIST: And now . . . how does that fit in?

ELIZABETH: I don't want to say it.

THERAPIST: Why?

ELIZABETH: (She lowers head slightly and looks out of the corner of her eye.)

THERAPIST: Check your ego state.

ELIZABETH: I'm in my Adult.
THERAPIST: Group?
FRANK: You're in your Child.
LISA: I think you're in your Child, too.
OTHERS: Yes . . . uhuh. . . .
THERAPIST: How do you know?
DAN: (Speaking to Elizabeth) You put your head down . . . like this. . . .
MARY: Your eyes went to the side. You were being tricky.
THERAPIST: What was going on, Elizabeth?
ELIZABETH: I felt caught . . . and I didn't want to be . . . but kinda did too.
THERAPIST: How's that?
ELIZABETH: You all are right. I am angry a lot. But I don't mean to be. It just happens. I can see there are some things I am doing but I'm not doing it all . . . I *know* that.
THERAPIST: And how is it you would like to be caught?
ELIZABETH: Sometimes I get very tired. (Tears begin to come.)
THERAPIST: Feel your feelings.
SANDY: (She offers Elizabeth a Kleenex.)
ELIZABETH: Thank you. I get tired having to make people love me. I wish they would just do it . . . but they don't!
THERAPIST: So how does getting mad at me and others help?
ELIZABETH: It doesn't help.
THERAPIST: My Adult agrees with your Adult. But your Child thinks it helps and that's what I'm asking.
ELIZABETH: I still don't see how it would help.
THERAPIST: How *might* it help?
ELIZABETH: You can't get in.
THERAPIST: How's that?
ELIZABETH: The anger keeps you out and I go on believing what I want to believe . . . and you can't get away either.
THERAPIST: Tell me.
ELIZABETH: I said it but I'm not sure.
COTHERAPIST: It makes sense to me, Elizabeth.
ELIZABETH: How?
COTHERAPIST: John *has* to pay attention to you if you are angry . . . therefore, he can't get away and, at the same time, as long as you are angry, he can't get through to you, through your wall of anger. You're right.
ELIZABETH: Thank you . . . and I see.
THERAPIST: What do you see, Elizabeth?
ELIZABETH: I am beginning to see how I use anger. I use it to manipulate people just as I did with my parents.
THERAPIST: Good insight. And so people can't get away from you and can't get through either . . . how does that help?
ELIZABETH: It sounds stupid, but it's better than nothing.
THERAPIST: What is?
ELIZABETH: Manipulating people to make them stay around.

THERAPIST: Why do you want people to stay around?

ELIZABETH: To keep from being alone . . . but I think we're going in circles now.

THERAPIST: I think you're right. Will you take a couple of minutes and do an experiment with me right now?

ELIZABETH: Yes, I guess.

THERAPIST: Let yourself relax . . . good. . . . Let yourself ease down in your chair . . . good. . . . Take a deep breath . . . good. . . . Now . . . feel your way into "being alone" . . . good. . . . Now, tell us what being alone feels like.

ELIZABETH: (She sighs.) It feels very lonely. And . . . I don't like it at all. I'd like to stop now.

THERAPIST: Good, Elizabeth . . . stay with it a minute more . . . OK?

ELIZABETH: OK.

THERAPIST: Look under the lonely and tell me if you see another feeling and what it is.

ELIZABETH: (Crying) It's scared. I'm afraid I'll be rejected if you really know me. (She continues to cry.)

THERAPIST: Good, Elizabeth. Let yourself feel the scared . . . the fear of being rejected.

ELIZABETH: I am . . . and it's right. That's where I am.

THERAPIST: Good . . . be easy with yourself. You're on it.

ELIZABETH: (She lifts head and sort of shakes the tears away.) OK, I'm through . . . for today. But I'd like to come back to it another time.

THERAPIST: Good . . . when you're ready, let's do it.

FRANK: Come to think of it, Elizabeth, I guess you did some of my work today. I really identifed with the lonely part under the anger. So, thanks.

ELIZABETH: Thank you.

DAN: (To the cotherapist) Margaret, is this what you call a racket?

COTHERAPIST: Looked like that to me.

DAN: And Elizabeth has been using her anger to cover her fear of being rejected.

COTHERAPIST: Does that make sense, Elizabeth?

ELIZABETH: Yes.

DAN: So maybe what I've been running is a "wordy racket." (He laughs.)

COTHERAPIST: Or maybe it's a confusion racket. What do you think?

DAN: Sounds right. But what am I hiding?

COTHERAPIST: You'll know, if it's there. What is it?

DAN: Anger, I think . . . even rage. I'd like to think about that.

COTHERAPIST: I think you're on target.

DAN: Thank you.

COTHERAPIST: When you're ready to go deeper, let's do it.

DAN: I will.

THERAPIST: We're at 7:28 . . . time to stop. Anybody have anything else that needs being said?

LISA: I'm going to be out of town next week on vacation so I won't be here.

THERAPIST: OK. . . . Thanks. . . . Anybody else? . . . Robert, this was your first evening in group . . . how was it for you?

ROBERT: Interesting . . . and scary . . . but I'm not as scared now as when I came tonight. I think I'm going to like it.

THERAPIST: Good to have you with us.

ROBERT: Thank you.

THERAPIST: So you all have a good week and we'll see you then.

COTHERAPIST: Mary, you and Elizabeth do a write-up of your work. Dan, you may want to put down a few words about what you're taking with you. And, Robert, if you want to write a sentence or two about your reaction to being in the group, do so.

(Cotherapist hands clip board with group note sheet on it to Mary . . . with Mary's name and Elizabeth's name already written on it. Dan says he will write something too. Robert says he'd rather not.)

The session has ended. Therapists leave. The group members may and often do stay in the group room or outside talking for anywhere from a few minutes to an hour.

STRENGTHS AND LIMITATIONS

An important strength of TA is its *intellectual clarity*. However, "pure" TA would be only partially effective, in that it would be limited to working with clients whose Adult was in charge. For others caught up in tragedy, failure, and emotional trauma, TA insights would help in understanding how the rackets, games and scripts worked without necessarily being able to help the client stop them.

Another strength of TA is its *simplicity* (O'Hearne, 1977). A few hours spent in reading or listening to a lecture on TA can give an individual a basic grasp of the subject. The theory is immediately applicable in the diagnosis of one's personal dynamics as well as the transactional dynamics of friends and relatives. At this point, the strength of simplicity can become a limitation if TA insights are used in one-upmanship or in a put down game of "Now I've Got You."

Finally, the very simplicity of basic TA theory which so easily recommends itself to the layman may put off the professional (O'Hearne, 1977). The use of colloquialisms and innumerable circle diagrams may not appear, on the surface, to be "scientific." The fact is, however, that TA is committed to the scientific method and has, in the process, created simple, usually reliable models for predicting and changing the behavior of individuals and small groups (Barnes, 1977, p. 28).

SUMMARY

TA is a philosophy, a theory, and a set of techniques which are fully integrated as a therapeutic modality. TA takes the position that people are OK in spite of the real tragedy of not-OK life decisions and not-OK behavior. TA intends itself to be easily available to professional and nonprofessional understanding and utilization.

The foundations of TA were laid by Eric Berne in the early 1950s. The furthering of the theories and their application continues in the work of some 6,000 therapists and members of the ITAA.

The thrust of TA is toward group treatment believing that therapy in the group setting is the most effective and the therapy of choice for the majority of clients.

Finally, TA does not see therapy as an end in itself but as an effective method to be used by the client in setting her life straight and as a set of problem-solving tools to be used in the promotion of the successful living of her life.

<h2>REFERENCES</h2>

Bader, E. Redecisions in family therapy: A study of change in an intensive family therapy workshop. *Transactional Analysis Journal*, 1982, *12*(1), 27–38.

Bandler, R., & Grinder, J. *The structure of magic I*. Palo Alto, CA: Science & Behavior Books, 1975.

Barnes, G. (Ed.). *Transactional analysis after Eric Berne*. New York: Harper's College Press, 1977.

Berne, E. Ego states in psychotherapy. *American Journal of Psychotherapy*, 1957, *11*, 293–309.

Berne, E. Transactional analysis: A new and effective method of group therapy. *American Journal of Psychotherapy*, 1958, *12*, 735–743.

Berne, E. Trading stamps. *Transactional Analysis Bulletin*, 1964a, *3*(10), 127.

Berne, E. *Games people play*. New York: Grove Press, 1964b.

Berne, E. *Principles of group treatment*. New York: Grove Press, 1966b.

Berne, E. Away from a theory of non-verbal participation. *Transactional Analysis Journal*, 1971, *1*(1), 6–13.

Berne, E. *What do you say after you say hello?* New York: Grove Press, 1972.

Bloom, W. Attitude changes during a four-week TA workshop. *Transactional Analysis Journal*, 1978, *8*(2), 169–172.

Bonhoeffer, D. *The cost of discipleship*. New York: Macmillan, 1963, 45–60.

Capers, H. Winning and losing. *Transactional Analysis Journal*, 1975, *5*(3), 257–258.

Dusay, J. M. *Egograms*. New York: Harper & Row, 1977a.

Dusay, J. M. The evolution of transactional analysis. In Graham Barnes (Ed.), *Transactional analysis after Eric Berne*. New York: Harper & Row, 1977b, 32–52.

English, F. Racketeering. *Transactional Analysis Journal*, 1976, *6*(1), 78–81.

Fetsch, R. J., & Sprinkle, R. L. Stroking treatment effects on depressed males. *Transactional Analysis Journal*, 1982, *12*(3), 213–217.

Fine, M. J., Franz, C., & Maitland, R. A transactional analysis of two kinds of consultative experiences. *Transactional Analysis Journal*, 1982, *12*(2), 159–161.

Gilmour, J. R. Psychophysiological evidence for the existence of ego states. *Transactional Analysis Journal*, 1981, *11*(3), 207–212.

Goulding, R. New direction in transactional analysis: Creating an environment for redecision and change. *Progress in group and family therapy*. New York: Brunner/Mazel, 1972.

Goulding, R., & Goulding, M. *The power is in the patient*. San Francisco, Cal.: TA Press, 1978.

Grimes, J. A dialogue between the New Testament and transactional analysis. Unpublished doctoral dissertation, Louisville Presbyterian Seminary, 1975, 73–84.

Groder, M. Guest editorial. *Transactional Analysis Journal*, 1976, 6(4), 366.

Groder, M. Asklepieion: An integration of psychotherapies. In Graham Barnes (Ed.), *Transactional analysis after Eric Berne*. New York: Harper & Row, 1977, 134–137.

Haley, J. (Ed.). *Advanced techniques of hypnosis and therapy—selected papers of Milton H. Erickson, M.D.* New York: Grune & Stratton, 1967.

Haley, J. *Uncommon therapy*. New York: W. W. Norton, 1973.

Harris, T. A. *I'm OK–You're OK*. New York: Harper & Row, 1967.

Holloway, W. H. Transactional analysis: An integrative view. In Graham Barnes (Ed.), *Transactional analysis after Eric Berne*. New York: Harper & Row, 1977, 169–221.

Horwitz, A. The relationship between positive stroking and self-perceived symptoms of distress. *Transactional Analysis Journal*, 1982, 12(3), 218–222.

Kahler, T., & Capers, H. The miniscript. *Transactional Analysis Journal*, 1974, 4(1), 26–42.

Karpman, S. B. Fairy tales and script drama analysis. *Transactional Analysis Bulletin*, 1968, 7(26), 39–43.

Martinko, M. J., & Luthans, F. An analysis of the effectiveness of transactional analysis in improving organizational effectiveness. *Transactional Analysis Journal*, 1981, 11(3), 229–235.

McClenaghan, J. C. *Transactional analysis research: A review of empirical studies and tests*. 1978.

O'Hearne, J. J. Pilgram's progress. In Graham Barnes (Ed.), *Transactional analysis after Eric Berne*. New York: Harper & Row, 1977, 458–484.

Prothero, J. C. TA with problem drivers. *Transactional Analysis Journal*, 1978, 8(2), 173–175.

Revised Standard Version of the Holy Bible. New York: Thomas Nelson & Sons, 1952.

Schiff, A. W., & Schiff, J. L. Passivity. *Transactional Analysis Journal*, 1971, 1(1), 71–78.

Simonton, O. C., Matthews-Simonton, S., & Creighton, J. *Getting well again*. New York: St. Martin's Press, 1978, 125–139.

Sinclair-Brown, W. A TA redecision group psychotherapy treatment program for mothers who physically abuse and/or seriously neglect their children. *Transactional Analysis Journal*, 1982, 12(1), 39–45.

Spencer, G. M. Effectiveness of an introductory course in transactional analysis. *Transactional Analysis Journal*, 1977, 7(4), 346–349.

Spitz, R. Hospitalism, genesis of psychiatric conditions in early childhood. *Psychoanalytic Study of the Child*, 1945, 1, 53–74. New York: International Universities Press.

Steere, D. Body movement in ego states. *Transactional Analysis Journal*, 1981, 11(4), 335–345.

Steere, D., Tucker, G., & Worth, A. Change in two settings. *Transactional Analysis Journal*, 1981, 11(3), 222–228.

Steiner, C. Script and counterscript. *Transactional Analysis Bulletin*, 1966, 5(18), 133–135.

Steiner, C. *Games alcoholics play*. New York: Grove Press, 1971.

Steiner, C. *Scripts people live*. New York: Grove Press, 1974.

Transactional Analysis Journal, 1982, 12(3), 233.

Transactional Analysis Journal, 1985, 15,(3), 244.

Wilson, B. D. Doctoral dissertations on TA. *Transactional Analysis Journal*, 1981, 11(3), 194–202.

Woollams, S. J. From 21 to 43. In Graham Barnes (Ed.), *Transactional analysis after Eric Berne*. New York: Harper & Row, 1977, 351–379.

Woollams, S., & Brown, M. *Transactional analysis*. Dexter, Mich.: Huron Valley Institute, 1978.

Woollams, S., Brown, M., & Huige, K. What transactional analysts want their clients to know. In Graham Barnes (Ed.), *Transactional analysis after Eric Berne*. New York: Harper & Row, 1977, 487–525.

GLOSSARY

Adapted Child. The part of the Child which adapts to the Parent in self and in others, either compliantly or rebelliously.

Adult. An ego state oriented toward objective, autonomous, data-processing and probability-estimating.

Angular Transaction. An ulterior transaction in which the originator of the transaction is aware of the psychological message.

Brown Stamps. Psychological stamps used to justify depression and sad racket behavior.

Business Contract. The contract between the therapist and client defining the professional relationship, including: (a) mutual consent, (b) valid consideration, (c) competency, and (d) legal object.

Change Contract. See Treatment Contract.

Child. An ego state consisting of feelings, thoughts, and behavior typical of children and spontaneous adults.

Complementary Transaction. A transaction in which the stimulus and response vectors are parallel—with only two ego states involved, one from each person.

Con. The invitation to game seen in the hidden message of the opening ulterior transaction.

Constant Adult. A form of pathology in which the Adult ego state dominates the person's behavior, characterized by little feeling and computerlike functioning.

Constant Child. A form of pathology in which the Child ego state dominates the person's behavior, characterized by always playing, entertaining, or being confused.

Constant Parent. A form of pathology in which the Parent ego state dominates the person's behavior, characterized by authoritarianism and preachiness.

Contamination. A form of ego-state pathology occurring when ego-state boundaries break down and the Adult becomes contaminated by the beliefs and prejudices of the Parent and/or the fears and old experiences of the Child.

Contracts. Clearly defined agreements between therapist and client, including the business contract, the treatment contract, and the working agreement.

Counterscript. See Subscript.

Critical Parent. The part of the Parent which controls, structures, protects, and states the rules for living.

Cross. The momentary feeling of confusion or being "crossed up" following the switch in the game process.

Crossed Transaction. A transaction in which the vectors from initiator and respondent cross.

Discounting. To make less than—to ignore or distort aspects of internal or external experience.

Drama Triangle. A diagram used to depict racket and game positions, role interaction, and role switch.

Drivers. Negative, restrictive messages received from the Parent of parents—summarized into five groups: Be Perfect, Hurry Up, Try Harder, Please Me, and Be Strong.

Duplex Transaction. An ulterior transaction in which two sets of transactions occur simultaneously, one on the social level and the other on the psychological level.

Eclectic. The selection of what seems best from various systems.

Egogram. A bar graph showing the relationship of parts of the personality according to the energy emanating outward from each.

Ego State. A consistent pattern of feeling and experience directly related to a corresponding consistent pattern of behavior. The three basic patterns are: Parent, Adult, and Child.

Electrode. The Parent in the Child—the location of the script which, when activated, brings about an almost automatic response.

Empty Chair. A Gestalt technique used to assist the client in contacting, clarifying, and integrating parts of the personality, ego states, thinking and feeling, and so forth.

Excluded Adult. A form of pathology in which the Adult ego state is virtually not used, seen perhaps in a kind of switching back and forth between Parent and Child with thoughts and behavior unrelated to objective reality.

Excluded Child. A form of pathology in which the Child ego state is virtually not used, seen perhaps in the person who has little fun, does not get close to anyone, and expresses few feelings.

Excluded Parent. A form of pathology in which the Parent ego state is virtually not used, characterized by a quality of irresponsibility and a lack of conscience.

Exclusion. A form of ego-state pathology occurring when one or two ego states dominate a person's behavior over a period of time.

First Degree. A light level of game playing that ends with merely uncomfortable feelings.

Free Child. The part of the Child ego state which reacts only to itself, according to its own needs without regard for the rules of Parents. It is also called the Natural Child.

Game. A series of ulterior transactions with a con, a gimmick, a switch, and a cross—leading to a payoff.

Gimmick. An attitude or weakness which makes a person vulnerable to a particular game.

Gold Stamps. Psychological stamps collected when a person feels a need to justify her behavior by doing good things.

Homework. A short term contract between therapist (and group) and client in which the client agrees to perform a specific task or behavior outside the group.

Injunction. A Parental command either intuited or consciously heard and recorded by the Child.

Intake. A beginning process and/or printed form used by the therapist to gather information from the client.

Invitation to Game. The beginning or "con" in the game process.

Life Change Circle. The process and diagram used to clarify the way a life pattern can be changed or preserved.

Life Script. See Script.

Life-Script Payoff. The ultimate destiny or final display that marks the end of a life plan.

Life-Script Questionnaire. A series of questions, usually in printed form, both subtle and direct, designed to elicit information about and insight into a person's script.

Little Professor. The Adult in the Child and the seat of intuition. During the early years, the Little Professor plays the primary role in the process of making decisions about how to get along in the world.

Loser Script. The script of a person who does not accomplish his declared purpose and who sets himself up to receive more negative strokes than positive.

Martian. An approach and attitude utilizing the innocence and intuition of the Child to see through accepted beliefs and images.

Medical Model. The traditional model for healing which emphasizes the active role of the therapist or healer in the diagnosis and cure of illness.

Miniscript. The concept and diagram used to describe the second-by-second process by which a person furthers her script.

Negative Conditional Stroke. A stroke which discounts a person for his or her qualities, accomplishments, and/or possessions.

Negative Stroke. A stroke which discounts self or another, carries a "you're not-OK" message, and tends to lessen growth and self-esteem.

Negative Unconditional Stroke. A stroke which discounts a person as a person without reference to qualities, accomplishments, or possessions.

Nonwinner Script. The script of a person who works hard just to stay even and who sets herself up to receive an approximately equal number of positive and negative strokes.

Nurturing Parent. The part of the Parent which is caring, concerned, reassuring, and warmly protective.

OKness. The sense that the nature of reality is OK, that is, belonging to acceptance and love.

Parent. An ego state borrowed from parental figures and containing the rules for living. The Parent may function in either a critical or a nurturing fashion.

Payoff. The outcome of a game or a script.

Permission. (a) An intervention offering the individual a license to disobey a parental injunction. (b) A parental license for autonomous behavior.

Positive Conditional Stroke. A stroke which affirms a person for his or her qualities, accomplishments, and/or possessions.

Positve Stroke. A stroke which affirms self or another, carries a "you're OK" message, and tends to encourage growth and self-esteem.

Positive Unconditional Stroke. A stroke which affirms a person as a person without reference to qualities, accomplishments, or possessions.

Potency. The power of the therapist within the therapeutic environment.

Protection. Physical and psychological protection for the client as he tries out new behavior, clarifies his script, makes a redecision, and changes old habits.

Provocation. The vengeful position in the not-OK miniscript sequence used by the individual to avoid painful feelings by blaming someone else.

Psychological Message. The hidden message in an ulterior transaction, heard at the emotional, out-of-consciousness level, and diagrammed as a dotted line.

Racket. An inappropriate interpretation of events and transactions used to support a main bad feeling as a substitute for other, less acceptable feelings.

Racket and Game Analysis. The analysis of transactions which comprise the running of a racket or the playing of a game.

Red Stamps. Psychological stamps used to justify anger.

Responses. Responses to the con and the gimmick in the game process as analyzed in Berne's Formula G.

Script. A life plan based on a decision made in childhood, reinforced by the strokes of parents, justified by subsequent events, and culminating in a chosen outcome or script payoff.

Script Analysis. The analysis of a life plan, that is, the childhood decisions it is based on, the reinforcement of parental strokes, the use of subsequent events as justification, and the culmination in a chosen alternative.

Script Matrix. A diagram used to simplify the voluminous material relating to an individual's script—clarifying the messages coming from parent figures and other important persons.

Second Degree. A medium level of game playing that ends with a socially embarrassing payoff.

Social Message. The overt message in an ulterior transaction, heard intellectually, and diagrammed as a solid line.

Stamps. Feelings or strokes collected and later used to justify racket or game behavior.

Stopper. The second position in the not-OK miniscript sequence. It is derived from the script injunction.

Stroke. A unit of social intercourse and attention.

Structural Analysis. The analysis of the structure of a personality in terms of ego states, that is, Parent, Adult, and Child.

Subscript. A secondary script derived from the less potent messages of the Parent of the parents. It was originally called the Counterscript.

Subscript Injunctions. Injunctions drawn by the Child from the messages of the Parent of the parents.

Switch. Part of the game process in which there is a switch in roles or ego states at the psychological level.

Third Degree. A heavy level of game playing that ends in tragedy and/or tissue damage.

Time Structuring. Six categories of the way time is structured in order to get strokes: (a) withdrawal, (b) ritual, (c) pastimes, (d) work, (e) games, and (f) intimacy.

Transactional Analysis. The analysis of a transaction to determine the specific ego states involved.

Treatment Contract. The contract between therapist (and group) and client clearly defining the issues and direction of change the client intends. Also called the Change Contract.

Ulterior Transaction. A transaction involving a double message, one overt and the other hidden.

Winner Script. The script of a person who accomplishes her declared purpose(s) and sets herself up to receive more positive strokes than negative.

Working Agreement. A contract, usually temporary, between therapist (and group) and client in which the client agrees to accomplish a specific task.

3

Encounter Group Therapy

FRANK JOHNSON

INTRODUCTION

One of the obvious innovations in the field of psychology has been the rapid and prolific growth of the placing of people into groups in which it is expected that the mutual experience of therapy will aid every person present. It is increasingly apparent that our psychological health depends upon our group membership—our ability to interact with others in a communicative and effective manner. The fastest way to learn to manage relationships is in a situation, such as a group, where the opportunities to learn, experiment, and practice such skills are both rich and varied.

DEFINITION

A group is a collection of persons who are gathered to interact with one another in order to satisfy some need in each person present, to accomplish some group goal, and who are in agreement as to who is and who is not a member of the group. If you are voluntarily cooperating with other persons to reach a mutually agreed upon goal from which each person derives a sense of satisfaction, then you are part of a group. Although there are many different kinds of groups in our life—the families we belong to, the work relationships among office personnel, task forces, committees, and teams, social groupings of short- or long-term duration, clubs, civic organizations in which we take part—all of these fall into the definition. A group is functioning when we participate together in face-to-face interaction based upon a commitment to cooperate with each other, each person aware of his or her membership in the group and each getting a sufficient measure of satisfaction from participating in the group's activities.

Frank Johnson • Department of Training and Management Development, Ethyl Corporation, 330 South Fourth Street, Richmond, Virginia 23217.

HISTORY

The history of groups is as old as the history of the human race. The first grouping that we experience is the one into which we are born. From this profound experience, we can picture group life as beginning the first time a wandering male begged to be allowed to share the shelter, fire, and protection of the female. The envy of and return to the Mother is certainly symbolic of the need for cooperative management of tasks for survival, warmth, and nourishment, as well as supportive, caring relationships. So groups formed for mutual protection and defense, for maximizing the benefits of food gathering, for religious ceremony, and for what became family life, then clan, then tribe, then nation. Learning to survive taught that cooperative effort was the fastest way to grow and learn and to maintain life.

From the beginning, then, civilization is expressed in the relationships between people as they voluntarily form into groups for mutual benefit. To ascertain the beginnings of group consciousness in terms of dates is thus impossible.

However, the modern field of social psychology does have its antecedents. The usefulness of group life to enhance the psychological insights and personal growth of an individual has been discovered and developed within this century. Many writers point back to the classes held by Joseph Pratt in Boston in the early 1900s as the beginning (Pratt, 1906). In classes held informally in the homes of tubercular patients, Pratt noted a marked improvement in the attitudes and moods of the patients. A group of about 25 persons met weekly and heard Pratt deliver lectures about the importance of rest periods throughout the day. Although a very heterogenous grouping, a spirit of common cause developed and a fine social time was had by all. Pratt published many papers describing his method, but the psychiatric community appears to have shown little interest in it at that time.

Another early observer of the phenomena of group life was Sigmund Freud. In 1922 he wrote an essay, "Group Psychology and the Analysis of the Ego," in which he remarked on the apparent loss by an individual of his own values and beliefs. Freud noted that some people in a group will behave in ways they would never countenance as an individual. He also noted that there was a strong identification of group members with the leader, and that group members apparently found it difficult to express feelings of conflict or feelings of caring toward one another (Freud, 1922).

Another early pioneer was Trigent T. Burrow, who had studied with Carl Jung. In his practice as a psychoanalyst, Burrow began to explore the relationship process at work between the analyst and the patient. This led to his postulating that the behavioral disorders he was treating could be traced back to the context of the social group of which the person was a part. He worked out some methods for identifying the group instead of the individual, but the adoption of his work was not widespread (Burrow, 1927).

Certainly an early pioneer of working with groups was Jacob Moreno. Before coming to the United States in 1925, Moreno had developed his concepts of group therapy. As he practiced these approaches he invented the psychodrama technique, in which an individual is encouraged to regress and relive certain scenes from his or her memory. Group members are coached to serve as voices for underlying feelings and messages, in order to help the patient gain insight into the influence of such "unfinished business" upon present-day interpersonal relationships. Moreno's emphasis on setting up and directing the scene has led to many other structured exercise approaches to enable participants in a group to experience new feeling situations and to practice new skills (Moreno, 1957).

The direct grandfather of the training-group (T-group) and the encounter group approach is Kurt Lewin. Born in Prussia in 1890, Lewin received his psychological training from Max Wertheimer and Wolfgang Kohler at the University of Berlin, where he later became a professor of philosophy and psychology.

When Hitler came to power, Lewin left Germany for the United States, where he first taught at Cornell University, then went to the University of Iowa, and finally moved to the Massachusetts Institute of Technology to become the director of the Research Center for Group Dynamics. A man of boundless energy and personality, Lewin's biggest contribution to the field of social psychology was not his theoretical base, but rather his fertile suggestions for research. He used his "field theory" to generate "action research," which employed moving from particular observations to general applications. He was deeply interested in how people learn to learn. He would film a young girl learning, by practice, study, correction, and repractice, how to back up two steps and sit down on a stump. Then he would drive his students (and himself) to analyze, instant by instant, exactly what she tried, what she thought out, how she gave herself information, and what she did with it. Out of such clinical observations, Lewin hypothesized that the process of change involved unlearning what one has known before, learning what is appropriate to the present situation, be it crisis, emergency, an unknown factor, or an undeveloped part of the self, and then transforming the new learning into rules for future behavior. He described this process as "unfreezing–learning–refreezing."

Lewin adapted the term *field theory*, to express his conception that each person is a part of his or her perceptual environment—what he termed a person's *life space*. Within this space is the psychological makeup of the person, which Lewin pictured as a complex set of interrelated cells. These cells are permeable with communication flowing between them unless, for some reason or other, the energy is blocked. When energy is balanced on both sides of a boundary, then the person is in a place of tension where the counterforce is equal to the force. When the energy flows once again in the desired direction, an individual can reach his or her goal and enter into a state of relaxation, having established an equilibrium.

If the energy continues to be blocked, then the individual either finds alternative goals which are easier to reach, increases the amount of energy to drive toward the original goal, or finds ways to reduce the strength of the blocking forces. A final alternative, should nothing else work, is to escape mentally or physically from the tension-producing situation (Hall & Lindsey, 1970).

Field theory, in summary, postulates that the behavior of an individual cannot really be studied apart from the context in which the individual is being studied. There is no noninfluencing observation post. How we perceive an object is determined by the total field in which the object is embedded, and we, as the observers, are a part of the field. Therefore, naturalistic study of behavior is at least as informative as the so-called clinical situations. Analysis of any behavior begins with the situation as a whole and then proceeds to the component parts. In opposition to this stands the famous phrase "the whole is more than the sum of its parts." Finally, it is possible, says Lewin, to conceptualize the concrete person who is a part of the situation by centering on precisely what is happening in the situation, making notes of what helps and what hinders a person from reaching his or her goal, and getting the person to remember what former learning experiences were responsible for behaving in this particular way in this particular (unique and new) situation. These "ah-ha" moments of insight and revelation often come to members of a group when someone is seen to be acting in a rote way in a unique situation and we wonder what forces caused the person to exhibit that particular piece of behavior (Lewin, 1951).

The story of the group movement is the story of the founding of the National Training Laboratories (NTL) for the study of group dynamics. In 1946, Lewin and three of his associates were conducting a summer biracial workshop. After class, Lewin and the others would meet to discuss what had taken place during the day and what would be the best approach to the next day's materials. Some members of the class asked to sit in on these after-sessions, and were encouraged to come along provided they did not interrupt while the summarizing and planning were taking place.

At the end of the course, Lewin gave out an evaluation instrument. The response which came back was intriguing. It suggested that as useful as the content material had been, the most profound learnings had taken place in the after-sessions. Far more understanding and behavioral change came from this process of analyzing the underlying group dynamics of the class than from the instructional content.

Being the kind of person he was, Lewin saw a possibility for further research. To build on the idea, a conference was planned for the next summer at Gould Academy in Bethel, Maine, in which educators, psychologists, and sociologists were to participate. Unfortunately, Lewin died suddenly before this conference took place. Out of that beginning however, came many more such conferences to study the dynamics of a group simultaneously with the events of group life, and to emphasize this "laboratory learning" approach. From Lewin, then, has come the development of *T-groups* (T = training), *L-groups* (L = learning), *D-groups* (D = discovery), *sensitivity training, encounter groups,* and practically everything else which has happened in the field since— in fact, the whole new field of experience-based learning—designated as *ap-*

plied behavioral science. This development has led to a particular approach to consultation called organizational development. To repeat, Kurt Lewin, lively, energetic, stimulating, was the grandfather of all of us who have "trained" or "facilitated" in groups ever since (Bradford, Gibb, & Benne, 1964).

At the time Lewin was working out his theories in the United States, Wilfred Bion had become interested in group phenomena at the Tavistock Institute in England. Bion worked with groups of military patients suffering from battle fatigue and began to notice some intriguing ways in which group members seemed to work against their own intentional goals. He postulated that although groups form for a rational reason, which he termed the "work" of the group, there was, nevertheless, a concerted effort by the group that was irrational and "anti-work." Like Lewin, Bion saw that many of the underlying needs in the individuals comprising the group obstructed the group's functioning effectively.

Bion further observed that different groups avoid work in different ways. Some avoided it by being so utterly *dependent* on the leadership that the group could not function with any initiative or autonomy. Just as a small child hollers for the mother to help get a shirt off or on, or to tie a shoe, so some groups can attempt no tasks unless the leader is around to encourage. What such groups expect of their leader is that he or she be a savior, someone who rescues them and makes everything right. But woe to the leader who betrays the group when inevitable imperfections appear.

Much of the early technique of the T-group was to put members into a time of "unfreezing," by deliberately not supplying them with any direction, structure, or sense of leadership. I once was the "leader" of a T-group where for 2 hours the group did not know who I was (and didn't ask), preferring to speculate that the man sitting next to me had to be the "psychologist," because he had gone to sleep. Such an approach (from which the leader who has denied the group gratification subsequently catches a lot of resentment) knocks the pins out from under a dependent group and leaves them to sink or swim. Some groups, who will not accept responsibility for themselves, prefer to sink.

A second life-style that a group can take, as observed by Bion, is that of *fight*. Such a group draws a tight definition of its membership boundaries and posts "keep out" signs to all the others. When one is in such a group there is a deep sense of "us" as over against the "them" which exists just beyond the group. Usually the "them" is seen as having power or authority which must be wrested away. Just as two teams in a sports event set out to prove who are the winners and who are the losers, so some groups see their basic existence as defensive, and all others in an adversary position. Such groups want the leader to exemplify the values of the group, that is, he or she must be the best fighter of them all, the shrewdest dealer, the one who can take on all others and emerge victorious. When the reigning champion is beaten, then the victor may be the new leader as far as the group is concerned and the loyalties all shift. The group has its new identity around this new strong one. Often in a group, the challenge to the leader is attempted by someone who is hoping to take over or by someone who is testing the leader's power over the group.

All of the stories of the new foreman or the new prisoner in the yard who must first win a fight before being respected are examples of this group character. I remember a group where for 4 days I could not relax because of one member who would attempt to attack anything I said or did. In another group I ended up arm wrestling with a younger male because of the same sort of dynamics.

The third way that a group can behave is to take *flight*—that is, to make the same sort of assumptions as the fighter group, that there is a powerful enemy outside the door. In this case the group has decided that it is too weak to fight the "them," so the obvious course is to escape. This group elects a leader who will be the most efficient in organizing the escape plan and mapping out the route. If the order to the day is retreat, then whoever can manage the retreat the best is the natural leader. I remember one group which suddenly, at a prearranged signal, rose up and marched out of the room. (They all came back in about 10 minutes later; their leader was evidently ambivalent about fleeing too far away.)

The fourth set of group assumptions that Bion noticed was what he called *pairing*. The main underlying need of such a group is to love one another. Those people who help provide this atmosphere are the ones to turn to. There is much discussion of what we all could do if we ever wanted to, but in the meantime change is postponed because it is more important that we remain in place and continue to work on our comfort level.

I once helped to lead a wonderful weekend simulation about community organizing with a group of mental health workers. We had given tasks and directions, but the people in this system were much too interested in building relationships to pay attention to any of the directions. When we announced that the time period for the simulation was now over, that the deadline had passed, that they had not gotten the task done, and that we wished them better luck next year, all hell broke loose. Far into the night some folks were still expressing their astonishment at our hardness of heart. A group with this particular illusion does not want leaders and the group will certainly dump the leader who is about to get them to accomplish something. They prefer to bask in the warmth of relationships and talk over what they could do if the world only knew.

Finally, Bion speculated about a *mature group*, which would find its meaning by dealing with all of the above illusions and the members would proceed to the task with an accurate understanding of what the group is to do and how they are relating to one another. Such groups are rare. They are characterized by a high degree of problem-solving, which includes self-dianosis as well as the ability to proceed to a solution based on relevant data. They also show a high degree of interdependence. The leadership can shift, subgroups can work on the task then regather to work as a whole—without the others in the group insisting on doing the subgroup tasks over.

I remember a workshop on advanced design skills which worked much that way. No matter whose job it was to design the next segment, they always organized for the task by electing a recorder and a time keeper, starting with the question: "What's the data about our workshop at this present moment?" In this case everyone was a skilled professional and had the same background in the design process. As Bion said, such mature working groups are exceedingly rare (Bion, 1961).

The first T-groups which were held at Bethel had a trainer who gave process comments to the group about what it seemed to be doing, but who refused the role of group leader, thus shifting all of the responsibility for decision making onto the group members. The purpose of these laboratory experiences was to study the group process while it was happening. I have already mentioned the way some of these groups began—with no direction or instruction. Typically, group members would feel uncomfortable in a new and strange situation and would attempt to become more comfortable by filling the leadership void with tasks such as introducing themselves to one another. I even remember one group whose members went around the room emptying all the wastebaskets. Of course, many early attempts are made to seduce the "leader" into solving the dilemma by taking charge. If such efforts are resisted, then the group must work on structuring itself until it comes up with something relevant, on the way to which it learns from its own experience about membership, leadership, decision making, and goal setting.

As the group method began to spread, there were many innovations and adaptations of the above process. In the Tavistock approach, for instance, the consultant does not function as a group member, but rather, addresses his or her remarks to the unconscious assumptions the group is making. The NTL leadership style acknowledges that the trainer is a part of the group process and that, after the group solves its leadership problem, he may enter in as a member. A dramatic example of this happened to a friend of mine. At a certain point in the life of the group, the members lifted him up, carried him over to the corner of the room, laid him down on the floor, and folded his hands over his chest. Then they all went back and sat down in a circle leaving one empty spot. The invitation was clear: he could join them, but was no longer needed as the leader.

The above illustration highlights the nonverbal communication aspects of group life. Shortly after the T-group was inaugurated, people began to request some kind of explanation as to what the experience was all about. Because it is next to impossible to describe verbally what one learns by experiencing, proponents of the theory decide to demonstrate the experience, and the *microlab* was born. This consisted of a series of structured exercises which would take anywhere from a few hours on up to a day. By careful design, the participants in the microlab could walk through the dynamics of membership, decision making, affection, and trust building.

One of the side benefits to the group process was the enhancement of their awareness of other people. More often than not, group participants discovered that they could work to understand the others in the group and feel a sense of caring for the personal struggles that others were going through. When the focus of some groups shifted to this goal, the name also shifted from the T-group to *sensitivity training*. Another aim of sensitivity training was to increase the awareness one had of one's self—thus, many experiments with creativity were used, such as eating a meal without utensils, or spending some time in movement expression or in finger painting (Gunther, 1968). Dick Byrd, for instance, established the Creative Risk-Taking Lab to encourage participants to set goals for expanding into areas where they had no previous experience, or thought themselves without aptitude (Byrd, 1970).

On the West Coast, the group movement took another turn. Carl Rogers had supported some of his students in applying to group sessions the same counseling techniques used for individual clients. In such groups, which came to be called *encounter groups*, the therapist would see to it that all of his or her interventions encouraged a supportive climate for group members and pro- vided as much acceptance of each person as possible. By providing a secure situation for group members to discuss any problem they might have, even those about which they feel ashamed, embarrassed, or guilty, the individuals would come to like themselves better, understand themselves more, and give themselves permission to experiment with ways of changing (Rogers, 1971).

William Schutz, who led groups at Bethel in the early days, established himself at Esalen in California and, with the publication of *Joy*, became a spokesperson for the Encounter Group movement. Schutz encouraged people to express feelings that they considered not nice, stressed the importance of each group member being responsible for him- or herself, and introduced a variety of consciousness-raising techniques such as psychodrama, Gestalt awareness exercises, bioenergetics, and massage (Schutz, 1967).

When I was first learning about the field of applied behavioral science, someone gave me a picture of the difference between the T-group trainer and the encounter group facilitator. It went something like this: the T-group tries in every way it can think of to involve the leader in the group, while the encoun- ter group leader takes the spotlight from the first moment the group meets and the group must do anything it can to get it away from him or her. Those are the two extremes, but there are ample illustrations of both styles since the late 1950s. The study by Lieberman, Yalom, and Miles (1973) compares different leadership styles to see which, if any, is more effective. In general, they found that groups respond more favorably to a leader who establishes a climate of nurturance and support, and who pushes the boundaries without being too confronting.

There are a lot of problems trying to research groups. It is difficult to isolate a single variable and very difficult to replicate any results, since the group, being new, has unique dynamics. About all one can say thus far about group leadership is that the best leader in the world can do little or nothing about a group which doesn't want to go anywhere, and a group which is moving, enthusiastic, and cares for one another can get a lot done in spite of having little productive leadership.

GOALS

What are the *goals* of the encounter group or T-group? As indicated in the foregoing section, there may be different goals at different times. There certainly may be recognized and unconscious goals which are incongruent. The sum total of each member's personal needs may be the goal of the group. Or members may submerge personal needs to attend to a group goal which they see as having priority. Some of the goals of a group session would be the same as any therapy—healing, wholeness, becoming more comfortable with one's self, increasing coping skills, demonstrating a higher capacity for problem-solving, and so forth. Some groups work hard for the attainment of insight and self-understanding. Other groups practice regressing the group member to the time of hurt, and beginning again. Most groups have goals that can be boiled down to an increased awareness of one's self and increased effectiveness in relating to other people.

Some of the reasons why people seek group experiences include the desire for open and close personal relationships, finding an acceptance which may be missing in other parts of their lives, learning to express and deal with strong emotions, gaining skills in conflict management, assertiveness, self-esteem, intercultural communication, and learning how groups function and work most effectively. Special group experiences have been devised to aid people in building skills in such areas as couples communication, leadership styles, power and conflict, and designing cooperative educational climates within the public school classroom. The rush toward groups may represent deficits in other parts of our society which prevent people from gaining the skills required for forming fulfilling relationships with others. With the breakdown of the extended family, the emphasis by institutions on numbers and bigness, and the increased mobility of the population, there are certainly good reasons for groups to become tools for learning how to initiate, build, and end personal relationships.

There are too many varieties of groups to list all of their possible goals in this chapter. For purposes of simplicity I am going to highlight some of the general goals of the T-group, and will use that term to refer to most of the other forms of group procedures.

First of all, the T-group has a goal of focusing upon the interpersonal phenomenon which takes place between group members. By doing so, a person within the group has the opportunity to hear from others how he or she is perceived. By requesting the information, a person can learn what behaviors are noticed and how they are interpreted by others. The flip side of this is that the group member commits himself or herself to providing that same information to others. Along with these reactions to others, group members may obtain insight into what factors in them create the reactions they are having. A third goal is to gain some understanding of the skills which enable interpersonal relationships to flourish. A fourth goal is, in addition, the gaining of concepts about how groups function, what helps them to work effectively and what hinders them from doing so. Another goal is to experiment with new behaviors and thus increase one's repertoire of possible actions or reactions in future interpersonal situations. Certainly another goal is to increase the awareness of what one observes happening in a group's interpersonal climate. In short, T-groups provide an experience designed to maximize the opportunities a person has to reveal his or her own behaviors, feelings, and reactions; to develop an awareness of self and others; and to learn the processes of good communication and effective group functioning (D. W. Johnson, 1986).

As mentioned before, a group meets with the general purpose of studying itself as it goes along, but otherwise is without an agenda. The facilitator may outline some procedural aids which will meet the above goals. In a group meeting for the first time, I often mention a number of expectations that I have:

1. We will stay focused on the present life of this particular group—staying in the here and now.
2. Anything may be discussed within the group, and whatever is discussed should remain the property of this group only, that is, the importance of confidentiality.
3. We will practice stopping from time to time to look at the process of what is happening in the group to learn as much as we can from the group experience.

The list could be longer. Gerald Egan (1973) has suggested that the first half of the group's time together be very tightly structured to teach the participants the skills of being a productive group member. After the skills are learned, group members contract with one another to practice the skills and received the group's opinion of how capable they are becoming.

If these were listed as goals, then they might look something like this:

1. Speaking for self—always say "I," never say "You."
2. Expressing feelings—all feelings, regardless of whether they are perceived as "good" ones or "bad" ones.
3. Listening skills, such as:
   a. Crediting—remembering who said what you quote later.
   b. Paraphrasing—putting into your own words by way of summary what someone else has just said.
   c. Reflection of feelings—indicating that you understand the emotional importance of what the other person just said.
   d. Keeping one's mouth shut during the time the ears are supposed to be open. It is often astonishing how few groups can allow someone to speak until his or her thought is finished.
4. Skills in giving accurate and nonevaluative information to another person who has requested reactions to his or her behavior. In the jargon of the field we term this *feedback*.
5. Leadership functions which enable a group to choose goals and make decisions.
6. Different styles of dealing with conflict.

These are some of the primary skills of group membership (for a fuller discussion see Johnson, 1986 and Johnson & Johnson, 1986).

There are obviously, then, many factors affecting the quality of the group experience. Besides the skill and personal style of the facilitator, there are also the assumptions that each group member (including the leader) has regarding the group, and the various learning goals of group participants. Fortunately, groups are usually flexible enough to manage to reach very disparate goals. Although one member may want to learn how to express anger, another may want to learn how to express warmth and tenderness. When the trust is high, all group members become resources to one another, and together the group meets the needs of each.

One of the basic assumptions of the group is embedded in the preceding paragraph. The group promotes a set of values that emphasizes cooperation, individuality, trust, and openness, and that builds an awareness of and concern for other people. The deepest experience within a group is characterized by a sense of being connected to all other human beings and understanding, indeed loving, the particular human persons collected for this experience.

Much has been said of the narcissism inherent in many of the self-discovery methods which are popular in our present-day society. The T-group, however, has its roots in just the opposite philosophy—that through the experiences which are usual within the life of the group there will come an increase in sensitivity to others, a heightened confidence in one's self, and a demonstration of the best democratic procedures. It was the hope of the founders of the method that enough small group training in time would lead to an increased sense of participatory citizenship.

Another major assumption of those who are committed to the group approach is that the experiential approach to learning is one of the best ways for people to learn. Through studying the various facets of their own experience, people draw more lasting learnings which are more directly relevant to other facets of their lives.

Experiential learning—the inquiry approach to learning goals—is based on three assumptions: one learns best from participating and being involved; knowledge which is truly meaningful is that which has been personally discovered; and the readiness for learning is highest when one is free to make a commitment to his or her own learning goals.

With the help of the group facilitator, a group often stops to "process" what has just occurred, that is, to study the process of the group's life rather than the content. Thus, at given points in the life of the group, the group deliberately stops the generating of interpersonal data and reflects upon the experiences is has had thus far. Typically, a group will choose one event to study, then group members will recall precisely what happened and further what were the feelings each person had as the experience took place. One of the unique qualities of this kind of learning process is that it provides an opportunity for affective and behavioral aspects to be studied simultaneously. Indeed "feelings are facts" is one of the earliest things emphasized by the trainer/facilitator (Johnson & Johnson, 1986).

Most often, participants discover that there has been an assumption of group-mindedness which is just not true. As members share their feeling reactions to a common event they discover that not everyone has reacted in the same way or is feeling alike at this moment. The next question for study becomes: "What is my own personal cause for selecting this particular feeling in response to the experience rather than the others which I have just heard mentioned?" In my experience with groups this is often the magical "ah-ha!" moment when someone makes a major self-discovery. There is an encouragement to expand one's selection of reactions with the support of other group members, to practice new behaviors, and to experiment with hitherto restricted feelings. I can remember someone saying in incredulous tones: "You mean that all I have to do it to give myself more credit?" and the group responding with a joyous "Yes"! It is a moment of pure discovery. For those of us who have been there, it is one of the major reasons to be involved constantly with groups of unique people who are living miracles with the power within themselves for survival, courage, growth, and love.

Finally, a new discovery about one's self or about group process needs to be practiced for a while until new behaviors feel as natural as old ones. I remember leading a group once when a young student suddenly stood up and said, "You mean you people can only be honest with one another when you're in a group like this?" I share her surprise. Unless the learnings obtained in a group setting can be applied to all other interpersonal relationships, the experience has been of no real worth. The test of a new learning is an increased range of options in the "real" world, not just in a situation where the rules are enforced by a facilitator/trainer. The application of new learnings to other situations is the real proof of the pudding.

This is true even when the general feelings of the experience fade. Many organizations have used T-groups as a management intervention into the system. A friend of mine did some interviewing of T-group participants in a big industrial organization 6 months after the event, and found everyone very vague about the names of the leaders, exactly who was in their group, and exactly what the group did. However, many of the interviewees described how the atmosphere of the work environment had changed, how the trust level was raised considerably, making it easier to relate to workers in other parts of the system, and how the communications seemed to be easier, making the whole operation more efficient and more pleasant. This is what I'm talking about. New skills had become so well integrated that the T-group was no longer even given credit. For me the transfer of "back-home" learnings are the most important part of group life.

To summarize, then, the experiential learning process is fourfold. First, there is an event on which the group decides to reflect more deeply. Second, each person shares his or her reactions in terms of behaviors and feelings around that particular event. Third, each person searches for causes of the reactions in her- or himself and in the group process. They may list the benefits and the negative consequences of the reactions they are noting. Fourth, group members begin to apply what they have learned to other groups of which they are a part and to work and family relationships. Each may take as goals to attempt alternative behaviors in the future.

I often ask members of a group to keep a journal. There are many approaches to what to put in the journal. One of my favorites, for situations where the emphasis is the learnings we can draw from group process, is to ask the participants to write a description of a back-home group on the first evening. Each following evening I have them return to that same group in thought, and to analyze its dynamics based on what they had learned about groups during the day. Often by the end of the week this has become a very valuable resource and people can't wait to get back into action with the application of their new insights.

Parenthetically, many group atmospheres seem to build the illusion that the only people who exist for the moment are those in the group. I believe that such a thought is a delusion, and that it is also unethical for the facilitator to encourage it. All members of the group have many complex relationships from which they came and to which they return. Any moment in the group ought to be lived out in that context. Although it may seem desirable to abandon all standing relationships and pretend that we are all on an island in a far sea, that is not actually true, and few learnings which relate to reality will come of such an approach. Many people who have felt "burned" by group experiences did not remember the reality from which they came and to which they would return. If they had, they would have been developing their coping skills instead of depleting them.

I do not mean by this in any way to put a damper on someone experimenting with new behavior. An experiment is conscious and is a moving forward to increased behavioral competence. What I am against is a rationalizing of unconscious needs which sometimes can be dangerous, but most often is just plain silly. It is important to remember in experiential learning that experiencing alone is not necessarily beneficial: one learns from a combination of experience and the conceptualization of the experience. Often trainers will add a bit of theory after the reflection/sharing time, to offer handles upon which people can build their own learnings. All of us who do counseling know that no one learns from experience alone. In fact, many people seem doomed to repeat their particular pattern over and over until they stop to give deep study to the assumptions and behaviors which are creating such a mechanistic response. Therefore, a series of experiences in a group setting is of little use unless it is accompanied by times of analyzing, drawing conclusions, deciding on changes, practicing new behaviors, and seeking others' reactions to whether the new behaviors are bringing the desired results. It is then that the group experience is of use to the participants and through them to the community of which they are a part.

Theory

Basic Concepts

The basic idea of the group is that it is a group. A group starts with a collection of individuals, but does not end there. The group develops a life of its own. In the group "gestalt," the whole is more than the sum of its parts.

One of the simplest methods of conceptualizing a group is that which was developed by William Schutz (1960), who hypothesized that individual needs are the strongest motivators we have. Such needs fall into three categories: our needs for membership or affiliation, our needs for leadership or influence, and our needs for intimacy or closeness. He termed these inclusion, control, and affection. In most groups these needs occur as stages each time they meet. One can see how the inclusion stage (membership concerns) affects the first part of group life. The second stage of control consumes the group's attention at the point of decision making, and the resultant feeling of productivity gives a glow of affection.

Every group, no matter what its task or composition, has to deal with these three needs. First comes the question of who is "in" and who is "out." Much of the time this concern is dealt with before the group actually "starts," in the cocktail hour, the conversation around the making of the coffee, the greeting of newcomers, introductions at the table, and so forth. In fact, all behaviors by group members can be seen as attention-getting mechanisms to solve the problem of feeling a part of the group.

Sometimes when a group member is discovered to be feeling particularly "outside," a structured exercise can be used to focus the group's attention on the phenomena. For example the group stand in a circle with elbows linked. The "outsider" is instructed to try to get into the circle. Observing how the person goes about the task: forcing his or her way, tickling someone, asking very politely, pleading, trying to crawl between legs—I once even saw someone vault over the heads of the circle—can give volumes of data as to what assumptions hinder the inclusion process so as to convince the person he or she is an outsider.

Just breaking into the circle, however, does not bring actual inclusion, although it does pinpoint what is going on. The question of how a group draws its boundaries may be a very complex one. I once saw a group in which every member had to somehow be in the center of the circle for one reason or other before he or she was accepted into the group. Little rituals of initiation develop—everyone must cry, or tell a joke or two before he or she feels definitely a part of the whole.

Many groups have existing boundaries—working for the same company, being a graduate student in a group dynamics class—while other groups make up the boundaries as they form. I am constantly amazed at how quickly a newly formed group can define itself into a "we" versus "them." Count off by threes and within minutes the Ones are congratulating themselves that they are not Twos and the Twos are thankful none of them got placed in the Three bunch. A very quick group-forming exercise is to count off, have the groups meet in various parts of the room, and then give them 5 minutes to come up with one thing that makes their particular group unique from all the others.

The need for *inclusion* is the need for keeping a satisfactory relationship going with the other members of the group, a feeling of belonging in this setting with these people. Because it has a lot to do with the beginning of relationships it comes usually at the start of group life. It is important to remember, however, that some method of inclusion is taking place every time the group meets. I recall one group which ended an afternoon session and came down a flight of stairs to decorate tables for the evening's banquet. They began to be frustrated by how disjointedly they were working together until someone said, "Oh, we haven't done inclusion." Taking a couple of minutes to huddle in the middle of the room to regard one another, they regained the group sense of task and finished the decorating in a few minutes with a minimum of fuss and bother.

Within the ongoing life of a group the inclusion question can be raised many times as it goes into deeper and deeper forms of relating to one another. At the outset my being a friend of a friend of the hostess is enough to get me into a party. By the end of the evening, however, I will have shared much more of myself and discovered kindred spirits, maybe even have made new friends. When an encounter group begins, it may be sufficient for inclusion that we are gathered together for a similar purpose in this same place. As the time of getting to know one another proceeds, each member works on the question: "How will I be accepted by these others?" A group facilitator will notice a shift from this when people start saying "we" instead of "I." Often the next stage of group development begins when someone says: "What are *we* supposed to be doing?"

Control problems are the next necessary process for the group to solve. Once the commonalities have been discussed and some sense of trust and safety is generated, the differences between people start to show. People will attempt to take different roles to aid the group in its task, and they will often be resisted by others who similarly wish to be seen as leaders. The members of the group have to work out a satisfactory solution amongst themselves regarding cooperation and the sharing of power and influence. This struggle is heightened (in its most frustrating aspects) when the facilitator abdicates any role-power he or she has, and refuses to bail the group out of this dilemma. Every person has the need to control his or her situation at least to some degree. When the expected leader does not give the expected help, then the situation becomes unpredictable and somewhat scary. It is similar to those moments in childhood when the reassurance of parental control is somehow missing and one is thrown in with one's siblings to work out, by trial and error, by force and manipulation, by anger and by tears, all of the power issues.

Even if the facilitator can be counted upon to give all sorts of directions, the control struggle will come up. In an analytical therapy group it may be a struggle over who gets the attention of the leader. In most groups, someone will eventually question the leader's authority, wisdom, credentials, and so forth. Who is he or she to tell us what to do? Groups can be expected at some point in their life in some manner to rework the need for a leader. Recently a weekend group demonstrated this perfectly by not needing me as facilitator for all of one afternoon. Once a young man said to me at the end of the group: "I really like you a lot better since you got down off that leader stuff and became one of us." In a termination meeting of a group of graduate students this spring, a young woman, saying something about the low energy level every- one seemed to have that day, reached over and crossed my hands over my chest.

The group needs to learn how to get along without the leader in order to mature and grow. Groups that solve this problem learn how to share the control so that every member feels an important and influential part of the group's proceedings. Some groups do not reach a solution. I remember a time I put a "heavy trip" on a group of people by asking: "How does this group make decisions?" The group then demonstrated for 3 days how competitive feelings were keeping it at a standstill.

Affection is based on the building of emotional ties. Various people show differences in the degree to which they want to allow closeness. In the inclu- sion phase, members meet one another and decide whether to continue to build the relationship. In the control phase, members confront their differences with one another and decide how to work together. To continue to build the relationships, ties of affection are formed and members must decide how strong an emotional bond is suitable for the relationship. Many times this awareness comes as the group completes some task and is conscious of warm, mellow feelings of being with good people with whom it would be fun to work again.

In the life of a therapy group, the need for caring deeply for one another can at times be quite high. The ability to maintain close personal relationships is often the key factor which has been lacking for those who opt for group therapy. In the context of the group, members can explore their fears of inti- macy by being a part of one another's lives. They can practice intimacy and closeness in a setting where they will receive instruction and feedback from one another. Couples therapy and family therapy often start with sorting out the power struggles, but end with the question of maintaining intimate relationships.

A group-phases theory was developed by Jack Gibb (1978), who saw the life of a group as a four-step sequential process of development.

The first step in group life deals with membership concerns. The question for the individual is, "Who am I in this setting?" When the group is not effectively dealing with this question, fear and suspicion are displayed. Con- versely, the working through of this situation leads every member to feel acceptance and trust in the group.

The next step of group building centers on decision making. To reach that stage, members must exhibit a high level interaction. All members must par- ticipate. (Silence never means consent.) A group can be diagnosed as not achieving this stage when it is noted that there is a lot of politeness and caution characterizing group meetings. Resolution of this awkwardness will be when lively, spontaneous interaction and the free flow of reactions and responses takes place.

The third step in group life is goal formation, which requires that the group have a clear target, a sense of direction, so that it may eventually have a feeling of completion. When a group knows what it is doing, then it demonstrates enthusiasm and agreement. If the goal is still undecided, then the observer will note competition on the one hand or apathy on the other. Clarity means enthusiasm and cooperation.

Finally, after having met, deciding how to decide, and selecting a goal that all group members can commit themselves to, the fourth step involves the group's need to organize for reaching that goal. The question here is one of control, and a successful group demonstrates shared leadership to set up mechanisms to accomplish its task.

To heighten awareness of these group process concerns, here is a checklist for an observer of the life of a group:

Process Questions

I. Acceptance in group

By what process were people given membership in the group?
Anyone left out? How?
Any who seemed hesitant to speak up?
Was anyone obviously withdrawn?
Did anyone make a sudden shift in his or her level of participation?
What could you do to build trust?
What did the group do to build trust?

II. Data flow

Were there a lot of interruptions?
Did people seem confused?
Did some folks seem misunderstood?
Did some folks seem to get no response or reaction from the group?
How could you build listening skills?
How could you improve the quality of the feedback?

III. Goal formation

Did anyone seem confused about the direction the group was heading?
Was there an obvious low investment in the task?
Was there argument about what the group ought to be doing?
What did you do to help the group pinpoint its differences?
How did you aid people in sharing their expectations?

IV. Control

How did the group focus on the question of who was in charge?
How did the group treat your leadership role?
Was there any struggling over leadership positions in the group?
What did you do to help the group focus on its decisions about leadership?

V. Closeness

> How were feelings expressed in the group?
> How available were you to the group?
> Did group members like/dislike the experience?
> Do you like/dislike the group?

The importance of conceptual systems for the group leader is that it provides a framework aiding her or him in making decisions about when and how to intervene in the life of a group. The findings of behavioral science offer facilitators a means of organizing their observations and perceptions, and a basis for communicating such observations to group members. Each person who attempts to lead a group should have explicit conceptual schemes they can systematically use to enable group members to learn. Even the methods of trusting one's intuition and acting on one's feelings can be communicated openly to group members as they seek to learn about themselves and group process. Both intuition and theory are useful in generating effective interventions within a group. It is a mistake to slight either method of understanding the group process.

The most prominent study of psychological damage resulting from T-group experiences is one which was conducted by Irving Yalom and his associates at Stanford University, where different groups were led using different leadership styles. In general, it was found that group members perceived a supportive, accepting leadership style as more beneficial than an aggressive domineering style (Lieberman, Yalom, & Miles, 1973).

Theoretically, the encounter group differs from the T-group regarding the philosophy of conflict between members and the confrontation of that conflict. If the expression of angry feelings is seen as positive, then striving for such feelings makes a good deal of sense. On the other hand, if establishing a safe learning environment is seen as the positive good, then expressions of acceptance and trust are those sought and those built upon. The theoretical stance of the leader affects the outcome. For instance, based on my understanding of what stage the group is in, I can exercise a lot of leadership or refuse any attempt by the group to get me to lead. It depends on my judgment of what is going on, based on my theories of group process.

A more analytical view is that the group itself represents a reenactment of the family setting for each group member. Therapy groups are often deliberate in providing symbols of both mother and father through the use of cotherapists. There have been many moments of powerful regression and rebuilding when a group member works to recreate his or her past family life. The modeling of a positive parental team can be a powerful force in opening up new options for someone whose childhood experience was constricted by fear and suspicion.

A schema which applies the previously mentioned work of Bion to the life of a group was developed by Warren Bennis and Herb Shepherd (1956). Basically, there are two phases of group life, with each phase having three subphases within it. The first stage represents a preoccupation by the group with authority; the second stage is characterized by a preoccupation with intimacy.

To some degree each time the group meets it relives some of its past behavior and forecasts its future. (In fact, there are interesting clues to the entire life of the group in the first 20 minutes of group time.)

According to Bennis and Shepherd's model, the movement from authority to personal relations, from relating in role ways to relating as persons, represents a change in emphasis from power to affection. In the first phase, the group struggles to handle the differences arising from the individuals which comprise it, while in the second phase the individual differences are celebrated by the group.

As stated above, each group phase consists of three subphases. The first of these is characterized by dependency. The group in its infancy needs the parental figure to orient it to the factors that make up its new world. Often there are people in a group who desire throughout the life of the group to be dependent. A leader working from this conceptual framework will usually think that it is all right, in the opening session, to give directions, set guidelines, and answer questions so that the group will have a sense of safety and trust.

Inevitably the dependent stage gives way to a counterdependent one. Someone in the group will challenge the leader's skills, authority, knowledge, or intentions. This person will, at that time, be speaking for the group as it needs to move away from the dependence upon the authority role. Sometimes there are people in a group who are always counterdependent and resent any and all suggestions made by a perceived authority figure. The conflict which develops within the group is based upon the two extreme positions of utter reliance on an authority figure and the instant rejection of everything and anything the authority represents.

If the group is to solve the problem, then those who are not in either extreme camp must assert leadership. These independents who can both receive leadership as well as handle it on their own represent the group's young-adult stage, which is capable both of handling its own affairs and of letting the person in authority be a resource to the group as it proceeds further in its life.

Having settled the question of authority, the group is ready to enter the second phase of its life. Again there are three subphases. The first of these is characterized by a kind of euphoria which the group feels, having successfully resolved the conflict about leadership. This stage is led by those who are able to be open and personal, who find it easy to express feelings, and who assume that what they feel is also what every member of the group feels and wants. Sometimes this subphase is called the pseudopersonal time. Everyone feels warm and nice, but underneath is fear of anyone rocking the boat. In fact, the group will attempt to overpower anyone who suggests that all is not as it seems.

Just as the dependents were challenged by the counterdependents, so the group changes when someone becomes spokesperson for those who are more cautious about relating personally. Someone may ask a person sharing, "Do you really want to reveal so much?" or "Won't you be sorry tomorrow that you allowed so much of yourself to show?" These counterpersonal figures make apparent the ambivalence of the group about intimacy. Revealing one's self to others is a risk and all of us feel uneasy about it. The push to achieve intimacy is counterbalanced by the fear of it.

A rule of thumb addressing this conflict is that the group can only become as intimate as its least intimate member. One group I was in was just reaching towards intimacy when one of its members became increasingly agitated and finally jumped up and left. In some groups that might have stopped the action; in this particular one we just drew closer and went on. In groups that meet weekly for a period of time, it is a common occurrence for people to drop out 2 or 3 weeks from the end—for two reasons, I think. First, the increasing intimacy is a problem; they feel pressure to reveal more of themselves than they are comfortable revealing; and second, they are aware of the upcoming termination and cannot live through saying goodbye.

As in the first phase, the resolution of this problem of ambivalence for the group comes from those who can manage closeness but do not desperately need it. These group members help the group achieve a satisfactory balance of caring for each person as he or she actually is, not denying differences, but accepting all in the group.

As mentioned previously, a group may be teased about one of its members, and, as is the case among family members, draw close: "He may strike you as strange, but he is one of us." In this last subphase of group life, the group is interdependent. The members know each other as distinct persons and rely on one another to be caring and trustworthy. Such a group has reached a level of maturity that is rare, has problem-solved some deep abiding problems, and is justified in its wish to continue to meet and grow with this circle of good friends.

A final group theory is based upon the work of Kurt Lewin (1951). His attempt to put personality theory into a framework where it could be mathematically measured is applicable also to group life. The group is challenged from within or without; energy builds up around the tension. A force-field analysis at that point would list the factors in the group which are motivating the group to change and reach its goal. Just as important are those factors which are hindering the group and keeping it stuck. At such times, the group atmosphere is often one of apathy and boredom. This generally means that the group is sitting on the lid, keeping the energy bottled up. An intervention is called for at this point. Then the energy is released and the group is unblocked and can move forward.

Often the clues for what is going on in the group can be found in its members' conversation, what Lieberman terms the *focal conflict*. One group I was leading came back from lunch talking of boxing and the style of Muhammed Ali. I asked them if there was a fight in the group which we were not addressing, and sure enough there was. Similarly, someone may speak of beauty or love or good friends and be subtly giving a message to the members of the group. All that is needed is to invite them to speak more directly in the here and now of the group life. (Rule for facilitators: the group conversation always addresses what is happening in the group.)

Assumptions about Human Nature

One of the cardinal ground rules of group life is to stay in the here and now. The group members, of course, are not used to such a requirement and need to be trained in how to remain only in the present. Often the reaction is, "How can we get to know one another if we can't find out anything about each other?" People are often amazed to discover all the data that they possess in terms of their own reactions and what has been thus far communicated, verbally and nonverbally.

Some leaders insist that group members, in their discussion, never stray outside the group. Although I am all for the principle, I think it is important to be somewhat flexible. For one thing, it is a difficult discipline to learn; for another, sometimes the pressure of outside difficulties is just too high, and some feelings must be ventilated. Another cogent reason for relaxing the rule is that the group sometimes needs the more conventional information to establish commonalities and build trust. They can find it all out over lunch, so why be too tyrannical about what kinds of statements are allowed? Moreover, groups usually figure out for themselves that stories from the outside are eventually boring because they are not directly related to everyone present. What is directly related is the events within the life of the group.

There is a similarity to Gestalt theory at this point. This similarity concerns staying focused on the present moment, starting with what is very obvious to everyone, and assuming that what people are doing in this situation, their process, is precisely what they do in any similar situation. So the focus is on the interpersonal interactions, as far as the group is concerned, but what is unconsciously being acted out are the angers, fears, apprehensions, suspicions, and coping mechanisms which are still unfinished business from the past. Thus, through becoming aware of what he or she is doing in the interaction, the person can often gain a great deal of insight into how he or she developed this particular set of behaviors, and how to change them.

Because of the phenomena that they focus on, the current event and all the responses to it in the present moment, T-groups are often very therapeutic for those who experience them. For years, the controversy has gone on about whether the learning group was therapy-oriented or education-oriented. In my mind, it really does not matter which way to approach the human being, because the results of self-discovery can be very much the same.

Many people come into therapy because they are so unskilled in relating to others. The frustration which this causes has led them to feel depression, anxiety, guilt, and anger. Sometimes they demonstrate conscious behavior to force interaction, always with less than desirable results. Their lives are different when they become practiced group members with skills of making personal statements, identifying and expressing feelings, giving and receiving support, giving and receiving feedback, directing messages straight to the other person with eye contact in a full and genuine way; such skill-building undoubtedly changes a person's life in very dramatic ways.

At the University of Maryland Counseling Center, one of my colleagues and I have conducted groups which are limited to working only on skills of interpersonal communication. The group lasts an hour and the last 5 minutes are set aside for processing the group. We emphasize that no one talk about outside matters, and that all statements be directed to someone in the group. We spend a lot of time studying each statement's impact on others. Our experience is that some people who have had years of personal therapy dramatically blossom in attaining new skills and a new image of themselves as socially competent.

Our assumption about groups then, is that people have a marvelous capacity for growth and can change in desired directions. We assume that each person is in tune with his or her own needs and can pace his or her own growth. I strive to have no expectations about what group members *should* do. If I did I would be acting as another parental figure against whom the person can rebel. It is important that all exercises are voluntary. This establishes that the participant is always in charge. Each person is responsible for his or her own learnings.

Sometimes group members need to be protected for some reason or other from the very real pressure that can build up to force them to perform some behavior the group has labeled as "right." My job, when that occurs, is to question the group about what it is up to and to direct the interactions away from the person under attack.

In general, I believe that conflict should go on between group members unabated to provide learnings about how we are in conflict. However, when group pressure appears too great, I check with the member under pressure to maintain the voluntary nature of the interactions—sometimes at the expense of getting conflict directed at me. In time, though, the group learns to be more sensitive to its members and to confront those who need confronting and support those who need supporting.

From the foregoing, it can be concluded that one of the basic purposes of group methods is to help participants achieve some kind of behavioral and cognitive change which will increase the quality of their relationships, the ability to cooperate with family, neighbors, and co-workers, and will produce an overall increased competency in managing their relationships. In so doing, people are enabled to live more self-fulfilling lives. The capacity of groups to provide corrective emotional experiences with peers sometimes borders on the miraculous.

In this chapter the approach to group therapy is definitely focused upon the client's interpersonal process. In order to aid clients in this task, there are questions the counselor should ask, such as what are the skills needed to function adequately in our society? (See Johnson, 1986.) Given a list of those which are helpful, then what specific skills are clients failing to utilize properly? And will the learning of behavioral skills reduce the pathological behavior of a client and increase his or her ability to create a more self-fulfilling life?

Within the group context, there are definite processes by which to teach interpersonal skills, many of which have been covered elsewhere (Johnson, 1986; Johnson & Johnson, 1986). The first teaching phase consists of the persons' becoming aware of what skills are lacking and of their need for obtaining them. As group members interact with one another, the apparent need of skills arises around the frustrations about the way the interaction is going.

The second phase is the conceptualization of the skill. If someone is to learn a skill, he or she needs to have a definite idea of what the skill is and how it is to be applied. This includes identifying the behaviors involved and putting them in proper sequence. Often this phase of conceptualizing calls for some didactic input on the part of the teacher. This input can be a formal presentation or it can be informal coaching within the group interactions on what aids and what hinders the process.

The third phase of skill building is practice. The life of the group offers many occasions for trying out a new skill and becoming more proficient in its use. It is not enough to explain a skill; the repeated use of it is necessary for it to be integrated into someone's available behaviors. I felt frustrated by the medical student in a group who once said to me, "Just give us a checklist of what responses to make when a person comes into the office and we will remember to use them. That is how we learn things." From my point of view, that is impossible. Cognitive learning is one thing, but behavioral skills firmly mastered are quite another—as I tried to explain to the medical student. Memorizing where organs are located is a far cry from operating on someone.

Finally, the fourth phase of skill building is receiving feedback about how well the new skill is developing. "Feedback" is a word that refers to the other members' perceptions of reactions to the behavior of the client. With this source of information one can assess the progress of the new skill. The purpose of feedback is to provide constructive information so that the client can correct errors, identify problems, chart progress, and compare the intention of the behavior with the actual reception of it by others.

Here, again, the group setting provides the richest and safest environment for the type of information needed to adjust behavior. The group can encourage the group member who perseveres in the learning process until he or she experiences success. Often group members come to subsequent meetings with exciting tales of having used the new skills to aid the family discussions or to initiate new acquaintances. When the skills began to spill over into the client's daily activities, then the behaviors are becoming natural and integrated into the life-style of the client.

Improving the client's interpersonal skills is a major key to reducing self-defeating attitudes and increasing psychological health, and the group setting provides the optimal locale for this to take place. If the counselor is thinking in these terms, then he or she can accomplish a great deal in effectively promoting increased positive attitudes about the self and attitudes about functioning effectively and competently in relationships with others (Johnson & Johnson, 1979).

Comparisons with Related Theories

I have already written of the close relationship I see between Gestalt theory and the T-group. The Encounter Group movement draws heavily upon the techniques of Gestalt awareness to enable people to make new discoveries about themselves.

The group (including the setting) constitutes a living organism, so by paying strict attention to what is obvious in the present moment, one can develop the group's awareness of its own life. Often there is an unconscious collaboration by the group to avoid dealing with something. In that event, the therapist may need to raise the level of the group's awareness by helping the group to exaggerate what it is doing, in order to get the energy flowing again— for avoidance almost always means repressing the energy and avoiding real contact with one's own feelings and with others. When the group releases its denied or pent-up feelings, then genuine person-to-person interaction can take place once again.

In my view, the only difference between the T-group, as I am describing it, and the Gestalt theory group is one of timing and degree. If the end goal is group process, then Gestalt awareness techniques may be sometimes useful to edge the group over a stuck place. If the personal therapy of the individual group member is the primary focus, then the group process may take a back seat to one-to-one interactions between the therapist and the group member. From my point of view that is often unnecessary. In the therapy groups I have experienced, members are often marvelous therapists to one another, requiring only minimal intervention from the therapist, at times, to call attention to what they are or are not doing as a group.

Rational–Emotive therapy asks the client to change his or her belief system—to act "as if" something other than what currently affects behavior were true. In the group, I might ask someone who states they are frightened to speak in front of so many people, to experiment with pretending that these people were family or best friends. Somewhere along the way, I picked up a rule of thumb: where the feet go, the body follows. By this, I mean that if one starts to behave in a different manner, then the results produce that which the person dreamed of but was too pessimistic to try. The confrontation: "What if the opposite of what you fear were true?" is worth exploring. And the group, as stated previously, is an excellent place to try out new behaviors, and receive feedback on them. With that kind of support, new belief systems about oneself become possible.

Another base for the encounter group is the Humanistic Psychology movement and Carl Rogers's approach to counseling. One of the most vital parts of the beginning life of a group is to build trust. This is done by raising the safety level for everyone enough to provide that sense of security that leads to sometimes dramatic exploration and risk taking. It is very important that the group member feel accepted as a person in a way that allows the self-restricted feelings which he or she perceives as awful or naughty or bad or not nice to also surface and be expressed. Under safe conditions one is invited, but not forced, to reveal one's self. The key to this approach is to reach a level of trust where genuine caring is given and received, and to thereby increase human potential.

The Transactional Analysis approach has often been especially useful in a cognitive way. Many of us find insight in reflecting on our inner child who is still very much with us, and an intentional choice of adult behaviors often brings out the adult behaviors of the other person. Both the cognitive map and the deliberate practice of transactions is important. However, I disapprove of the jargon, which often seems too superficial to me. I have talked with people who can label every single bit of their behavior, but are still in deep pain and are still messing up their lives and others! Somewhere, for them, the labeling has fallen short.

The analytic approach to group counseling has often in the past not been *group* counseling at all. A therapist would place people in a group and proceed to behave as if each was in a one-to-one relationship with the therapist. Of the analytic contributions to interpreting what is happening in a group, the recognition that the group's unconscious is a powerful force is especially valuable. When someone "acts out" in a group (or a family or a classroom), then that person can be seen as expressing that energy for the group, as being used by the group so that other members need do no work. The group needs to face what it is doing to create the conditions for this acting-out behavior. It is important not to blame the individual for expressing the group unconscious.

Analytic approaches suggest that the therapist is a member of the group and is a vital force affecting the field. One can note the transference, but not deal with it often in the group—mainly because the transference is spread to other members of the group and to the group as an entity in itself. My cotherapist and I certainly symbolize father and mother, and the other members of the group symbolize the siblings, and there is a richness to be worked out there too.

Rather than discussing transference, the T-group operates mostly on the conscious, rational level. The group is asked to study the interactions and experiences of the group which everyone can see, hear, taste, touch, and smell. Further, group members are encouraged to share their feeling responses to the group and to the different members within it. In so doing, the group usually stays on a level of cognitive understanding, but each member becomes aware of his or her projections onto others. At times, especially with a growing feeling of warmth and support, there are profound moments of pain and rebirth which seem almost miraculous.

THERAPY

Theory

In the theory section I have already described many models and conceptual frameworks which can provide the basis for a facilitator to understand what is going on in the group. To summarize that discussion, the assumption is that the group is an entity, not just a collection of people. There are definite stages of development in the life of the group, and much can be learned by paying attention to group process. In the T-group or encounter group, the focus of the group's attention is on the interpersonal interaction between group members. By studying the events of the group life, group members will learn interpersonal skills, will increase the possibilities of self-expression, will become more autonomous individuals, and will gain insight into how their past experiences are creating patterns for their present interaction. It is also possible for someone in the supportive, caring climate of the group to regress to a very early state and to begin again, this time with nurturance and wisdom. In other words, the group has a healing capacity which makes major changes possible.

Process

The process of the group is the major focus for the learning experience. The group leader may set ground rules, such as keeping the conversations direct and responding only to what is present in the room, or may let the group begin on its own with accompanying consternation, in order to heighten the awareness of what group members need, in the way of skills, to relate to one another. This beginning usually means that the group will be well motivated when it learns something that it has discovered itself. If this method is chosen by the facilitator, then he or she may want to make group norms and standards explicit as they emerge by writing them up on newsprint or at least by stating them and expecting the group subsequently to enforce them.

For me, the choice often revolves around the time frame. If a group meets 90 minutes per week for one semester, then I usually start it out with some suggestions as to how to begin together. If it is a week-long residential group, then I often rely on the group's discovering what helps it get the job done as it goes along.

After the decisions made by the trainer about how to start the group are solved, then comes the middle part of the group life. One way or another, my interventions are around group process, "what are we doing now," or about communication, "let us look at that dialogue between John and Sue again to see what we can learn from it." Part of the training function is to teach the group how to process—that is, what awareness questions to ask in order to learn from the experiences. Some approaches to this have been outlined earlier in this chapter.

Another vital skill for group members is how to give feedback. Because the benefit of learning a new interpersonal skill is greatly enhanced if there is feedback about one's behavior, the quality of the feedback is very important. The rules of good feedback are to be well timed, specific, observable, behavioral, and, especially, nonevaluative. A feedback practice statement would go: "when you did _____ (describe the specific behavior you observed), I felt _____. (For a further discussion of feedback see Johnson, 1986.)

Another set of skills which is emphasized are those regarding listening. In some groups there may be a low-key approach, just pointing out that one should not interrupt, for instance. Other groups may have didactic input and practice sessions around such things as paraphrasing and making an understanding response (Johnson, 1986).

Also involved in group life are the different attempts to provide leadership for the group. Certainly letting the members in on what to observe about participation and influence is something that happens either as the result of the leader's modeling or through practice sessions. The distributed leadership functions within the life of the group can be highlighted by postmeeting pencil-and-paper instruments asking who filled what function during that meeting. A discussion of this may lead to increased understanding of what is missing in group life (see Johnson & Johnson, 1986).

To help the group focus on the problems of influence, an exercise I particularly like to use is to have the group members line themselves up according to who is most and who is least influential in the group. In a few minutes one can see the struggles which are taking place around control and can process the exercise for a long time. This exercise is used to help the group focus on the struggles which are taking place for leadership within the group.

During the middle phase of the group there is a lot of time, of course, when no skill building in a formal way is going on, but the interaction of the group members flows. Unless the group is diagnosed as needing something specific, it is better for the facilitator to stay out of its way. Even at points of apathy and increasing frustration it is best not to jump in to "rescue" the group, but to let the hidden feelings surface themselves. In fact, *especially* during periods of inactivity is it important not to intervene.

The boring parts are a normal and necessary part of group life. Maybe the group needs a rest; maybe it needs to really experience that no leader is going to save it, that passivity will not be reinforced, and it is up to each group member to help the group move.

The last set of decisions for the group concerns termination. It is important to reach some sense of closure. It is also important that the rush to closeness not set up conditions for group members to act inauthentically. Sometimes the group spontaneously wants to express itself in a group hug, but certainly not every time. Sometimes one needs to have a last round of member participation to articulate the unfinished business and plan for next steps to complete that business. Sometimes there is a lot of grief work, and denial, anger, withdrawal, and acceptance can all be seen to be happening in a very compressed period of time. My tendency at the end is to direct the process toward the back-home application of what has been gained from the groups.

Many varieties of endings are possible and, once in a while, the only thing that is possible is just to declare that the time is up. In any case the facilitator will indicate interest in any follow-up needs. A couple of other endings are: a last round of feedback, maybe with some growing-edge wishes for people; or a final chance to express appreciations and resentments. Many groups receive evaluation forms to fill out near the end of the sessions. In any case, the facilitator has several decisions to make about how to have the group deal directly with its terminating.

Mechanisms

Many methods of aiding the group to discover itself have been outlined. I find most of them very valuable, at certain times, to highlight certain aspects of group interaction. Over the years, many exercises have been developed to enable groups to do their work. These exercises fall into roughly five categories:

1. Intrapersonal—the awareness exercises, for example, which reveal to a person more parts of himself or herself
2. Interpersonal—to focus the attention of the interaction going on between people
3. Skill-building—to teach concepts and allow practice of specific group-member skills
4. Intragroup—to focus the attention of the group on what the group is dealing with at the moment or to enhance team building, and group cohesion
5. Intergroup—exercises designed to highlight systems communication issues, power and authority assumptions, competitive/cooperation assumptions, to focus on "we–they" attitudes, and so forth

What are the purposes of using structured exercises in the life of a group:

1. They may be one way of dealing with a group need—such as getting acquainted, team building, conflict management, closure.
2. They may be used to highlight and deal with interaction concerns between group members, as when two people are uneasy about confronting one another and the group sets up a structure to support each of them.
3. They may deal with individual concerns. This is especially true of the Gestalt experiment, but can also be a payoff for a management training exercise.
4. They may introduce and practice skills needed by group members for more efficient group functioning.
5. They can energize the group which has been working intensely for a long period of time.
6. They can generate data for the group to process. (The processing time following any exercise is very important. A rule of thumb is that the reflection period be at least as long as the exercise. In fact, it may be much longer. The 5 minutes used in setting up a line as to who is most and least influential in the group may lead to hours of interaction and learning. Another rule of thumb is that any exercise will lead naturally into at least twice as much unstructured time. The exercise is to focus

on something or unblock something, so if too many exercises are required to keep the group going, the group is just entertaining itself and
not really dealing with its own dynamics. If a facilitator discovers that
he or she is using exercises as much as one-third of the time, then
something is wrong.)

7. The use of exercises can speed up the group process. (I have already
   mentioned how the microlab developed to demonstrate experientially
   the processes which take place in a long-term group. Similarly, the use
   of exercises to generate data can enable a short-term group to get to
   more learning issues than entry. For example, the semester-long
   groups run by most university and college counseling centers are just at
   the point of being ready to begin when the semester is suddenly over.
   This results in negative learning. The group ends up disbanding at the
   worst possible moment in its life, just as the differences between people
   and the control conflicts start to emerge. The solution to this is to use
   exercises judiciously to speed up the group process and reach some
   sense of completion rather than abandonment.)

I have encountered two extreme positions in teaching students. One position is taken by those who are very distrustful of group exercises and see them
as always manipulating the group in negative ways. I think the danger of
manipulation is certainly one to be considered, but to toss down a good tool
because it can be mishandled is silly. Besides, most groups can stop a leader
from becoming too directive. In other cases, it may be silly not to provide some
structure to enable the group to function more effectively.

The other extreme position, also bad, in my opinion, is characteristic of
leaders who do not have the patience for any unstructured time; as soon as a
group gets through with one exercise they are on to the next. It keeps everyone
busy, but it also leads to an unreal set of illusions. Just because the group has
done six inclusion exercises does not mean that it is time to move on to control.
The group may have broken the ice, moved around a little, and gotten to see
who is here. It may even have learned names, but it is nowhere near knowing
the fears and reactions of those who feel "in" and those who feel "out."
Inclusion is still to come. Those who believe that something has been accomplished may be surprised when the group breaks down later.

Any group involves choice about structure. The silent beginning of a T-
group is just as much a decision of the facilitator as is a get-acquainted game.
Either silence or an exercise can be manipulative. The question is not whether,
but how. With openness on the part of the leader and enough time to process
the experience afterwards, group members should not be too confused.

PRACTICE

Problems

One of the outstanding features of the encounter group or T-group is that
the manner of using the group process has by this time become very much

enriched by awareness exercises, Gestalt methods, bioenergetics, structured group exercises, body therapies such as Rolfing, Feldenkreis, Lomi, Aston Patterning, and meditation. Group leaders have become so eclectic that they can freely draw on a variety of approaches according to the needs and the direction of the group.

The approach to problem solving is often an unfamiliar process to those in a group. If the ground rule is to remain in the present, attending only to the interactions which are currently taking place, then the problems to be solved are immediate ones. Through this demonstration, group members can learn to apply the skills to other situations of which they are a part.

The encounter group approach, in general, is to allow interpersonal data to flow, trusting that as a person gets to know the others in the group, there is a growing recognition that what he or she is noticing is definitely related to parts of the self—that these other people are doing things, feeling things, being aware of things in common with the observer. Thus, personal growth occurs in a broadening of understanding about what it is like to be oneself and in a growing respect for the complexity and strengths of others.

The T-group leader, while certainly practicing any behaviors which would lead to the above, may also work with the group to delineate behaviors which are helpful and to practice them deliberately so that problem-solving mechanisms can be applied beyond the confines of the group.

One danger that can occur in a group is that most of us have a natural tendency to give advice. Someone just *has* to give a member with a problem advice about the best solution, what the person ought to do, what kind of assertive responses the group member ought to make. Often the participant who has shared a problem only ends up feeling more dependent and more weighted down with "shoulds."

Advice giving usually results from a concern for the individual, but the facilitator needs to discourage it and perhaps confront the group about what they are doing. A good question is what is in it for the group? Why so much energy around solving the member's problem? When the interaction is processed, perhaps it is discovered that the problem is symbolic for the group in some way. It may even be a substitute task for a similar problem that exists within the group. In any case, the place to practice skills which will solve problems is inside the boundaries of the group.

Sometimes the energy of the group is drained around someone who has what the group considers to be enormous problems. This is certainly true in some cases, but I am suspicious when the group starts to feel drained. If we are really caring for a person, then the energy would be flowing—replenishing all of us as we meet one another. If the reverse is true, then the group needs to look at its process to see what is blocking the energy flow: perhaps it is that most group members have been holding back their own needs because they do not seem as dramatic, somehow. Maybe the person who is receiving so much attention is really making insatiable demands or is busy rebuffing the group's concern.

If I get a chance to screen ahead of time I often screen such people out of a time-limited group. They waste too much time and the group does not immediately recognize this. In addition, such people often use the group as long as the group can stand it, and then drop out of the group rather than be called upon to give to others. It is true that they are narcissistic and deeply wounded, but an encounter group or T-group focus may not be helpful to them unless they really want to change; if this is the case, then they need to commit themselves to the group long enough to learn to care for others.

Evaluation

The expectation surrounding the interpersonal growth group is that almost anyone will benefit. Analytic categories may have some possible use in directing the facilitator's thoughts about a certain person in the group, but unless the group experience is counterindicated, those labels seem of little use. Some group members may have quite severe problems, while others may come to a group motivated mainly by curiosity and a desire to have the experience. Some come to share themselves with others, to broaden their knowledge of self, to have new experiences, and to enjoy the companionship; others come for specific gains in behavioral goals such as overcoming shyness, learning to initiate relationships, to share grief, or to learn to be more assertive. There are those who are driven by unconscious stirrings—needs of nurturance or power or attention. Whatever the reason, groups have almost always been open to everyone. Once the group gathers, whatever happens after that is a part of the group dynamic. Groups have an amazing capacity to heal.

Sometimes, though, a group experience is enhanced when the members are less needy and prepared beforehand for taking part in the group. I usually screen people—always for therapy and often for other kinds of group interaction. A couple of times, not often, I have asked someone not to become a group member. When I sense someone is going to demand an inordinate amount of the group's energy, then I am apt to question the wisdom of the individual's being in a group. As most groups have a limited amount of airtime, it may be harmful to the person who needs more and to the group.

The opposite is also true. Groups provide a very intensive experience which requires a good deal of hard concentration and a lot of energy. It is best to warn people ahead of time and discuss with them the serious commitment of group life. There are times in our lives when none of us should be in a group; we just are not up to it.

Another factor which should be considered is whether or not the prospective group member is already in therapy. Personally, I believe that the best of all possible worlds is to be in both group and individual therapy, but many therapists prefer those whom they are seeing in individual counseling not to split their energies between two places at once. By all means, entering a group is something that should be talked over between the client and the counselor before such a step is taken.

As in any therapy, perhaps the most important question to ask is whether the person has a focus. If someone has a clear motivation or goals for the experience, then the person will know when the group process is beneficial or detrimental to such goals. Part of being in the group is learning how to ask for and receive what one wants. Without such clarity, little progress can be achieved.

A before-group contracting session will include all of the above, enriched by the interpersonal experience between the candidate and the interviewer. I trust my feelings and intuitions in such a session. In addition, it is important to be clear about all the expectations of attendance, length of contract, cost of the group, procedures for paying, place, and time. All expectations of the facilitator and the possible participant should be introduced and discussed; then the ground rules of the group come as no surprise.

Treatment

The treatment approach has been amply covered in the foregoing sections. All of the grist for treatment is inherent in an individual's methods of interacting with others. By using the group process, a skilled facilitator can help each person in the group to recognize assumptions he or she has made about self, others, and the world. In giving and receiving feedback, a person can learn to understand the impact he or she has on others, and by practicing new behaviors a person can progress toward desired goals of change.

Management

It is often the case that most management questions are brought into the group for a group decision to be made. The more one believes in group process the easier this is to accomplish. The group can decide whether or not to add (or subtract) members, when and how often to meet, what kind of commitment is necessary to maintain group membership, whether differential payment plans are possible, and so forth. Indeed the only question for the facilitator is, "What limitations do I have about group decision making?" The important thing to remember here is not to deceive the group. Any vagueness is unfair. Either give the group the decision-making power or keep it. Whichever approach is used, process the whole experience so that group members can learn first hand all of the terrors of responsibility or the rebellions against authority that are present around management issues.

APPLICATION

Group Selection and Composition

The ideal situation is to have a heterogenous grouping with variety of age, life experience, coping styles, and gender. While this is not always possible, it is wise not to have such an imbalance that makes one or two individuals deviants in the eyes of the group.

Coleaders can help in this situation. Again, there are all sorts of combinations possible, but the usual approach is to have team members of opposite genders. If this is a balanced team, then there is good parental transferences and a good modeling source for coequal relationship which is rare in our society. Care must be taken that the balance of power is not too unequal, as when a "senior" trainer is always working with a trainee, because this models a theme of being one-down. It is also quite possible for coleaders to be of the same sex, but less desirable. It means part of the group will lack an identity figure in the power team. If coleaders choose to do this, then they might raise the issue in the group. A little survey by NTL interns a few years ago (1974) indicated that same-sex combinations are best in groups where the behavioral goals are clear and the group members are not new to the group process. When it is a first Basic Human Interaction experience or when it is Advanced Personal Growth or Therapy, then opposite-sex coleader teams are preferred.

Group Setting

Once I was told by a kindergarten teacher that a "good" group needed only two things, a comfortable setting and refreshments. After many years, I think she is almost right. The site must be accessible, it should be easy to maintain the temperature range, and, for my taste, there should be a padded carpet and large pillows to sit on. The reason many groups sit on the floor is that it allows one to move in many different ways, and, therefore, is less tiring than a more formal seating arrangement. However, the purpose is comfort. There is no rule. If someone is better off in a chair, he or she should be encouraged.

Group Size

The ideal number of group members is between 8 and 12. When the group is fewer than 6, then the pressure is high for everyone to participate all the time, and there is little chance for quiet withdrawn periods. When the group approaches 15 members, then it becomes a difficult task for the facilitator to be aware of all the dynamics, and anything larger than 15 is actually impossible because of the difficulty of having real input from everyone.

Therapy Frequency, Length, and Duration

Once a week for 1½ to 2 hours is the most widely employed schedule for group therapy. T-groups and encounter groups have used many different approaches, from a 1-day workshop or a nonresidential weekend to a residential week-long or 10-day laboratory. Month-long or 3-month training programs are not unknown. Along with the once-a-week schedule, a group can often be greatly enhanced by having periodic 1-day or weekend sessions. A 5-day residential experience is advantageous, because group members work, eat, and play together, and because there is no need to climb in a car after a session and immediately return to work or family responsibilities. Such a setting can allow a great deal of regression and still reach some resolution and closure before the end of the week, so that people leave with higher coping abilities and a new set of behaviors to facilitate a new image of self.

On the other hand, the once-a-week session offers both a secure climate to explore one's self and a steady support for changes through the course of many years. I would not allow anyone into a long-term therapy group unless the person were willing to commit him- or herself to 6 months or (better yet) a year. As in individual therapy, some clients may find the group setting useful for a number of years.

Media Usage

A very scary form of feedback for group members is the video camera. When one sees oneself from the external view can be quite a revelation as to what one is communicating to others. However, the playback takes a lot of time, and stopping to process the reactions to the visual replay requires additional time. For that reason, I have always been somewhat disappointed with the results of videotaping, even though it seems like such a good idea. I think the best use of tape is for the training of new leaders, for specific segments of group life which the group decides is worth the time to study, or for data about how new behaviors are being practiced.

Leader Qualifications

First of all, someone interested in leadership should be a participant in as many groups as possible; one learns by experiencing group process. I am always shocked when the Counseling Center has an intern or advanced practicum student enter the program, who is expected to be supervised in coleading a group without ever having been in one. Many schools have group courses, but the majority of those courses still pretend that group dynamics can be learned by reading certain books and hearing lectures on styles of group leadership.

For me, the main body of knowledge comes from experience. Sometimes I have group leaders that I am teaching come up with their own theories about group process based on their own field observations. The data of group experience are the same for them as it was for Bion and Lewin; they may find a better way of explaining it. At least they know, from the inside, about the issues of trust and inclusion, of confrontation and tenderness.

For the group leader, a minimum of experience would be received in 5- or 6-week-long residential workshops, with time to study the theories in between. As one works on becoming a group facilitator, one needs the time to reflect, to let the process sink in, to mull over the feedback received, to note what is puzzling, and to set new learning goals.

One organization of which I am a member requires a weekend, then a week-long, residential Human Interaction Workshop (HIW). Following that is another week-long HIW, but one in which the group members focus much more on the group process. The third week is comprised of didactic input and experiential sessions which are focused around design skills. Finally, there is a week-long workshop in "Advanced Personal Growth."

At this point, a person is ready to start the training to be a cofacilitator. Along the way, he or she, to qualify in this system as a trainer, must attend a week-long leadership workshop directed at giving supervision and feedback in facilitating interpersonal groups.

I belong to two professional organizations which have put considerable effort into analyzing what skills and attitudes a facilitator needs and into providing a professional recognition process for those who so desire. There are nearly 100 such skills. The process of recognition asks the would-be facilitator to get feedback from peers and from clients on how well he or she uses these skills and to ponder the feedback to ascertain strengths and weaknesses.

Although there are very few frauds in the field, there are some persons who purport to know more about the group process than they really do. In choosing a group to join, one should ask six questions about the qualifications and orientation of the trainer.

1. Does he or she have adequate training in a behavioral science? A trainer should have a background of knowledge in personality theory, psychopathology, group processes, and interpersonal dynamics. We would never let a person operate on us who had merely been through an operation once (as the one operated upon). Similarly, one should not attend a group led by someone who was in a group and decided it would be a good experience for others.

2. How much experience has the trainer had as a participant and as a leader? In general, the more experience in each of those categories, the less danger of mishandling the process.

3. What is the personal level of self-awareness and self-understanding of the trainer? The personal qualities of the trainer, especially his or her ability to care for and be sensitive to others will make the crucial difference between a good experience and a bad one.

4. Is he or she certified by a professional organization? The best known of these on a national level is the International Association for Applied Social Scientists and the Association for Creative Change. Both groups publish a list of those trainers who have completed the professional recognition process which each has established.

5. What is the trainer's style? In the early groups, the trainer was a participant-observer who refused leadership. In more recent times, trainers may often perform more active and directive styles to put pressure on participants to behave in certain ways. One danger of this is that these trainers may force individuals into expressive experiences, such as anger or affection, for which the individual is not prepared.

6. Does the trainer offer the possibility of follow-up? Many issues begin in

the life of the group, especially a weekend or week-long one. Any qualified trainer will be willing to discuss postgroup reactions with a member and help him or her choose any follow-up steps necessary to maximize the learnings from the experience.

Ethics

All learning activities require a code of ethics. One of the primary goals of the field of behavioral science is that such ethical expectations be explicit.

One set of ethics involves the contract between the facilitator and the individual group member. A group member has the right to expect that the facilitator is portraying himself or herself honestly, that he or she has the competencies to aid in the achievement of group goals, and that he or she will freely announce if the group is asking something of the leader for which he or she is not prepared.

A major ethical stance undergirding any therapeutic relationship is the right of the group member not to be exploited sexually (or any other way) by the therapist. Unfortunately, the human capacity for self-deception is so high that an occasional counselor or therapist can rationalize sexual behavior as being an act of love and for the client's own good. The transference issues are so complex that such a decision is simply impossible. The only ethical stance is "never." A client has a right in the counseling relationship to safely explore any behaviors without fear of ruining the working alliance.

In the group, the facilitator should have a bona fide reason to lead any experiment or structured exercise. Further, he or she ought to be able to back up any process observations with the relevant theory and concepts. In fact, the trainer must have competency in making observations and skill in giving feedback to the group about what is occurring. In leading an exercise or experiment, the facilitator should respect the group members' freedom to participate or not. I tell group members that I may push them at times to confront more about themselves, but that I will stop instantly whenever they say they want to stop. And if I don't my coleader must remind me of the necessity of proceeding at the pace that the participant is in charge of.

A qualified facilitator will be very aware of the impact of his or her behavior on the group and will often deliberately use that as part of the learning possibilities for the group. It stands to reason that the facilitator will be very open (and eager) to receive feedback from group members to help evaluate his or her performance. We all have our blind spots, and the group is the best place to discover more about them.

Finally, as mentioned before, the facilitator should be able to spot symptoms of psychological distress, help such a person pursue the best course of action, and provide follow-up possibilities for group members after the group is ended.

The professional organizations in related fields have developed ethical guidelines. In some of them, a peer review panel exists to purge the field of those who do not meet the qualifications or who deliberately misuse the power of the facilitator to their own ends. Many states are reviewing legislative guidelines which will give even more protection to the group member. However, the best ethical safeguard is in the person of the trainer. As long as his or her behavior is based upon caring, respect, and genuine regard for the group members, there will be no necessity to raise the spectre of ethical violations.

RESEARCH

During the past decade or two there have been many comprehensive reviews of the hundreds of studies about group member/leader behaviors, group communications, group problem-solving abilities, group conflict resolution, and the processes of group development. Ever since the first conference at Bethel, Maine in 1948, which engendered interest in the "laboratory method" of learning, there has been a deliberate and persistent effort to validate group process generalizations through research. Today there are quite a few journals dedicated to communicating the findings of such studies, such as the *Journal of Applied Behavioral Science,* published by NTL. A recent review of over 1,000 such studies (Dies, 1979) reports a definite leap in the study of various sorts of groups in the past few years.

In the early years of deliberate use of the small group process for educational and personal growth purposes, there was a usually pessimistic or hostile viewpoint expressed by the mass media. Many fantasies were engendered by returning participants who used metaphors such as "we were utterly stripped of all our usual masks," and were misunderstood to mean that nudity was a requirement of group pressure. These misunderstandings—in some cases deliberate distortions—were further exacerbated by the real inability of anyone to describe the impact of an experience. It is easy to describe behaviors, "we sat around and talked to each other in an honest way," but not easy to share the impact of the behavior. Many a spouse or business associate has replied, "you spent all that money just to sit around and talk." The only way to share an experience is to experience the experience.

An additional pressure on those who were using a group approach was the rumor of psychological damage being linked to the group experience. It is quite verifiable that the group process is often emotionally intensive for group members, but it is very uncertain that harm can result. There have been various studies following up participants, and the conclusions are mixed: some studies show damage (Back, 1973), others conclude there is none that can be attributed to the particular group episode that the person attended (Smith, 1975). A strong feeling was engendered that group experience led to acute pathological reactions, but little direct evidence was being given. Obviously this was a crucial question and required research by persons who were not too biased either for or against groups.

One of the major studies has been presented by Lieberman, Yalom, and

Miles (1973). They concluded that 16 out of 175 members in continuing groups of various types suffered psychological hurt; on the basis of those numbers, a pretty high 9% of those attending groups get hurt somehow. One of the problems in the study cited, however, is a rather broad definition of hurt. Five people dropped out of the groups after feeling attacked either by the group or the leader. Does that fall into the same category as the two who needed emergency psychiatric aid? And perhaps those two received needed help, as well as the eight who decided to go into therapy after the conclusion of the group. Is not such a decision positive?

William Schutz (1975) raised many good questions about the methods used to gather the data. At least these questions point to the need for further sophistication of group research techniques and the replication of the various studies done thus far.

The difficulty in doing research on a group is how to manage the multitude of variables that contribute to any one group session. Factors of group composition, the setting, the time of day, the expectations of the leaders, the expectations of the group members—all could be taken into account, including the act of filling out questionnaires or being taped. The task of differentiation is overwhelming because the list is almost endless.

In the beginning, the research about groups focused mainly on the aspects of group process which were inherent within the group. Separate approaches to research findings can be seen here. On the one hand, the quantifiable systems count numbers of times that participants do something. The approach that Robert Bales (1950) has developed to observing the interactions between members of a group has 12 major behavioral categories. Trained observers watch (many times through one-way mirrors) and record units of interaction by checking such behaviors as: gives praise, asks for information, gives orientation, disagrees, shows tension or withdrawal, behaves competitively. Bales arranged his behaviors into categories of positive reactions and negative reactions, postulating that the group with more positive interactions will proceed more effectively than one with more negative behaviors (see chapter on "Joining Together," pp. 49–51).

The influence of Kurt Lewin on research is seen in the question: "What effect does the observer have on the object he/she is studying?" The act of observation is a part of the whole group process. No one can acutally find a place on which to stand where "objective" observation is possible. Nor, ethically, should any group be under observation without this being known to the members. When it is known, the observer is affecting the groups' boundary and is, therefore, a part of the group. One way to respond to this problem is to become a participant-observer, to acknowledge that the group is making the observer a part of its life, and to conduct clinical observations from this post within the group. The "field theory" approach to group research, then, is to collect data from experiencing, along with the rest of the participants, what it is that the group does, and to test out any hypothesis from that vantage point. This applied behavioral science methodology is very much in keeping with Lewin's work, but is open to the charge of bias in terms of generalizations. As number of group studies increases, however, patterns do emerge. And, secondly, the "pure" scientists are just as open to charges of biased results from the manner in which they approach the "field" as are the clinical or naturalistic observers.

In recent years group research has focused more on outcomes than on the group process itself. A good many studies have attempted to measure personality change in the context of the group, such as increased flexibility (or decreased rigidity) stemming from the group experience. Another set of measures is around more effective performance of certain skills (such as listening or dealing with a conflict) because of the identification and deliberate practice of those skills in the life of the group. Another set of studies points to how well cooperative, heterogeneous groupings in a school situation teach content and social skills, and enhance self-image (Johnson & Johnson, 1986).

Through the years, I have been involved in many research studies. A usual methodology is to administer some measure before and after the group: such tests as the FIRO-B, the California Personality Inventory, Personal Orientation Inventory, and the Affective-Sensitivity Scale. In some studies it is a simple adjective checklist. All are attempts to catalog changes which occur to individuals within the group. Most of the results for those studies I know personally indicate that there are short-term changes, but that long-term changes are harder to perceive. However, one interviewer I know, doing a follow-up study on the use of T-groups in an industrial organization, noticed that many new skills had become integrated in employees' behavior even though they could not, at that later time, state clearly the effects of the T-group on their work situation. Perhaps there is a point where people no longer remember when new behavior began, because these have now become their normal methods of interacting.

I remember one group, led by a psychiatrist, in which blood pressure was taken before and after and a urine sample was analyzed to determine the somatic effect of group life. As stated previously, when all of the variables are considered along with all of the possible ways of looking at a group, the research problems are difficult.

A part of the group structure which has received little consideration so far is the effect of coleaders on a group. The perceived interaction between two coleaders has a lot of impact on how the group members express themselves in the group. Sometimes the group can induce the coleaders to become the split-apart scapegoats for whatever the polarization is within the group. It is certainly true for cofacilitating teams that open, disclosing styles of communication plus expressions of warmth and the ability to openly disagree are important positive factors in group development (Dies, Mallet, & Johnson, 1979).

There are two major approaches, then, in the conducting of research on the process of a group. The first approach studies the developmental changes in group process and structure; how a group is born, goes through infancy, states independence, enjoys maturity, and ends. A related category of studies would show how the group develops leadership, handles controversy, rewards the members, practices exclusion, and interacts with a wider environment.

The other approach is to study the direct effect of different sorts of leadership interventions. Why do some groups have satisfaction and some feel badly? In spite of the variable that each group is unique as a collection of persons, are there certain patterns of leadership which aid a group in its process? Is it the personality of the leader? The style? The method? Is it role authority or expertise? Which behaviors have beneficial outcomes and which drive a group crazy?

Research can focus on studying those elements of group life which are quantifiable. There is a danger here of losing out to minutiae. With a large mass of checkmarks about this or that some things become clear—like who is speaking most of the time—but it may demand an unwarranted leap of imagination to suggest group truths by adding up group particulars.

On the other hand, much of the study of groups has been conducted by clinical observation. The danger here is conceptualization from only a few members, thereby leaving it to future research to validate these pointers. The assumption such research makes is that there are universals in human behavior which can be relied upon to explain all cases. Perhaps this is true for a genius—Sigmund Freud based his theories on 22 patients. Would conclusions from such a small N sample pass a doctoral committee in one of our modern universities?

The task of future research will be to come up with a means of investigation that will allow for great flexibility in the life of the group, will not interfere with the group's boundaries, will not result in a mass of numbers which mean little, and which will give solid data on the best ways for a group to grow and to function. In the past 25 years much has been learned about the effects groups have on their individual members. We are able to predict group reactions with a fair degree of reliability. An ethical question arises as to the extent someone can deliberately manipulate group process to create specific states of mind—even leading to mass suicide. In the years to come we need to continue to learn more about the effect of the group on personal growth.

GROUP SESSION ILLUSTRATION

The group enters the room. One person, Laura, has been away for a couple of weeks. She murmurs, "Do I dare show my face?" The group members welcome her back and ask politely about the meetings. They say that they missed her.

As the group progresses, there are references to things that happened during the past 2 weeks. One member talks of being absent the next week and states it is his opinion that absent members should not be brought up to date, since they are choosing to be away. I wonder about the effect of this on Laura.

One member, Norman, deciding to move away from a fairly intellectual discussion, turns to Laura and says: "I heard you say a while ago that you were not feeling a part of the group."

LAURA: Yes, and now after what Sue said I am thinking that I should not ask the group about what happened the last 2 weeks. However, I am curious, but I don't suppose anyone wants to take the time to fill me in. When I left here 2 weeks ago, a number of things were left hanging, it seems to me. Now they do not appear to concern the group much, so I don't know what happened.

FACILITATOR (to Laura): Would you like to check out with other members how they feel about filling you in?

LAURA: Oh, yeah, I guess so.

MARYANN: I don't mind taking 5 minutes to catch you up.

LAURA: Well I wouldn't feel right being the center of attention. It is probably best for the group to go right on and I'll catch up with you.

FACILITATOR: How about trying something?

LAURA: OK.

FACILITATOR: I want you to stand here in the center and have the rest of us stand in a circle around you.

LAURA: That's exactly what I didn't want to happen. (She stands, the rest stand around her.)

FACILITATOR: What are you experiencing?

LAURA: It's not so bad. I kind of like it. Feels good to be in the center. I'm wondering, though, what everyone else is thinking. (She moves back to seat and we all sit back down. I ask the group to share what reactions they were having.)

CURTIS: I didn't want to do it. When you first suggested standing my reaction was to not go along with your suggestion. I waited to see what the group would do.

FACILITATOR: So in this particular decision you decided to go along with the group.

CURTIS: Yes.

MARYANN: I liked doing it. I felt like I was supporting Laura.

PAT: Me too!

SUE: I feel good about welcoming Laura into our circle. We have been excluding her some today—nobody filled her in on what went on last week.

RICHARD: I felt uneasy when you asked us to stand. I wondered what else you would want us to do; wondered where all this would lead. Is this what you had in mind?

FACILITATOR: You thought something would happen that was more intense.

LAURA: The main thing I learned from this is that I really wanted to be in the center, even when I said that was the last thing I wanted. I think a lot of times I want to be the center of attention, but I don't think I should ask that of anyone, so I end up feeling frustrated.

NORMAN: I'd like to give you some feedback around that. I was unclear as to what you wanted when Frank asked you to check out whether the group would fill you in on what had gone on when you weren't here, and you decided—it seemed on the basis of not deserving it—to not specifically ask the group to do this for you. It seemed to me you were trying to hold both sides of the conversation in your head. You didn't want to believe that we would do this for you.

LAURA: Yes, I guess that is what I do all right . . . not only in here.

SUMMARY

In this chapter we have traced the history of therapeutic works in groups. We focused on the group as a social unit holding great promise for support, resources, and relearning social and personal awareness skills. I attempted to describe the multiple approaches that are possible within the broad category of growth groups. I am aware that the T-group, the encounter group, and the therapy group are all different animals, but I have put them all under the one roof of interpersonal groups. This does not do justice to the nuances of difference between them, but this chapter would have had to become a book in order to cover them all. There were times when I thought it was becoming that long!

Another polarization which makes itself felt throughout this chapter is that of the focus of the group facilitator! Kurt Lewin viewed the group's energy as directing itself toward growth and learning. The trick for the group is to avoid bottling up this energy, to allow it to flow. In the view of Wilfred Bion, the group's energy is all too often directed unconsciously toward stopping the flow, not going anywhere. The challenge for the group is to work out of the present state of affairs by striving for an understanding of what we allow to stand in the way of meeting goals. Because these reasons are unconscious, they are difficult to discover. As group leaders we are called upon to be able to walk both sides of the street—at times reassuring ourselves that the group is working in a manner which will lead to discovery and growth and, at times, challenging the group on the devices it is using to stop itself from doing and knowing more.

Always groups are exciting. Each is unique and offers us clues as to how it is doing, what it is doing. We who are the leaders have the privilege of adding up the clues, and bringing the group to a heightened awareness of itself. It is an exhilarating experience at times, and that is undoubtedly the reason we all go back to commit ourselves to the people and the process once again.

REFERENCES

Back, K. *Beyond words: The story of Sensitivity Training and the Encounter Movement*. Baltimore: Penguin Books, 1973.

Bales, R. F. *Interaction Process Analysis*. Reading, Mass.: Addison Wesley, 1950.

Bennis, W., & Shepherd, H. A Theory of group development. *Human Relations*, 1956, 9, 415–457. Reprinted in G. Gibbard, J. Hartman, & R. Mann (Eds.), *Analysis of groups*. San Francisco: Jossey-Bass, 1976.

Bion, W. R. *Experiences in groups*. New York: Basic Books, 1961.

Bradford, F. P., Gibb, J. R., & Benne, K. *T-group theory and the laboratory method: Innovation in re-education*. New York: Wiley, 1964.

Burrow, T. The group method of analysis. *Psychoanalytic Review*, 1927, *14*, 268–280.

Byrd, R. Self-actualization through creative risk taking. Unpublished doctoral dissertation, New York University, 1970.

Dies, R. Group psychotherapy: Reflections on three decades of research. *Journal of Applied Behavioral Science* [NTL Institute], 1979, *15*, 361–373.

Dies, R., Mallet, J. & Johnson, F. Openness in the co-leader relationship: Its effect on group outcomes. *Journal of Small Group Behavior*, 1979, *10*, 523–546.

Egan, G. A two-phase approach to human relations training. W. E. Pfeiffer & J. Jones, (Eds.), *Annual Handbook for Group Facilitators*. La Jolla, Cal.: University Association Press, 1973, 225–232.

Freud, S. *Group psychology and the analysis of the ego.* (Complete works, Vol. 18). London: Hogarth Press, 1922.

Gibb, J. *Trust: A new view of personal and organizational development.* Los Angeles: Guild of Tutors, 1978.

Gunther, B. *Sense relaxation: Below your mind.* New York: Collier Books, 1968.

Hall, C. S., & Lindsey, G. *Theories of personality* (3d ed.). New York: John Wiley & Sons, 1978.

Hirsch, C. Trainers sexuality and participants' self-acceptance. *Graduate Student A.B.S. Newsletter* [NTL Institute for Applied Behavioral Science], Summer, 1974.

Johnson, D. W. *Contemporary social psychology.* Philadelphia: Lippincott, 1973.

Johnson, D. W. *Reaching out: Interpersonal effectiveness and self-actualization* (3rd ed.). Englewood Cliffs, N.J.: Prentice-Hall, 1986.

Johnson, D. W., & Johnson, F. P. The use of counseling groups to improve interpersonal skills. *Journal for Specialists in Group Work*, 1979, *4*, 211–215.

Johnson, D. W., & Johnson, F. P. *Joining together: Group theory and group skills* (3rd ed.). Englewood Cliffs, N.J.: Prentice-Hall, 1986.

Lieberman, M. Group methods. In F. Kanfer & A. Goldstein (Eds.), *Helping people change.* New York: Pergamon Press, 1975.

Lieberman, M., Yalom, I., & Miles, M. B. *Encounter groups: First facts.* New York: Basic Books, 1973.

Lewin, K. *Field theory in social science.* New York: Harper & Bros., 1951.

Mullen, H., & Rosenbaum, M. *Group psychotherapy* (2nd ed.). New York: Free Press, 1978.

Moreno, J. L. *The first book on group psychotherapy.* New York: Beacon House, 1957.

Pratt, J. H. The "Home Sanitorium" treatment of consumption. *Boston Medical and Surgical Journal*, January–June 1906, *154*, 210–216.

Rogers, C. *Carl Rogers on encounter groups.* New York: Harper & Row, 1971.

Schutz, W. C. *The interpersonal underworld.* Palo Alto, Cal.: Science & Behavior Books, 1960.

Schutz, W. C. *Joy: Expanding human awareness.* New York: Grove Press, 1967.

Schutz, W. C. Not encounter and certainly not facts. *Journal of Humanistic Psychology*, 1975, *15*, 7–18.

Smith, P. B. Are there adverse effects of sensitivity training? *Journal of Humanistic Psychology*, 1975, *15*, 29–47.

GLOSSARY

Encounter Group. The group is encouraged to know itself through a high level of openness and direct personal contact between members. The group sometimes relies upon the facilitator to give stimulation through the use of fantasy trips, body awareness exercises, or nonverbal structured experiences. The focus can be on the interpersonal or the intrapersonal realm. Participants are encouraged to identify parts of themselves in how they perceive others.

Group. A collection of persons in face-to-face interaction aware of belonging in the group, the purpose of the group, and gaining satisfaction from participating in the group.

Interpersonal. The communication and relationship which takes place between people. The study of normal human interaction.

Intrapersonal. The focus on the inner motivations and awarenesses of a single person.

Laboratory Learning (Experiential Learning). Learning from experiences by reflecting upon an event, analyzing why it happened as it did, what various reactions were present toward the same stimulus and checking out the observations of others in the group. The final step is to generate some alternative approaches for the next similar situation. It is sometimes called the "discovery" method of learning.

Process. How the group does what it does. A much different focus than the content of what group members are saying or the task to which they are assigned. The manner in which the group members interact with one another.

T-Group. Training group. Refers to a group process involving a leadership vacuum and an atmosphere of stopping to reflect upon the group and leadership dynamics as they occur in the present and observable life of the group. Focus is on the interpersonal events.

Therapy Group. The focus here much more on the intrapersonal. Member interactions are studied to reveal the unconscious processes at work, to identify the transference, and to take back the projections. The therapist may take a very active role in directing the group to face its own process.

4

Rational–Emotive Therapy and Related Cognitively Oriented Psychotherapies

RICHARD L. WESSLER and SHEENAH HANKIN

INTRODUCTION

Rational–Emotive Therapy (RET) was originated by Albert Ellis (1962), a clinical psychologist and psychotherapist who published extensively on RET and its application to human problems. This chapter presents not only Ellis's ideas about RET conducted in groups, but also extensions and elaborations of Ellis's ideas, as well as related conceptions and practices found in other cognitively oriented psychotherapies.

DEFINITION

Ellis has used the term Rational–Emotive Therapy in two ways: first, to refer to the set of concepts and procedures he typically uses with his own clients; second, as a synonym for the broader field of cognitive-behavior therapy (CBT). He has called the more restrictive use of the term RET "elegant" or "preferential" RET, and the broader use of the term "general" or "unpreferential" RET (Ellis, 1980). Other writers have made a similar distinction between narrow or classical RET and comprehensive RET (Walen, DiGiuseppe, & Wessler, 1980; Wessler & Wessler, 1980). Unfortunately, Ellis has not always clarified which of the two meanings of RET he intends in his writings.

In this chapter, RET will refer to the more restrictive meaning. The broader field of cognitive-behavior therapy will be called CBT, and the authors' own work will be identified as Cognitive Appraisal Therapy (CAT) (Wessler &

Richard L. Wessler • Psychology Department, Pace University, Pleasantville, New York 10570.   **Sheenah Hankin** • Cognitive Psychotherapy Associates, 68 East 91st Street, New York, New York 10128.

Hankin, 1986). The "cognitively oriented psychotherapies" referred to in the title of this chapter include the various psychological approaches to explanation and treatment that share the theoretical assumption that "learned misconceptions (or faulty beliefs, or mistaken ideas) are the crucial variables which must be modified or eliminated before psychotherapy can be successful" (Raimy, 1975, p. 186). In addition to RET and CAT, most of CBT falls under this label (including the work of Beck, Mahoney, Maultsby, Kelly, and Bandura); excluded are those approaches that employ cognitions to control behavior without assigning importance to cognitions in the creation of emotions and behaviors (Wessler, 1982).

Cognitively oriented group psychotherapy is conducted with groups of people rather than with individuals. The aim is to help people modify their goal-defeating emotions and actions by identifying their self-disturbing beliefs and assumptions, and by showing people how to modify such ideas and actions or to induce such changes. The focus is on the individual; the therapy group serves to help its individual members discover and modify self-disturbing cognitions. Among the prominent disturbing cognitions Ellis has identified are those of making unrealistic demands on oneself, other people, and the world, and especially that of demanding perfection of oneself.

The cognitively oriented psychotherapies are partly based on an educational model rather than a medical, emotional release, relationship, or conditioning model. In addition, at least RET and CAT are partly based on an attitude-change model (Wessler & Ellis, 1980). People who are neurotically disturbed may not readily relinquish their self-disturbing cognitions even when they know what they are. Therefore, the therapist and group members often direct persuasive messages to the focal client in an effort to get him to adopt more realistic perspectives on self, other people, and the world in general. The group is frequently able to muster influential opinion better than the therapist could do in an individual session, and to encourage people to attempt new actions which often precede cognitive change.

HISTORY

Albert Ellis originated RET at the beginning of 1955, after experimenting with several forms of psychotherapy. He trained in and practiced psychoanalysis for several years before becoming disillusioned with its results. To create RET, Ellis called on philosophy, which had become his hobby during adolescence, and his own personal experiences of social anxiety. He began to directly confront patients with their self-defeating philosophies, actively argue against their ideas, and assign homework activities for them to perform.

Ellis has made only minor changes in RET since the publication of his classic *Reason and Emotion in Psychotherapy* (Ellis, 1962). From its inception, when it was known simply as Rational Therapy, RET has given a central place to perceptions, semantic meanings, appraisals, and philosophies of living as mediators of action and experiences. Relying heavily on such philosophers as Bertrand Russell and Robert Thouless and on the ethics of humanism, but relatively little on psychological thought prior to RET, Ellis created a theory of disturbance with a pronounced philosophical emphasis and humanistic-existential outlook. Some authorities (e.g., Davison & Neale, 1982) describe RET as a system of ethics, and it is certainly true that Ellis rejects culturally prescribed, especially religious, values stated as absolute imperatives, and sees them as a major source of neurotic disturbance. In its place, he advocates a position in which each person decides for himself, through the use of reason, what values will most likely maximize his own individual survival and happiness.

Ellis has had considerable influence on psychotherapy and counseling in America. One survey showed him to be one of the two most influential psychotherapists today (the other being Carl Rogers), although less than 2% of the respondents cited RET as their theoretical orientation (D. Smith, 1982). This same survey found that CBT was the predominant representation among the top 10 most influential therapies, and that CBT is one of the major trends in counseling and psychotherapy. Ellis's influence is even more remarkable considering the fact that he worked alone, except for an occasional collaborator on an article or book, was not a regular faculty member of a university graduate school, and has conducted virtually no research in support of RET.

His influence derived from his numerous books and articles about RET, as well as frequent lectures and other public appearances. His Institute for Rational–Emotive Therapy in New York City has offered extensive training programs since the early 1970s. Ironically, these training programs never presented pure RET as Ellis conducts it. Due to the efforts of the Institute's directors of training, and with Ellis's tacit approval, the broader version of RET (i.e., CBT) was taught to participants.

Training in RET was aided by the appearance of several books that describe its methodology. Bard (1980) and Hauck (1980) have produced books that stick closely to Ellis's version of RET, as does the bulk of the book by Walen, DiGiuseppe, and Wessler (1980). Ellis and Abrams (1978) is more an account of what Ellis claims is done in RET as opposed to what he actually does in therapy sessions. His actual work is better represented in verbatim transcripts (see Ellis, 1971). Wessler and Wessler (1980) and Dryden (1984) advocate and illustrate creative uses of RET that depart in significant ways from Ellis's approach. Grieger and Boyd (1980) include a great deal of Maultby's Rational Behavior Training along with RET.

Maultsby's (1975) Rational Behavior Training and Tosi's (1978; Tosi & Baisden, 1984) Rational Stage Directed Therapy are direct outgrowths of RET. The authors' Cognitive Appraisal Therapy (CAT) is an attempt to preserve the best features of RET while substituting principles based on social learning theory and cognitive social psychology for those of humanistic philosophy. CAT seeks a union of RET-inspired principles and tactics with recent developments in CBT (Wessler, 1984a,b; Wessler & Hankin, 1986).

The cognitively oriented therapies developed independently of RET, and for the most part have their historic tradition in behavior therapy. Unlike radical behaviorism, the cognitively oriented psychotherapies are based on the general assertion that humans respond primarily to cognitive representations of their environments rather than to their environments *per se,* and that thoughts, feelings, and actions are interrelated (Mahoney, 1977). The most prominent examples of CBT are Beck's (1976) cognitive therapy, Bandura's (1977) social learning theory, Lazarus's (1981) multimodal therapy, Mahoney's (1974) cognitive learning therapy and Meichenbaum's (1977) cognitive behavior modification. All of these can point to Ellis's RET among their proximate intellectual predecessors.

Goals

The goals of RET and related cognitively oriented psychotherapies do not differ from psychotherapy and counseling in general. These include enabling the individual to experience less subjective distress and to engage in fewer maladaptive actions. For convenience we say that the goals of RET and CBT are to reduce neurotic disturbance and to solve problems of living, or at least to reconcile oneself to problems, for example, illness, that have no immediate solutions. Neurotic disturbance is a deliberately loose term that ranges from clearly diagnosable patterns of behavior to nonclinical but nonetheless psychological dissatisfactions.

It might appear that the cognitively oriented therapies take cognitive changes as goals. In a sense this is so, for they posit that no sustained affective or behavioral change will occur without alterations of maladaptive belief systems, faculty cognitions, negative thinking, or misconceptions. Raimy (1975) claims that cognitive change is the goal of therapy, and that affective and behavioral changes will follow. However, other advocates of cognitively oriented approaches do not agree, and view cognitive change as a subgoal or a means to the end of affective and behavioral change.

The cognitively oriented therapies also take a degree of self-help as a goal for therapy. Clients are not only helped to modify dysphoric moods and maladaptive behaviors, but to concommitantly learn how to help themselves continue to do so after the termination of therapy. In particular, RET holds that humans can learn to solve their problems more effectively and to rethink self-defeating assumptions about themselves, other people, and the social, economic, and physical environment.

Ellis often identifies the goal of RET as elegant philosophical restructuring or the elegant solution to human problems. Inelegant solutions include modification of specific cognitions and appraisals, that is, something short of pervasive philosophic change. Ellis calls the adopting of a new philosophy of life the elegant solution when the new philosophy consists of (a) nondemanding desires; (b) self-acceptance without conditions; (c) nondamning attitudes toward other persons; (d) stoic acceptance of reality that cannot be changed by the individual; (e) tolerance without complaint of frustrations, deprivations,

and discomforts; (f) willingness to work at improving one's life c
increase personal enjoyment.

THEORY

Basic Concepts

The central assumption of RET and other cognitively oriented psychotherapies is that "cognitions control emotions and feelings; disruptive affect is
the result of faulty perceptions, beliefs, and convictions. . . . The alternative
point of view, that emotion or affect is somehow an independent entity which
can be modified or eliminated only by expressing it, is an outmoded doctrine"
(Raimy, 1975, pp. 195–196). Cognitions include thoughts, meanings, images,
and beliefs. They serve as mediators between stimulus events and psychological and behavioral responses; they are organismic variables in Woodworth's S-
O-R paradigm. A quotation from the philosopher Epictetus summarizes this
view: "It is not things themselves that worry us, but the opinions that we have
about those things." The American sociologist W. I. Thomas echoed this
thought with his famous dictum: "If people define things as real, they are real
in their consequences."

The main task of RET and the cognitively oriented psychotherapies is to
identify clients' cognitions, beliefs, meanings, images, and perspectives, to
help them understand their role in personal distress, and to help them modify
their dysfunctional cognitions. The cognitions have been learned, and individual are either aware of them or can easily become aware of them, either
though personal experience or direct feedback from therapist and/or group
about their verbal and nonverbal behavior. RET, Beck's cognitive therapy, and
CAT give great importance to certain types of cognitions—appraisals or evaluative cognitions. Appraisals are crucial to several contemporary theories of
emotion (Arnold, 1960; Beck, 1976; Izard, 1972; Lazarus & Folkman, 1984;
Plutchick, 1980).

Ellis calls his theory of emotions and of disturbance the *ABC* theory. *A*
stands for activating event or experience, that is, one's observations of what
has happened, or thoughts and images of what might happen; *B* stands for
belief system; *C* stands for emotional and behavioral consequences. Emotion is
conceived of as part of an ongoing process of perceiving, thinking, evaluating
or appraising, and behaving.

There are two major categories within the belief system. Rational beliefs are
accurate cognitions and evaluations that express a preference, desire, wish,
want, or liking for something. They may lead to either positive or negative
experiences, depending on whether one's preferences are met or not. They are
defined as nondebilitating, even when negative, and as contributing to the
individual's survival and happiness; for example, a negative emotion might
motivate persons to take actions which are productive of their personal goals.

There is little therapeutic emphasis in RET on modifying rational beliefs, although clients might be advised to change their goals if they seem unattainable.

Irrational beliefs are by definition those that do not promote the individual's survival and happiness. This definition shows RET's roots in psychoanalytically influenced thought; here are Fromm's (1977) definitions: "I propose to call rational any thought, feeling, or act that promotes the adequate functioning and growth of the whole of which it is a part, and irrational that which tends to weaken or destroy the whole" (p. 352). In one sense, they are escalations of rational beliefs; the person can escalate preferences, desires, wishes, wants, and likings, to absolute requirements, demands, needs, and imperatives. They are good ideas perverted by exaggeration. Irrational beliefs are, according to Ellis, absolute shoulds, oughts, musts, demands, and commands instead of realistic preferences and wishes. All other irrational beliefs are derived from absolute must-statements. While he sometimes distinguishes between absolute musts and preferential musts, Ellis blurs this distinction in his writings and therapy sessions. He has coined a word, *musturbation*, which means thinking irrationally; and he tells clients to "look for the must" when they experience disturbance, because RET theory states that disturbance is determined by one's must-statements. Thus, clients who say "I *must* not feel a high degree of anxiety!" make themselves quite anxious about their anxiety and create a secondary symptom (anxiety about anxiety), just as they are presumed to have created their primary or initial anxiety by a must-statement, "I must be perfect!", or some other absolute must-statement.

This simple *ABC* model is usually presented to RET clients in both individual and group therapy. Although it can be taken merely as a mnemonic device to help clients learn the therapist's orientation, Ellis has stated that the *ABC* model forms a theory of personality as well (Ellis, 1974, 1977, 1978). There is ample evidence that perceptions, evaluations, and other cognitions largely determine human emotional experience (Beck, Rush, Shaw, & Emery, 1979). What is not so clearly supported by empirical evidence is the fundamental assumption that distinguishes RET from other cognitively oriented psychotherapies, the axiom that irrational beliefs determine inappropriate emotional and behavioral consequences. (Consequences are deemed to be inappropriate if they block the pursuit or attainment of one's goals, and thereby become dysfunctional for the individual. Such emotions as anxiety, hostility, depression, shame, and guilt are considered dysfunctional in RET, as are behavioral patterns that defend against them.)

ABC theory is very sketchy and does not account for other factors in the determination and maintenance of emotions, for example, reinforcers from the social environment and decisions about one's actions. The term "emotional episode" (also termed the cognitive-emotive-behavioral episode) has been introduced to present a more detailed account of the process, and to show cognitive, emotional, and behavioral interconnections (Wessler & Wessler, 1980). Even this more complex model recognizes that any arbitrary division of human processes is artificial, and that no model can fully represent human complexity.

We have adapted the new model to CAT by making two significant departures from Ellis's RET. First, we do not assume that exaggerated evaluations derive from must-statements; must-statements may show the strength or extreme degree of appraisal, but are not necessarily their source. Second, we drop the dichotomy of rational–irrational in favor of one single continuum of appraisal, closer in spirit to contemporary theories of emotion (Lazarus, 1982) than is RET.

The new model consists of nine steps which begin with a stimulus and conclude with reinforcing consequences. The mediating steps include stimulus detection, four types of inferred cognitive processes, and emotional and behavioral responses. This model is theoretical, but should be taken as a guide for clinicians rather than a systematic set of propositions ready for empirical testing. The model resembles Plutchik's (1980) theory of emotions, although it was developed independently, with emotional and behavioral responses assumed to be multidetermined through several covert or cognitive processes.

The model is derived from the basic clinical theories of Ellis (1962) and Beck (1976) with additions from social learning theory and attribution theory. In addition to the work of Beck and Ellis, the model adds an interpersonal dimension in its account of reinforcers, and incorporates Woods's (1974) taxonomy of instrumental conditioning.

The model consists of the following steps arranged in more or less sequential order:

Step 1: Stimulus. A cognitive-emotive-behavioral episode starts with a stimulus in the external or internal environment. An overt stimulus might be other people's actions, an object, or the loss of something tangible. Examples of covert stimuli are bodily sensations, for example, nausea or autonomic arousal, or any of the cognitive steps in the model.

Step 2: Detection. Stimuli, in order to have an impact, must be detected and discriminated from other available stimuli. The failure to detect stimuli may be conceived as defensive (as in psychodynamic theories) but may simply due to the lack of conceptual categories to pick up information (Neisser, 1976).

Step 3: Description or Symbolic Representation of Stimulus. This step is cognitive and can be divided into definition (observation) and description (or symbolic representations) of observations. Observations are temporally contiguous with stimuli, but descriptions need not be; they can occur after the fact or be about *images* that have no overt stimulus. Therapists do not deal with clients' observations, but with their reports of observations, which are taken as reports of clients' phenomenological awareness. Inaccurate descriptions may be labeled "distortions of reality."

Step 4: Inference and Interpretations. This step includes such logical and illogical operations as reasoning, developing forecasts and expectations, making causal and motivational attributions, and other nonevaluative meanings ascribed to one's observations. For example, the loss of a job might be taken to mean that one will never get another. Beck (1976) has extensively discussed how such false and arbitrary conclusions may be involved in emotional disturbance.

Step 5: Appraisals of Observations and Interpretations. Several accounts of emotion emphasize that cognitive appraisals of stimuli are essential to emotional experiences (Arnold, 1960; Lazarus, 1982; Plutchick, 1980). If an appraisal is neutral, ambiguous, or indecisive, no affective response occurs. The sight of blood may be appraised as very bad if flowing from your open wound, but appraised as very good if received as a transfusion following surgery. Appraisals may be implicit rather than explicit, but signaled by the connotative meanings of words one chooses to use, for example, labeling one's spending habits as either thrifty (positive appraisal) or stingy (negative appraisal). Much of Ellis's work has been to attempt to get clients to reappraise themselves, other people, and the events in their lives.

Step 6: Emotional Response. The arousal of the autonomic nervous system is hypothesized to follow nonneutral appraisals of stimuli. This step is partly cognitive in that changes in the central nervous system result in changes in the endocrine system and in proprioceptive bodily changes which may be labeled with emotional words.

Step 7: Behavioral Response. There is a general tendency for action to accompany arousal, for example, to approach that which is positively appraised, and to avoid, escape, modify, or freeze in the presence of stimuli appraised as highly negative. This is what Beck calls the "flight, fight, or flop response." Defensive behaviors may be seen as the seeking of conditions which bring relative comfort, especially immediate relief of discomfort, even though they may be only slightly more pleasant than alternatives. The acting on hostile thoughts and feelings, the avoidance of anxiety-arousing situations, the helplessness of depressive cognitions and feelings are captured at this step.

Step 8: Functional Consequences of Behavior. Reinforcing consequences of actions, including self-satisfactions, are postulated to affect subsequent emotional experiences and behaviors. Of special importance are social reinforcers—other people's reactions to behavioral responses—when they provide the satisfaction of having one's expectations about self, others, and social situations confirmed. Some, perhaps most, neurotic behaviors may be viewed as distorted transactions between two or more persons; indeed, this is the foundation for the family systems approach to therapy. The security of obtaining a predicted response to one's actions may outweigh negative aspects of the interpersonal reaction. Neurotic or defensive behaviors may result from the reduction of anxiety due to its reinforcing value. Experiences of mastery and personal efficacy may occur when positive results are obtained.

It is an oversimplification to speak only of punishments and rewards, as Woods (1974) shows in developing a complex classification of instrumental behavior. There are, according to Woods, eight basic possibilities formed by combining the consequent events (desirable or undesirable), the operation performed on the consequent event (present or increase versus remove or decrease), and whether the consequent event is contingent on response emission or omission. Thus, the failure to obtain a reward is not the same as a penalty or punishment; a penalty involves giving up what one already has, and a punishment involves the presentation of an aversive event. Woods

(1985) has recently expanded his taxonomy to include prior cognitive expectations regarding the consequence of behavior.

Special Additional Step: Decisions. Behavior, in this model, is conceived as controlled by decisions and self-directions. No corrective experiences or therapeutic progress is possible unless one refuses to act in ways that bring immediate relief and instead pursues a course of action that brings a delayed gratifying outcome. Decisions, then, are special instances of action based on instrumental expectancies or anticipations of Step 8 (Bandura, 1977; Woods, 1985). Of special therapeutic importance are decisions to think and act that are inconsistent with one's emotional response, for example, acting in spite of anxiety in order to demonstrate self-efficacy.

To further understand this model, consider the following analysis of public speaking anxiety. The crucial variables from the perspective of Cognitive Appraisal Therapy are not the speech (Step 1) or the person's knowledge that the speech will be given at a scheduled time (Steps 2 and 3). The person probably anticipates poor performance or poor audience reaction (Step 4) and appraises this anticipated outcome as highly negative (Step 5). The subsequent anxiety (Step 6) may be reduced by choosing (Special Step) to procrastinate (Step 7), which brings immediate relief (Step 8) but is a neurotic choice if the person's goal is to make the speech. The CAT focus is upon Steps 4 and 5: help the person make new forecasts about performance and audience reaction or both, and to reappraise the outcome, for example, modifying the appraisal "highly negative" and regarding it as slightly or moderately negative.

This model contains several different types of cognitions. The evaluative-nonevaluative distinction has already been discussed; it is the difference between what one "knows" about something and how one "feels" or appraises it (Moore, 1983). A second distinction is that between accurate and inaccurate cognitions; an interpretation or inference might be accurate, but one cannot know without obtaining additional information. What one "knows" can be subject to verification, but one's appraisals, strictly speaking, cannot, for they are based on one's personal values. Personal values can be subjected to a test of utility (i.e., whether one's values are personally helpful), but not to a test of accuracy.

A third distinction is between general and specific cognitions. Abstractions about events and behavioral data are general; specific thoughts about particular situations are derived from these general assumptions about self, people in general, the world, and similar abstract concepts. A generalization, for example, "people cannot be trusted" can lead to a specific thought "Joe cannot be trusted." Likewise, evaluative cognitions can be generalized and used as premises for reaching specific evaluative conclusions (this point will be discussed later in this section). Further, generalized appraisals can influence specific nonevaluative cognitions; for example, a woman who spoke of her hatred for men falsely inferred that a man's faulty directions were the cause of her friend's arriving late for an appointment, when in fact, the friend had simply chosen to delay her departure.

A fourth distinction is between conscious and unconscious cognitions.

The use of the term unconscious should not be understood as endorsing a Freudian model with its emphasis on hidden motives and ego-protecting mechanisms. Generalized cognitions may be unconscious in the sense that they lie outside one's awareness and are taken for granted. Specific evaluative conclusions may be based on unconsciously held evaluative premises that have not been labeled or verbalized (Guidano & Liotti, 1983).

The final category of cognitions is decisions about one's behavior, without which this model would seem very mechanistic and radically behavioral. Instead, the addition of decisions retains the existential orientation of RET. Further, the cognitively oriented psychotherapies emphasize the thinking about one's actions (as opposed to mindlessly repeating dysfunctional ones) and making self-instructional statements to carry them out (Meichenbaum, 1977).

The model of the emotional episode is too complicated to present to clients. The authors have developed a simpler approach for use with clients. Its central concept is that of "personal rules of living." The notion of rules comes from the work of Beck: "The person uses a kind of mental rule book to guide his actions and evaluate himself and others. He applies the rules in judging whether his own behavior or that of others is 'right' or 'wrong'. . . . We use rules not only as a guide for conduct but also to provide a framework for understanding life situations" (Beck, 1976, p. 42). Rules are prescriptions of morally desirable behavior (or values), stated as what one should do, and appear to be involved in the socalled moral emotions—hostility, guilt, shame, jealousy, social anxiety, and some depressions (Sommers, 1981). Such prescriptions are seldom unqualified musts as Ellis claims; they are conditional rather than categorical statements: If I want to act morally, I must do certain acts. (A close reading of Ellis [e.g., Ellis, 1962, p. 63] reveals that his examples of unqualified musts are actually conditional, qualified statements, "I must achieve *in order* to consider myself a worthwhile person.")

Personal rules of living and the appraisals they generate can be illustrated in minimodels of three typical neurotic processes: hostility, anxiety, and depression.

In hostility, there is an inference that a personal rule has been, could be, or will be broken (Beck, 1976). If the person holds a tolerant personal rule of living, for example, "I will not damn people even though they break my rules and I don't like that," the person will react with a degree of anger that falls well short of rage. Empirical support is suggested by the work of Berkowitz (1969). When the individual holds personal rules that express extreme, exaggerated negative appraisals of persons who break one's personal rules, enraged hostility is hypothesized to result. We explain this to clients in the following manner:

> Enraged anger begins when we create rules for other people to live by, observe that they are breaking or have transgressed against our rules, and then invoke another rule that says they should be condemned for what they have done. Your anger at your friend (spouse, child, etc.) is based on your rules about how other people should act and your punitive attitude toward them for not acting that way. Now, let's examine the angry thoughts about them in your mind.

In this manner we discover what people deem their important rules to be, what their (perhaps, nonconscious) evaluative premises or values are, and whether they accurately observe other people's actions as either rule-breaking or rule-conforming.

The minimodel of anxiety also involves observations, inferences about them, and appraisals. Following Beck (1976; Beck & Emery, 1985), anxiety is seen as the result of cognitive processes, not as an outcome of simple conditionings or autonomic responses to stimuli, nor due to the threat of unacceptable impulses breaking into consciousness. Our explanation to clients sounds something like this: "Anxiety occurs when you define something as threatening or potentially dangerous to your physical or psychological well-being, or to someone or something you identify with. Now, what dangerous or threatening event are you anticipating, and what makes it seem so dangerous or threatening to you?"

Ellis has usefully distinguished between two forms of anxiety: ego and discomfort. In ego anxiety, the threat is to one's self-esteem or self-acceptance. Anticipation of events that will result in one's making exaggerated negative self-appraisals result in this form of anxiety. Discomfort anxiety is simply the fear of discomfort, including inconvenience, strong emotional experiences, boredom, and so forth. The personal rule of living states something like: "Discomfort is so bad that I will do whatever I can to avoid it." Any given example of anxiety may contain both ego and discomfort components, and it is often the latter that impedes therapeutic progress.

The minimodel of depression begins with observations or images about actual, hypothetical, or anticipated loss (Beck, 1976), which are then appraised as extremely negative. The loss may be anything from one's personal domain or anything one identifies with, for example, people, causes, material possessions, or self-esteem. Themes of hopelessness emerge when the individual thinks of the loss as permanent or irreplaceable. Themes of helplessness follow from thoughts about personal inadequacy or lack of ability to remedy the loss. If the person focuses on personal inadequacy or self-condemnation for incurring the loss, ego depression (similar to ego anxiety) results. If the person dwells on the deprivation and enages in self-pity, a sort of discomfort depression occurs.

By using these minimodels, one can infer reasonable guesses about the client's cognitions when the client cannot readily identify them. By thinking of evaluative premises as personal rules of living, potential problems can be uncovered. For example, if people define money as a condition of self-worth and have never considered that they might not have money at some future time, they may not recognize that they have a potential anxiety/depression problem. By understanding the personal rules of living, the therapist can work prophylactically with the client as well as on current problems.

Assumptions about Human Nature

Ellis's assumptions about human nature are rooted in the humanistic philosophy he has advocated for most of his life. Humanism as an ethical system should not be confused with humanistic psychology. Ethical humanism rejects

God-given moral codes, holding humans responsible for their actions and capable of reasoning about the relative rightness and wrongness of their actions. Ellis advocates ethical codes based on enlightened self-interest. Self-interest is enlightened when one takes into account (a) long-term as well as short-term pleasures, and (b) that harming other people is disadvantageous in the long term because they will most likely boycott or retaliate against an offender.

Humans are not born good or evil, nor do they become good or evil persons, for these are global labels. People are not good or evil; they are simply people, who at times do good and at times evil.

Humans are biological organisms and have human biological potentials. Ellis (1976) states that the capacity for rational *and* irrational thinking are two human potentials. He has argued that humans are not simply taught irrational beliefs about their own perfection; they would learn them anyway because they are predisposed to do so. The tendency to self-denigrate is assumed to be innate and the practice quite easily learned, rather than acquired as a result of passive conditioning or failure to receive positive regard from others. Self-control through self-judgments about the breaking of group rules certainly would make the group's task of rule enforcement easier, and so there may be evolutionary significance to self-denigration tendencies that facilitate social control (Wessler, 1977). Humans are also conceived of as having the potential to overcome their tendencies to think irrationally, to work against their natural tendencies to demand, self-judge, damn others, complain about what displeases them, and prefer inactivity to activity.

In short, humans are assumed to be blank slates on which certain messages can be rather easily written. They acquire the content of their values from their culture, but easily distort values into unrealistic, magical, absolutist demands and the irrational conclusions that follow. They resist thinking for themselves and easily follow the dictates of culture or religion or political forces. While they are capable of reasoning about ethical decisions that promote their values, they readily rely upon social institutions or other people to do this for them.

In addition to assumptions about human nature, Ellis makes certain assumptions about the nature of nature. Because no Judeo-Christian God is postulated, there can be no certainty without a creator, and only probabilistic statements can be made about the future. People, when they demand perfection and predictability, are irrationally asking for that which nature cannot provide.

Personality Theory

Although Ellis claims that the *ABC* model is a theory of personality, it is difficult to discern how it qualifies. Even a sympathetic critic notes that the "theory can be criticized not so much in terms of what may be wrong with it but rather for its apparent narrowness. As yet it may not be considered a fullblown theory of human nature. . . . The A-B-C theory does not cover the total person's growth and development" (Corsini, 1977, p. 419). The theory lacks a propositional structure, does not lend itself to the deducing of testable hypotheses, and has generated no empirical research either by Ellis or by others.

In a specially prepared paper on an RET theory of personality, Ellis (1978) does little more than repeat his faith in cognitive mediators of behavior, and his probiological and antienvironmental position: (as much as) "80 percent of the variance of human behavior rests on biological bases" (Ellis, 1978, p. 304), he claims, but offers no empirical support for this assertion. The main thrust of his position paper consists of repeating his reason why other personality theorists go wrong—they are irrational thinkers: "Given a beard and a doctoral degree, one can make any assertion without any proof" (Ellis, 1978, p. 310).

The other forms of the cognitively oriented psychotherapies are not based on either grand or explicit personality theory (with perhaps one or two exceptions). Beck has written extensively about depression, but has yet to produce a theory of personality. Some forms of treatment are consistent with a very limited theory of disturbance (Lazarus, 1981), and assume no personality theory at all. Others have stressed a need for theorizing about disturbance (but not necessarily about personality as a whole) and for techniques derived from theory (Meichenbaum, 1977), but have not offered completely worked out theories. Because the various forms of CBT evolved from behavior therapy, it should not be surprising that they have not sought or offered grand theories of personality; noncognitive behavior therapy has done quite well without them, too. Perhaps the lesson here is that grand theory of personality is not a necessary condition for the development of an approach or system of treatment, and certainly not for the development of specific procedures; a limited theory of disturbance will suffice.

Exceptions to these observations about personality theory might be Bandura's (1977) and Rotter's (1954) social learning theories. Both give central importance to cognitive variables and present research data to support their contentions. Bandura specifies strategies of treatment in extending the behavior modification paradigm, and asserts that cognitive changes are most likely to occur when a person performs new behaviors and observes his or her own efficacy.

In developing our own RET-inspired conceptions of treatment (CAT), we have drawn on Bandura's and Rotter's theory and research, plus attitude theory, attribution theory, and other cognitive social psychology theories. Contemporary theories of emotions, as mentioned earlier in this chapter, stress cognitive appraisals, and provide the emphasis for Cognitive Appraisal Therapy (CAT). In general, but not in exact detail, CAT resembles Plutchik's (1980) theory of emotion. The main features of this theory are (a) stimulus event, (b) cognitive processing, (c) feeling, (d) behavior that (e) results in satisfaction of a motive, or adaptation that promotes survival of the organism. Though developed independently of Plutchik's work, the model of the emotional episode presented in this chapter corresponds to it closely. This model serves to articulate the various theoretical inputs to CAT; for example, when we speak of cold cognitions (Steps 3 and 4), which are descriptive and inferential statements, and distinguish them from hot cognitions (Step 5) or appraisals, we do so because both cold and hot cognitions are implicated in theories of emotion and in the cognitively oriented approaches to treatment (Wessler, 1982). As Plutchik (1980, p. 73) says, "Each emotion is triggered by some stimulus in the environment that must be evaluated cognitively by the animal affected by that stimulus."

Neither RET or CBT or CAT is based on full-blown personality theory. Instead, they rely on theory and research in several different fields of psychology, fields that are joined by the common cord of cognition. Both RET and CAT hold that personality is holistic. Thinking, emoting, and acting are in most responses inseparable, although separations can be made for analysis and discussion. Persons have core or central beliefs around which other beliefs are organized. Of special importance are one's beliefs about self, other people, and the world.

Comparison with Related Theories

Although Ellis has made many statements about personality, and claims that the *ABC* model is a theory of personality, the authors regard it as a theory of disturbance. Therefore, comparisons made in this section are to other theories of disturbance. We shall specifically compare several accounts of anxiety with the RET version.

RET is most closely allied to the cognitively oriented approaches to treatment of which it is a member. One of the earliest cognitive accounts of disturbance is that of George Kelly (1955), although he himself resisted attempts to categorize his theory. In both RET and Personal Constructs Theory, a few central cognitions account for behavior and experiences. These cognitions result from the individual's trying to make sense of experience, to organize observations. This is the human-as-scientist theme, a notion to be found in several other largely cognitive accounts of disturbance (and personality), enamored as they are of information processing and of that ultimate information processor, the electronic computer.

For Kelly, the experience of anxiety results from one's becoming aware that one is making wrong predictions about events and has no alternatives within his set of constructs to take their place. For Ellis, anxiety results from anticipated self-downing (ego anxiety) or "awfulizing" about discomfort (discomfort anxiety). What Kelly termed "threat" is probably closer to Ellis's notion of ego anxiety; threat is an awareness of an imminent pervasive change in the core structures which govern one's sense of personal identity and integrity. Both Kelly and Ellis take an ahistoric view of the person and disturbance.

Predictions about events, or expectancies, are important concepts in the theories of Bandura and Rotter. One learns expectations, either through direct experience or vicariously, for example, injury or failure, and thus anxiety arises. Through the performing of new behaviors one learns to defend or cope more adequately, and thus learns new expectations about one's own performance (the new learning may occur through other mechanisms as well, but new behaviors is the most likely mechanism). This necessarily sketchy account of anxiety differs from RET in some minor respects, but shares an emphasis on cognitions and anticipations. Ellis would also insist that cognitive change can occur through self-indoctrination, but like Bandura, he would endorse action as a powerful method as well.

Dolliver (1979), Wessler and Wessler (1980), and Nelson-Jones (1982) discuss RET in relation to psychoanalysis, person-centered counseling, transactional analysis, and Gestalt therapy. The main points will be summarized in the following paragraphs.

RET is theoretically close to Adler's position, but departs from it in treatment techniques. Both cite beliefs about worthlessness, inadequacy, and inferiority as sources of anxiety. RET does not use the Alderian concept of "social interest," although Ellis claims that it is inherent in the RET notion of self-interest. We disagree, and find social interest in the Adlerian sense to be missing in Ellis's RET; RET advocates putting one's own interests first, and having concern for others in order to avoid their thwarting one's pursuit of personal happiness.

Karen Horney's theory of disturbance is very similar to RET. Horney (1939) wrote of the "tyranny of the should" and generated a list of "neurotic needs" that is quite similar to lists of irrational ideas later published by Ellis (1962 and elsewhere). For Horney, neurotic need was a defense against basic anxiety stemming from infantile helplessness. Ellis reverses the relationship by postulating that the irrational beliefs are acquired first and the risk that they will not be fulfilled creates the anxiety—the irrational demand that one *must* get love and approval leads to the fearful anticipation that one might be ignored or rejected.

Sigmund Freud is a favorite target of Ellis's most vigorous attacks, and yet, as Dolliver (1979) notes, Ellis once acknowledged an "inestimable debt" to Freud's ideas. Both emphasized hedonism in motivation, rational control over emotions, and religion as childish dependence. Freud's account of neurotic anxiety features the threat of id impulses breaking into consciousness, whereas Ellis's source of neurotic anxiety (a term he does not favor) is irrational "awfulizing" and demandingness. Ellis rejects the Freudian notion of childhood determinants of adult behavior, insight as sufficient to change behavior, and the highly structured model of the unconscious.

RET and the person-centered counseling of Carl Rogers are poles apart in techniques, but similar in their goals. Ellis urges self-reliance in ethical issues, no moral condemnation of self or of other people, and tolerance for reality; Rogers believes that a person's innate goodness will lead to correct decisions and self-regard without self-imposed conditions of worth. Both make self-image a central theme in their theories of disturbance. Rogers's statements about anxiety, not unlike Freud's, give a central role to the awareness of threatening material. In Rogers's case, the threat is that one will become aware of the discrepancy between phenomenal actual self and the ideal self one creates from the conditions of worth imposed by parents and other socializing agents. The Ellis version is very similar in that irrational demands (e.g., "I must be loved and approved," or "I must be perfect to gain the love and approval I demand") must be fulfilled in order for one to feel worthwhile; that they might not be fulfilled leads to anxiety. The person-centered approach is one of gradual gaining of self-regard with diminishing conditions of worth; the RET approach is one of active advocation of a philosophy of self-acceptance, of the illegitimacy of any form of self-rating, and of challenging people to prove the truth of their self-rating statements. True to his de-emphasis of childhood experiences, Ellis believes that people teach themselves self-rating schemes and that they are not externally imposed. He also rejects Rogers's forming of close relationships with clients as a condition for successful therapy. Ellis equates relationships with warmth, and believes warmth is iatrogenic. He firmly believes that any but the most subtle communication of his empathetic understanding will show warmth, closeness, and thereby reinforce clients' irrational demand for approval.

Berne's Transactional Analysis (TA) is very similar to RET in concept, as they should be because both were derived from Adler and Horney, among other earlier theorists. Both are very cognitive, and both aim to help people become aware of their cognitions. However, RET stresses intrapersonal dialogue (or what Meichenbaum [1977] calls the "internal dialogue"), and TA an interpersonal dialogue.

Nonetheless, much TA jargon can be restated as RET jargon. Irrational must-statements about personal conduct can be thought of as TA's Parent ego state. Irrational must-statements about immediate gratification echo the Child ego state. Rational beliefs, by definition, correspond to the Adult ego state. Berne's explanation of anxiety is that persons with a "not-OK" life position create anxiety when they focus on the future and develop negative expectations; Ellis might refer to these persons as chronic self-downers who anticipate getting rejected, failing, because of their presumed inadequacy.

Where Berne and Ellis differ is in their accounts of how people come to become losers or self-downers. Berne hypothesized that losers develop a not-OK life position when, due to a lack of response to childhood dependency needs, they remain dependent on the environment. Ellis rejects such a developmental notion in favor of his hypothesis of biological diathesis for easily acquired irrational beliefs, especially through self-indoctrination.

RET, TA, person-centered, and Gestalt therapy share an aversion to the "should" and its tyranny. They stress individual responsibility, the here and now, and at least Gestalt and RET share the philosophical ideal of putting oneself first.

Perls's Gestalt therapy and Ellis's RET differ greatly in goals and techniques of therapy. Perls took an anti-intellect stand, Ellis a prorational thinking stance. Perls saw emotion as something to be attended to, Ellis as something to be reduced or eliminated (Dolliver, 1979). Perls said that anxiety is produced when persons fears not receiving or losing outside support they need because they lack integration, that is, are only in touch with a part of themselves. Perls held that self-awareness and integration produce wholeness and self-sufficiency, which eliminates anxiety; whereas Ellis assumes that self-acceptance and realistic thinking will accomplish the same result.

It should be apparent from this short survey that RET has many near relatives among theories of disturbance, as well as its own distinctiveness. RET resists easy classification, partly because Ellis has borrowed both theoretical concepts and techniques from various sources. For a while it seemed that almost anything anyone else was doing could become part of RET by Ellis's adding the word rational to it. Thus we have rational encounter marathons, rational sensitivity training, rational–emotive imagery, and, we daresay, rational group therapy. RET has been characterized as a behavior therapy, an existential therapy, a humanistic therapy, a phenomenological therapy, a cognitive therapy, an insight therapy, an active-directive therapy—with roots in psychoanalysis, humanistic philosophy, and general semantics. And as simple as ABC.

Therapy

Theory

RET and the cognitively oriented psychotherapies share a main assumption about the treatment of disturbance. It is this, that if people modify their maladaptive cognitions and behavior, they will experience less subjective discomfort and more positive enjoyment. In RET, evaluations of self, of other people, and of the world in general are the major targets of cognitive change. In CAT, the personal rules of living as well as cognitive distortions are the targets of change. There is no assumption that some deep or mysterious forces prevent people from changing their philosophies of living. Ellis (1976) hypothesizes that people have innate tendencies to retain or readopt their dysfunctional ideas, especially those for which there is widespread social approval, but this view is not crucial to the conduct of the cognitively oriented therapies.

Because people may resist or fail to change when new information is presented to them, persuasive attempts other than information giving are advocated in RET and CAT but not necessarily in other forms of CBT, for example, Beck's Cognitive Therapy of Depression. These persuasive attempts are better labeled "dissuasive methods," because their aim is to help people give up, reappraise, or reformulate their dysfunctional thoughts and to adopt more helpful ones (Wessler & Wessler, 1980). Dissuasive methods are based on attitude theory and research. The evaluative component of attitudes (often called the affective component in social psychological literature) is the particular target of change. Information giving is directed at the knowledge component, not the evaluative component, of attitudes; because many attitudes are not based on knowledge, information giving has limitations.

Attitudes are usually conceived of as having three components (knowledge, appraisal, and action) in an interdependent relationship; a change in one component may result in a change in the other two (Petty & Cacioppo, 1981). Several theories of attitude formation and change, called the cognitive consistency theories (Brown, 1965), propose the principle that changes in evaluations will follow changes in knowledge or action or both. The RET theory of treatment makes use of this principle by offering arguments against rigidly held beliefs (knowledge component) and assigning behavioral homework to be performed between therapy sessions (action component). Homework usually consists of the clients' acting in ways that are inconsistent with their cognitions and/or appraisals, thus inducing dissonance or imbalance among the components. People tend to adjust their appraisals to fit what they have done, or to fit what they have learned, or both.

In the therapy groups he has conducted for many years, Ellis relies heavily on strong cognitive disputing as the single most important factor in persuading group members to change what he deems to be their irrational beliefs. If, as often happens, clients resist his attempts, he actively confronts them with statements about their low frustration tolerance and insisted that they challenge their own ideas even more forcefully. When working with him as associate therapists in these groups, the authors often heard this typical Ellis intervention, "Unless you give up your nutty ideas you will continue to suffer and act crazily for the rest of your life!" His homework assignments for clients were more cognitive than behavioral, and aimed at reinforcing the disputing Ellis had begun during the therapy session. He assigned members the task of tape recording discussions with themselves in which each attempts to talk himself out of his rational beliefs. Clients brought the tapes to the next group session for evaluation and comment.

The authors agree with Ellis that it is the exaggerated evaluative conclusions which people draw from their own cognitive representations of reality that mediate most emotional responses. They disagree, however, with his chief method of obtaining the required cognitive modification and change. As previously stated, CAT has its roots in cognitive social psychology rather than humanistic philosophy. People very often have faulty attributions and predictions of the responses, reactions, and feelings that will occur if they act in ways that are out of tune with their present erroneous and overly rigid rules of living. The main focus of group therapy is to provide a setting in which members may have or make plans for having corrective experiences (Goldfried, 1980), and can observe their own efficacious behavior which results (Bandura, 1977). A therapy group can be an ideal setting for this to occur, in that it can provide an environment of perceived safety—a small, unusual version of the often feared outside world.

Process

A member of a therapy group may test out different ways of behaving and begin to experience and reevaluate the cognitive structures which are the predictors of human behavior (Mahoney, 1977). Between group sessions, a member can continue to build on his experiences by undertaking carefully planned homework assignments. The group can also provide direct feedback on his in-group behavior, proposed homework assignments, and how they were carried out.

Skillful and inventive leadership can make the group much "larger than life," in that feared stimuli, either internal or external, can be introduced in the members' experiences, and the normal anxiety-reducing avoidance and escape from such situations can be overcome. This approach is a direct contrast to the directive, argumentative style of Ellis, who verbally confronts and disputes their irrational beliefs of each client on a highly structured time-sharing basis (exactly 30 minutes per client).

The authors suggest that as each group member can reliably forecast what will occur in the next group session, an atmosphere of unrealistic predictability and dependence is created. One can anticipate that 30 minutes will be devoted to a focal client's problem, some verbal disputing will occur, suggestions on practical problems given, and interpretations of low frustration-tolerance made about clients who either do not do their homework assignments or who report lack of progress. And then, attention shifts to the next client who wants to present a problem in the group.

The authors attempt in their CAT groups to mirror and exaggerate the real world by creating a dynamic atmosphere in which a variety of different opportunities and unexpected situations are presented. Like an Ellis RET group, we help members to work on their presenting concerns and conscious disturbances. We also attempt, unlike Ellis, to help them to uncover their nonconscious and "right brain" experiences. We agree with Lazarus (1977) that images which a person creates are often the direct cause of emotional disturbance and that many streams of images lie buried in nonconscious thoughts outside one's awareness. By the use of imagery and guided fantasy, we attempt to clarify the clients' cognitions and to illustrate vividly the interrelation of cognition, affect, and behavior. We also attempt to create for the group members situations in which they may imagine themselves having new experiences and reappraising their thoughts as a result. Such reappraisals lead to less dysfunctional emotions, we believe. The members may, as a result of this experience, become more motivated in their attempts to change and develop more commitment, which will increase the attractiveness of the chosen course of action (Janis & Mann, 1977). (Some specific examples of these methods and other dissuasive maneuvers will be presented later in this chapter.)

Before describing how RET should proceed in its ideal form, a few caveats are warranted. The authors separately worked with Albert Ellis as associate therapists in weekly group sessions at the Institute for Rational–Emotive Therapy in the early 1970s and 1980s. Although we noted a high degree of consistency in his conduct of therapy, it does not correspond to Ellis's own description of his work (Ellis, 1982). He claims to invariably use a variety of cognitive, emotive, and behavioral methods, as well as the "dynamics of the group" to treat clients (Ellis, 1973, 1977; Ellis & Abrams, 1978). In fact, he almost never used any technique other than the cognitive disputing of irrational beliefs, and by his own admission not even much of that: "I do not devote the bulk of my therapeutic effort to combating irrational beliefs" (Ellis, 1979a, p. 98). The version of RET he demonstrates for professional and lay audiences routinely includes rational–emotive imagery, behavioral homework assignments, and self-administration of rewards and penalties, in addition to cognitive disputing. Yet, as Becker and Rosenfeld (1976) showed in their analysis of Ellis's initial individual therapy sessions, he did no imagery nor self-administration of rewards and penalties; his homework assignments consisted of a single statement—and to 25% of clients he assigned no homework at all. "Ellis spent a large portion of the session utilizing didactic teaching of a general nature, which was supplemented by frequent concrete examples" (Becker & Rosenfeld, 1976, p. 875). (Note that this is a sympathetic analysis: Becker coauthored with Ellis a self-help book, *A Guide to Personal Happiness.*)

In broad outline, RET should proceed as follows: the individual client identifies his goals or desired changes, although this may be done implicitly rather than explicitly. The therapist shows the client that emotional and behavioral changes can attained by cognitive changes, that is, teaches the basic *ABC* model. The therapist goes on to show the client his maladaptive beliefs, how they are invalid, and how they can be changed. The therapist instructs the client to work on making these cognitive changes, and to do so forcefully and vigorously.

This process can occur over one session or many. Some people never change much despite genuine efforts. Why their thinking is so difficult to change is not known, but Ellis holds that it is due to their biological tendency to crooked thinking and inertia. The antidote is to work harder and more vigorously at disputing their irrational beliefs.

There is no assumption in RET that any special relationship must be established between therapist and client or therapist, client, and other group members. However, as Dryden (1984) has noted, for treatment to proceed a sound therapeutic alliance between the group leader and members should exist. Wessler and Wessler (1980, see p. 255) have attempted to specify what constitutes an effective therapeutic alliance. The alliance seems especially important in a therapy like RET, in which the leader takes an active, directive stance, focuses on the individual, and makes no attempt to meld the members into a cohesive group structure.

In order to establish an effective therapeutic alliance, the client probably has to perceive the therapist as credible and accepting of the client as a person. The literature on attitude change and persuasion (McGuire, 1969; Zimbardo & Ebbeson, 1969) and on effective counseling (Janis, 1983) supports this notion. Perceptions of credibility are promoted when the therapist shows expertise and trustworthiness. A confident manner and belief in what he does tend to communicate expertise (cf. Frank, 1978), as do educational degrees and professional reputation and recognition.

The therapist provides a model for the group. In order to be seen as trustworthy, the leader will try to build warm, empathetic relationships with group members and to create an atmosphere in which clients' improvement and welfare are seen as goals of therapy. Clients develop when the therapist is perceived as genuinely interested in helping them, and not in meeting his own views of what constitutes change. This represents our position, not that of RET.

There are many other therapist variables that can color clients' perceptions. A leader who is energetic, highly motivated, and appropriately enthusiastic will help to encourage optimism among group members. Credibility is promoted when clients feel understood by their therapist. Good diagnostic skills seem essential to good understanding, including understanding what the client does not know. For example, if group members do not comprehend the underlying theory of emotional disturbance used by the therapist (in RET this is the *ABC* model), they cannot cooperate in the process. One way in which confusion and loss of credibility can occur is when a group member is encouraged by the therapist (and often by other group members) to change an irrational belief (or in CAT to modify a personal rule of living) when such cognitions are in fact not the real basis of disturbance.

That a therapist might misconstrue clients' lack of comprehension of the therapist's orientation for lack of cooperation or resistance is illustrated in the following example. A man who was both highly anxious and depressed was asked to change his belief that he must be perfect. He continually failed to undertake homework assignments in which he was to make several errors and to accept himself as a fallible human being though erring. However, the therapist did not ask this man about the secondary gains or payoffs for his perfectionistic philosophy (a functional analysis of behavior is seldom done in pure RET). This client attempted to perform perfectly, especially at work, because he feared negative criticism and demanded approval. The therapist did not attend to the reinforcers for not performing the homework assignments, which was instead attributed to low frustration tolerance. The client felt misunderstood by his therapist and even more negative about himself because of the defect his therapist had supposedly detected. CAT, like most CBT approaches, advocates functional analysis of behavior and other features of accurate assessment. With such information, the therapist can assist group members to reappraise, and through corrective experiences, to revise their personal rules of living that contribute to their maladaptive emotional and behavioral responses.

The therapeutic alliance is important for another reason quite unrelated to any presumed curative aspects of the relationship. Therapist characteristics that are irrelevant to clients' beliefs probably influence the acceptance of alternative ways of thinking. This point is supported by studies of attitude change (Strong & Claiborn, 1982). In other words, clients may change their minds for reasons other than evidence and logic. Clients may believe a therapist because they like him or her, or reject statements because they do not feel positively toward the person making them. If the individual does not like, respect, or trust group members and therapist, the chances of helping are greatly reduced.

The process of group therapy requires attention to the dynamics of the therapy group. The individual is the focus of change in RET groups and dynamics are important insofar as they affect the individual's thinking, feelings, and actions. The norms of the group, its communication patterns, and emerging leadership roles can be used therapeutically, or they can encourage continued maladaptive thinking, emoting, and acting. There is a risk that group members may reach a tacit agreement (group norm) not to confront each other, or to offer only practical problem-solving suggestions, or substitute commiseration for help. An experienced leader-therapist will recognize such actions, comment on them, and try to prevent their recurrence.

Cohesiveness of group members, which is a usual prerequisite for the development of group norms, is allowed, promoted, or discouraged, depending on whether therapeutic aims of individual group members are helped or hindered by group cohesiveness. It is not a primary aim in RET and other cognitively oriented psychotherapies, but if used wisely, cohesiveness can significantly facilitate the therapeutic process.

Group therapy, even more than individual therapy, provides opportunities for observing clients' interactions and making comments about them. Goldfried (1980) identifies two common features of all verbal psychotherapies: corrective experiences and direct feedback about clients' behavior. The group process provides material and the group setting a forum in which both the leader and members can give useful information about clients' belief systems and behaviors, especially social behaviors. These observations can be valuable when changes are contemplated. A woman who complained that she was only approached by men who treated her as though she were immediately available sexually, was surprised by feedback she received from the group about her overtly flirtatious manner and appearance. Using their feedback and information about new venues where she might meet more suitable men, she was able in subsequent group sessions to practice her new image and to rehearse new introductory conversations with two or three male members of the therapy group. Such teaching of interpersonal skills is rarely done in RET groups, despite its desirability. One reason is Ellis's almost exclusive reliance on cognitive disputation and practical advice, but another is that skills training improperly focuses on successful performances rather than philosophical change. Ellis (1977) holds that the teaching of assertive communication skills may aid a person in his everyday life, but in itself it is palliative—assertive skills may increase the chances of getting what one wants, but do not by themselves reduce the exaggerated evaluations about the catastrophe of not getting what one wants.

The process of therapy varies greatly, from the educative and confrontative position which Ellis normally uses in his RET groups, to the plethora of direct and indirect methods which the authors favor in their conceptualization of the effective group process. The procedures are different, the goals are the same—to aid clients in their attempts to live more effectively in their own social environments.

Mechanisms

Several mechanisms have already been discussed while explicating and illustrating processes in the previous section. We have noted that Ellis mainly uses a dialogue with focal client (to whom other group members may also freely direct messages), to uncover irrational beliefs, to dispute them, and to instruct the client to continue this process until change occurs, and even longer, to insure that reversion to old thinking habits does not occur. For example, a man who is unhappy because the woman he loves rejects him might be said to hold an irrational demand for love, and his belief restated as, "I *must* have her love! I need her love! I can't stand it if I don't have the love I require from her!" Ellis typically opens the disputing of this idea by asking "Where is the evidence that you *must* have her love? *Why* do you need it?" He argues against any reply the man makes in defense of his beliefs by saying, in effect, "You don't need her love! There is no law of the universe that says you *must* have her love! There are no *musts* in the universe!" The man will then be instructed to repeat these questions and answers to himself several times a day with vigor. The aim is to surrender the irrational demand and the neurotic unhappiness that it creates, according to RET theory.

Relatively little time is needed for implementing these mechanisms. The remaining portion of the 30 minutes Ellis allots a focal client may be taken up with additional examples and reasons why humans do not need love (even though they may highly desire it), and with practical advice about how to meet new women, where to meet them, and, perhaps, how to see his rejection as an opportunity for developing new relationships.

In its ideal form, RET in groups begins with an assessment of individuals' problems. Assessment here means inventorying the person's main cognitions, appraisals, emotional difficulties, and patterns of behavior, and how they interrelate. Facts about an individual's social or marital status, birth order, height, weight, age, and other demographic information are relatively unimportant. Treatment interventions should be based on assessment, otherwise the process might proceed like a dentist's randomly grinding teeth and filling cavities without regard for data a thorough examination can reveal.

Assessment involves the obtaining of an understanding of clients' cognitive appraisals and patterns of behavior, as the therapeutic process must begin here. Other nonpsychological problems are usually revealed in this procedure; it is convenient to think of clients as having practical problems of living and psychological disturbances about those practical problems. Direct assessment methods involve the therapist and group members in an active dialogue with the focal client. They ask questions, probe answers, offer comments, and test hypotheses inferred from a focal client's self-reports of thoughts, feelings, and actions, as well as his behavior in the group.

Group discussion in applying RET to the solving of personal problems generally follows the *ABC* model. The focal client usually begins with material that can be classified as either *A* (activating experience) or *C* (emotional consequences). Sometimes both *A* and *C* are contained in a single sentence about a specific problem, for example, "I got very angry at my husband last night when he asked why dinner wasn't ready on time." The focal client, in this example, reports material that can be classified as *A* (husband's asking why dinner wasn't ready on time) and *C* (hostility). The therapist then asks and urges group members to ask and discuss questions about A and C, for example, "What reasons did he give for asking that?" (an A-probe). "Does he always do this?" (another A-probe). "What did you have to do instead?" (another A-probe). "How did you let him know you were angry?" (a C-probe). These questions clarify the report and are especially helpful to the client who has difficulty recognizing and reporting emotional experiences.

Using the minimodel of anger presented earlier in this chapter, the therapist directs questions about the cognitive appraisals the client made of her husband's statement ("He shouldn't nag me about having dinner ready on time"), including blame ("He's a rotten bastard for nagging me"), intolerance ("He shouldn't be married if he is going to be so inconsiderate"), and grandiosity ("He has no right to expect me to cater to his demands"). One by one the client's thoughts about the situation are uncovered, and their role in her upset specified. Ideally, the group stays on target, but in fact it can easily sidetrack into matters that are irrelevant to the client's cognitive appraisals, including joining the client in condemning her husband (which is usually antitherapeutic) or simply offering ill-timed practical advice (e.g., about how to manage her time more efficiently). The therapist has the dual responsibility to work with the focal client and make sure that the group's efforts are helpful rather than sabotaging or irrelevant.

The group members vicariously learn the model employed by the therapist, not only by experiencing problem assessment, but also through direct teaching that cognitive appraisals (or irrational beliefs in RET) create their negative emotional experiences. In RET groups, they are also encouraged to read such books as *A New Guide to Rational Living* (Ellis & Harper, 1975), to reinforce their understanding.

We accept that direct methods can be effective ways to teach RET principles, but we often prefer to use indirect, experiential methods for this purpose. Our preference is based on the conviction that people assimilate new information better when they actively participate in the learning process rather than passively absorbing material through listening and reading. Indirect methods include exercises, games, and guided fantasies, each of which is specifically designed to make a certain point. In the early stages of the group's existence, we use games and fantasies which illustrate connections between cognitive appraisals and resulting emotions. Later, the process of cognitive change is undertaken in guided group fantasy in which each member can work on his or her own problem areas and can afterwards process the experiences in the group.

Here is an example of an exercise designed to produce quite strong and diverse emotional consequences (usually anxiety, guilt, shame, but sometimes joy). Defenses are exposed and a new group can be introduced to the principle CAT shares with RET, that thinking, especially strongly evaluative thinking, largely determines emotional experience, and that a great deal of such thinking is automatically done without much awareness. A great deal of information can be quickly gained in an indirect and nonthreatening way. Humor acts as a

"loosening up" procedure for a tense, new group, and the subsequent processing of the exercise involves a large measure of self-disclosure. Many less
responsive, reticent, and unassertive group members can respond more easily
because everyone is involved in the process.

The exercise: The therapist begins by inducing an atmosphere of calm. He
asks members to relax, to remove their shoes if they wish, and to close their
eyes. Speaking quietly and slowly (those skilled in hypnosis use induction
techniques), the therapist says, "You are all feeling relaxed. Check your bodies
for tenseness. Does your neck hurt? Relax your tense stomach muscles and let
your hands rest loosely in your lap. It has been a busy week, but it is over and
the weekend is here. You are invited to visit friends who live in the country.
You have not seen them for a considerable time and do not remember them
well. (Pause.) All you really remember is their warmth and familiarity.

"You travel to their country house—choose your method of transport—
drive your car or take a bus or train. Look at the countryside as it passes by—
trees, fields, and hills. It is a calm, warm day, and you will soon arrive.

"You see the drive to their house. (Pause.) And build a lovely house in
your imagination. Fill in the door and the windows and set in the garden of
your choice. Watch it grow.

"The front door is welcoming and open. Go in. Pause in the beautiful hall.
No one is there, but you feel relaxed and sense that your friends will return
soon. Enter the living room. There is a large comfortable sofa—a tray of drinks
and food—flowers, and perhaps a fire in the fireplace. Lovely china, silver,
and furniture surround you. (Pause.)

"Go upstairs. You know where the guest room is. Go in and look at the
luxurious bed—the comfortable chairs. Walk to the windows and look at the
beautiful garden. Next door is a magnificent bathroom. Furnish this room in
the way you prefer. Perhaps mirrors, soft lights, warm towels, or a whirlpool
bath and wooden furniture. Build your perfect bathroom. (Pause.)

"Go to the washbasin. It is sparkling clean and a large, shining mirror
faces you. (Pause.) Lying on the basin is an extremely large new tube of
toothpaste in its box. Take it out and feel it—it is new and unsqueezed. Hold it
in your hand. Slowly remove the cap—unwind it carefully and place it on the
basin. Taking your time, begin to squeeze the toothpaste all over the bathroom. Squeeze wherever you want to—walls, drapes, bath, mirrors, every-
where you want to. (There is a long pause while this image is created.)

"When the tube is completely empty, look around you carefully. Examine
your feelings. What are you feeling now? When you are ready, leave your
imagination and return to the group."

When everyone is ready, the therapist asks them to reveal what they are
now experiencing. Some usually report anxiety, others anger, and some joy.
Usually one or two people will have no particular feelings to report as they
refused to engage in the imaginary toothpaste squeezing. Occasionally, someone reports refusing to enter the empty house! As discussion of feelings gains
momentum, it soon becomes obvious to the group that it was *not* the imagined

action of squeezing toothpaste over an imaginary room that led to the different reports of emotional responses. Each member appraised the event and drew an idiosyncratic conclusion. Some typical responses are:

"I am very anxious. I think my hosts will return and be very angry. They will never speak to me again."

"I am angry. You (the leader) forced me to defile that lovely room."

"I feel happy. I have always wanted to do something like that but never had the nerve."

"Depressed—that's what I feel. I was really enjoying myself but predictably it had to end badly—things always do."

"I have no particular feelings. I only squeezed the tube into the bathtub and the washbasin. I cleaned it up immediately."

Further discussion may show people their defensiveness and self-protectiveness:

"I simply couldn't do it—even though I know it wasn't a real situation."

"I blame you—you made me do it. I am not responsible for the mess."

Group members who had similar emotional experiences find that they had similar cognitions, while others might be surprised that some persons responded in ways which they would not have predicted. The task of the therapist at this point is to keep the discussion (which is often enthusiastic and spiked with humor) focused on the cognitive descriptions, inferences, and evaluations that occurred during the experience. Attempts to describe the house, the journey, and so forth, are deferred for later enjoyment; although happiness and pleasure are important therapeutic goals, the therapist should maintain a professional, work-oriented atmosphere. "Is your reaction typical of the way you usually act when faced with a difficult task?" is a question to test how responses are generalized to other life situations.

This is but one example of the ways an imaginative and inventive group leader can use almost any exercise in the group. The art of the therapist is in processing the experience based on the specific purpose for which the exercise was designed.

One of the basic tenets of RET philosophy is Ellis's contention that humans cannot be judged or rated holistically because they behave badly. The behavior itself is subject to criticism, but the person is not a fool for acting foolishly. Many group members present problems of anxiety and depression which result from their damning themselves totally for acting, or sometimes even thinking, in stupid and unrewarding ways. Such ideas lead to attempts to *be* perfect, further self-damning, and even more anxiety and depression for failing. The following exercise was conceived to demonstrate both the idea of human complexity and the illegitimacy of self-evaluation.

The exercise: The chief participant can be a group member who has made some self-deprecating remark. The therapist points out that the client is globally denigrating himself, and asks the group to join in a research project which will discover which of two group members is better, more valuable, and therefore to be preferred.

To set the scene, the therapist asks a third group member to process all the data collected, and—to promote group involvement—asks everyone to imagine that the room is completely wallpapered with graph paper for recording the results. The question, "Where shall we begin this research project?" is usually met with silence. "How about your jobs? John (the focal client), on a scale of 1 to 10, how well do you perform at work?"

JOHN (after some thought): "I'd say a four."
JANE (the other group member): "I'm a seven."
THERAPIST: "What's next? Let's see who is better at driving a car."

Other performance are measured and added to the list. Group members quickly get into the spirit of the exercise and make suggestions. The therapist endeavors to treat the topic in a more lighthearted manner, "Who is the better dancer?" (This question once resulted in an impromptu Charleston contest, with the remaining group members forming a dance contest committee.) After several activities have been measured, someone usually asks, "Where will this stop?" The therapist replies, "When we have measured everything in the universe that these two people can do and feed the data into our computer." Most group members quickly see they have embarked on an interesting, often amusing, but quite impossible task. Many clients have reported using this graphic illustration in real life situations when they are attempting to measure themselves, usually negatively, against some other person.

As mentioned earlier, the authors prefer to employ a range of didactic and experiential techniques in group therapy. The rationale for using such diverse techniques is simply that we attempt to provide conditions in which members can immediately experience thinking and acting differently within the group. The use of guided fantasy is economic. With a group of 10 participants, the time spent on an individual is necessarily limited, although vicarious learning may occur from listening to and attempting to help others. With these CAT techniques, all participants who decide to participate are involved almost all of the time. They work internally on their concerns: thus defensiveness and resistance, due especially to interpersonal fears, are reduced to a minimum. Only during the processing of the exercises are the participants asked individually to discuss the experience. It is important that adequate time be available for processing.

The final exercise to be described is one which uses all nine steps in the emotional episode. It is a guided fantasy and requires about 50 minutes. No previous preparation is necessary, and group members do not have to understand the details of the emotional episode. Details are included here for clarity.

The exercise: Steps 1 (stimuli), 2 (detection), and 3 (description) of the emotional episode. The leader evokes a peaceful atmosphere and encourages group members to relax in silence. Everyone is asked to look back into their memories and uncover some loss experience, for example, the end of a special relationship, a death of family member or close friend, a transition period in life when we move from one close group into a new situation from college friends to work, or perhaps leaving home or getting married. "Maybe the memory of a child, once so small, and now grown up and gone." The therapist asks the group to remember the face or faces of the person or people in their past, and to recall some of the very special times that occurred then. "Remember both the quiet and hectic experiences, the laughter, tears, unique moments." Several minutes of silence are allowed for reflection.

Step 4 (inference and interpretations). Here are some samples of questions which are helpful in moving the clients' thinking to Step 4.

"How did you feel about yourself at that time?"

"What plans were you making for the future?"

"Do you remember some of your wishes and expectations?"

"How many of your hopes were fulfilled?"

"This person or group of people no longer plays a central role in your life. What are your thoughts about that?"

Provide adequate time for the group to consider the questions and to answer them silently. (Step 5 occurs later.)

Steps 6 (emotional response) and 7 (behavioral response). A high degree of affective response often occurs at this time. Several group members may cry and others exhibit nonverbal behaviors that indicate anxiety, discomfort, sadness, and dejection.

Step 5 (appraisals of observations and interpretations). This is a crucial step in delineating the emotional problem, and the therapist asks questions which are intended to help members to become aware of their evaluative thinking:

"How has this loss affected your thinking?"

"What conclusions have you drawn from this experience?"

"How do you judge yourself, the person concerned, and yourself, as a result of what happened?"

Some typical appraisals which have emerged during the later processing of this exercise, are:

"I'll never get over this loss—I can't stand it."

"I always fail in relationships and always will."

"I am a mean, spiteful person for treating him so poorly."

"People cannot be trusted and will always treat me badly."

The leader, at this point, has helped the group to generate enough material, and now attempts to encourage members to reappraise their experiences (Steps 1 through 7). Group members usually make a decision to modify or change some of their descriptions, inferences, and evaluations with a resulting reduction in negative emotional responses. The fantasy, however, continues as follows:

"You are alone on a quiet, country road. It is warm, calm, and very beautiful. The road winds down a hillside. You see a slow, wide river and a bridge ahead of you. You are carrying a very large, very heavy suitcase. You are hot and tired. Your arm is hurting. Progress is slow and difficult. Finally, you make it to the apex of the bridge.

"Put down the case and rub your sore arm. Look at the river. The suitcase contains all your memories—everything—about the loss experience.

"In your pocket you have a small plastic shopping bag. Take it out. Open the huge suitcase and look at all the contents. Slowly and carefully select what you really want to keep from this huge store of memories. Be extremely selective. Ask yourself, 'Do I really want to keep this—do I need it?'

"The contents of the suitcase are many, yet the shopping bag is small. Some of the memories are unhappy. Remember them and choose to keep some of them, too. Slowly fill the plastic bag and then proceed to throw everything else into the river. Discard them and watch them slowly float away. Now, throw away the suitcase, too."

(Allow several minutes for this procedure.)

"When you are ready, pick up your plastic bag. Feel your arm. It no longer hurts. The bag is light. You can easily take it wherever you choose to go.

"Walk down the other side of the bridge. A narrow road curves away in front of you and merges with the horizon. This is the road to your future. How are you feeling now?"

At this point, the leader and group are ready to process the exercise. This begins with each group member relating his experience. The therapist reinforces the conceptual connections between cognitions and emotions, and shows individuals how they respond more appropriately and functionally when they change or modify their descriptions, inferences, and evaluations. Some typical responses are:

"I realize that I only remembered the good times, and I also recognize that I didn't just behave badly. I do not need to cling to the past. I learned from it and now feel less guilty and more relaxed."

"From the group experience I now realize that many others have had similar tough times. I am not different and I was not singled out for this treatment. I feel relieved—less angry."

During the processing of the exercise, the therapist introduces Step 8 (reinforcing consequences), and does a formal functional analysis when appropriate. For example, persons who have remained depressed and guilty might reveal that they see these as suitable self-punishment for bad behavior. Someone with a personal rule of living that states, "people are untrustworthy," might become aware that this is a defensive response designed to protect the believer from possible future rejection. Good processing of the group experience is the key to successful outcome. Typically, a lively and insightful discussion ensues in which the therapist has many different examples to use in order to aid the process of change.

The authors attempt to be inventive when working with groups, and advocate the creation of new exercises that seem responsive to the concerns expressed by group members. The foregoing exercises should be taken as representative of our work, not a full description of it, as well as an encouragement to others to innovate whenever possible. The authors use the phrase Cognitive Appraisal Therapy (CAT) to identify their work and to make clear that it is not what Ellis does or would do. Although CAT evolved directly from RET, the influence of other psychotherapies should be apparent. The work of Beck, Lazarus, Meichenbaum, and other cognitive-behavior therapists has already been acknowledged. In addition, CAT incorporates ideas from Gestalt therapy, TA, reality therapy, and Greenwald's (1973) Direct Decision Therapy.

Along with inventiveness, therapists should have flexibility. Flexibility can occur when the therapist is well informed, inventive, and imaginative, and seems essential in order to effectively with a wide range of different people and problems. In turn, a diverse, creative atmosphere can encourage clients to become more flexible (and therefore less rigid) in their attitudes, and more creative as they seek solutions to their personal problems.

In addition to mechanisms outlined thus far, there are several others that are characteristic of RET. Homework has been a characteristic feature of RET since its inception, and Ellis recommends setting individual tasks for each group member to perform between sessions. When he sets assignments, they are intended to encourage clients to cognitively dispute their irrational beliefs with force and vigor (Ellis, 1979b). These activities include bibliotherapy, in which clients are encouraged to read Ellis's books and articles, and written homework using printed forms on which irrational beliefs are recorded and immediately disputed. These forms follow an *ABCDE* format (*D* for disputing, and *E* for effects of disputing), and differ from the Rational Self-Analysis form routinely used in Maultsby's (1975) rational behavior training (RBT). Ellis rarely assigns the use of these forms, but some clients use them on their own initiative.

In CAT, cognitive methods may be employed as homework assignments, but we very much prefer experiential assignments. Clients are less likely to change long held philosophies of living simply by deciding to do so. Better results can be achieved when the individual acts of differently and witnesses at first hand the consequences of behavior (Bandura, 1977; Goldfried, 1980). A woman with a forceful personality believed that she had destroyed a close relationship by attempting to control the life of the partner who had rejected her. She predicted that she would always act this way and was depressed, seeing her future as empty and unrewarding. Her homework task was to attempt to test out her own hypothesis by issuing detailed instructions to several friends and colleagues, and therefore effectively taking control of their lives. Some people resisted some of her suggestions by not carrying out her instructions. Others would not do as they were told. Many laughed at her dictatorial manner. She discovered that she did not have magical powers of control and at the same time that few people actually rejected her totally for her efforts. After this experience, she modified her attitudes and felt less depressed.

We have found that these corrective experience activities are usually more effective when the client decides on the task to be undertaken. Unlike Ellis, who originates and assigns the homework as a teacher would to a pupil, we prefer to increase motivation by asking clients to suggest assignments which they see as appropriate to the maladaptive rules of living which they are attempting to modify. If they cannot, we make suggestions and, in either case, negotiate an assignment both client and therapist can agree is likely to prove beneficial.

Very occasionally, Ellis will ask for behavioral homework to be under-taken. For example, to aid a client to get rid of the irrational ideas that lead to shame (which Ellis considers central to emotional disturbance), he might request a participant to complete a shame-attacking exercise. To attack the shame that upposedly underlies interpersonal anxiety over a real or fictitious inadequacy, a client might be asked to do something foolish in public. Recently, a young aspiring artist who had never sold a picture was set the task of walking into several fashionable galleries in Manhattan, and very assertively insisting that the owners look at her pictures and comment on her genius. The point of this assignment was not to sell pictures, but to overcome anxiety about showing her highly self-criticized pictures.

Risk-taking exercises are activities that the individual defines as "risky." Because the "risk" involved in psychological, what is "risky" is both idiosyncratic and objectively nondangerous. In the final analysis it is not truly a risk but the discovery of this fact that is the main purpose of risk-taking exercise.

Often these assignments involve clients' acting in ways which they may regard as daring. To behave in a daring way usually involves "stepping out of character" (this is the CAT adaptation of Kelly's fixed-role procedure). This exercise is used with individuals, but all members of a therapy group can be asked to "step out of character" as well. The basic instructions are simple, but can be elaborated and discussed with clients as needed: "For a short period of time act like the type of person you imagine you may like to be." A shy young man who envied his more assertive friends decided to ask several women in his office for a date. To his surprise, he actually enjoyed the experience. Most of the women refused his invitation, but seemed unoffended by his request, and one of them agreed to go to a concert with him. He found that he was not uniformly rejected as he had feared. We think of "step out of character" as doing something positive and desirable for oneself, and "shame-attacking" as doing something negative—doing something one wants to do versus doing something generally recognized as socially unacceptable.

Cognitive and behavioral rehearsal within the group are techniques which can give the person psychological preparation to withstand anticipated attacks in the outside world. The young man who stepped out of character first rehearsed his dating techniques in the group, to help him overcome his initial anxiety. He was encouraged to reevaluate his ideas about rejection (cognitive rehearsal). Behaviorally, he benefitted from direct group feedback when he simulated dates with two of the female group members. Although this activity often has amusing results as the group gains enthusiasm for cognitive and behavioral rehearsal, the intent is serious. A group provides a unique pool of experience which can prove to be very influential—a safe, shallow pool where, under the caring vigilance of experienced supporters, a person may learn to swim and develop style before plunging into the deep end of the real world.

Cognitive and behavioral change can be strongly reinforced by informative group feedback. The therapist encourages group members to comment on each other's problems, to share common experiences, and to give appropriate advice and information. In a fast-moving, increasingly complex society, a therapy group can provide the kind of service that troubled people used to receive from parents, grandparents, priests, and peer groups.

Feedback does not provide rewards in itself. It can be very uncomfortable to be the focus of negative or even positive opinion. Reinforcement of one's performance often leads to reevaluation of failures and accomplishments and the setting of new goals (Janis & Mann, 1977). As the client attempts to act on new decisions and to observe the consequences, the group can provide an encouraging, motivating forum. Often the reactions of significant other to changes made outside the group can be unhelpful, perhaps because they dislodge long-standing patterns of interaction.

A husband whose marriage was "in trouble" decided, after receiving extensive feedback from other members of a group, to talk more openly with his wife. He told of his warm loving feelings for her and of his fears that their marriage of 12 years seemed to be failing. His wife was confused by his new, unexpected behavior, and accused him of being weak. "You are having an affair and feeling guilty," was her angry response. He had decided to give up his new behavior when a woman in the group who had recently been divorced, told him how much she respected his efforts and regretted that she and her former husband had not had intimate conversations. Other group members added their encouragement and he decided to try again, this time prefacing his remarks with the information that he was seriously trying to improve their life together. Eventually, his wife began to respond more positively, and they talked about their problems and felt closer than they had for years. Feedback from the group gave this man new information which initially helped him to decide on a course of action, and to test its effectiveness. When he did not receive the response he had hoped for, he retreated. Further feedback then encouraged him to modify his plan, give more complete information, and again strive to reach his subgoal—better communication with his wife. This decision paid off, and he had a basis on which to work for his ultimate goal—a happier, more rewarding marriage. Both he and his wife had corrective experiences which modified their pessimistic attitudes toward change.

The reduction of defensive communication is an important goal in therapy. We prefer to confront this issue directly, and help convince group members that by disclosing personal information, and thus risking criticism and rejection, they can not only survive but live better. "Who believes that 'keeping oneself to oneself' is a good idea?" "Is it better to be polite or honest?" are questions that usually afford lively discussions. Often the emotional consequences of living by such rigid norms and values are revealed.

In many approaches to group psychotherapy, leaders, or rather "facilitators," attempt to develop a warm, loving, supportive climate in which people can trust each other, because the approach assumes that such a climate is in itself therapeutic. The authors share Ellis's view that such a climate is not therapeutic by itself, but unlike Ellis we believe that a warm, loving, supportive climate is not antitherapeutic, and can promote conditions by which other therapeutic interventions can prove effective.

It may be desirable, and at times necessary, to encourage people to reveal facts about themselves and to trust each other, but it is seldom necessary to continue this practice for very long. "Trust" is a term which is regularly raised in the early stages of group therapy. The so-called need for trust is often overemphasized, and requires clarification. Logically, some group members may refuse to trust the group and refuse to reveal intimate details about themselves because they could easily be disadvantaged by others' having knowledge of some privileged communication. Dissatisfied employees and unfaithful spouses come into this category. There is no guarantee that group members will not reveal secrets; despite careful security screening, the CIA regularly experiences such leakage. No promises of confidentiality can be made and invariably kept—and this is the definition of trust in this case. However, the therapist can firmly request that no group business be discussed outside the group setting, and can show how this is unhelpful.

More often, personal information is withheld for psychological rather than practical reasons. The experiencing of guilt and shame may lead to avoidance reactions. Skeletons that are silently concealed in closets are especially hard to exorcise. Here the therapist would best concentrate on the maladaptive cognitions which relate to these emotions. "I don't trust the group; if I confess that I sleep around they will say I am promiscuous, and I will be sexually harassed as a result," one young woman claimed. In CAT, the therapist would focus on the clients' rigid rules of living, which in this case include ideas such as: "It is wrong to enjoy sex and be sexually active. I am a hypocrite for thinking it is wrong and then doing it anyway. If men know that a woman likes sex and is available they will treat her like a whore." Each of these statements is extremely evaluative in tone. The dissuasive tactics employed in this example included helping the woman adopt a more self-accepting and less critical self-attitude for choosing (and choice is emphasized) to act in certain ways. Later, through assertiveness training, the woman learned to refuse unwanted sexual overtures.

Fear of psychological attack is yet another problem which hovers around the shaky trust issue. Some clients fear revealing their personal problems because they suspect that there might be some undiscovered psychological cause for their disturbance—that their difficulties may be much more serious than anyone has yet declared. They fear having their fears confirmed, and expect they will suffer at the hands of other people. Of course, there is nothing to trust other people with, in a very important sense, as psychological reactions result from their own cognitions and symbolic representations of reality, not from other people's words. The group members might more usefully ask, "Can I trust this therapist and these other people to help me with my problems? Do they have the necessary skills and information?" This issue, which seems much more realistic, is rarely mentioned in therapy groups.

Lack of trust is not the only reason that clients cite for remaining silent when it would be in their own interests to work on their problems. Ellis (1979c) states that low frustration tolerance (LFT) or discomfort anxiety is the main reason that clients fail to cooperate. "It's too damn difficult! You can't stand it!" are two of his favorite phrases to direct at "resistant" clients. The authors disagree with Ellis's notion that LFT is wholly maladaptive; it is a question of degree. An easily frustrated organism is far more likely to quickly generate alternative ways of thinking and behaving, which are important early steps in decision making (Janis & Mann, 1977). Many depressed persons are not only passive in the present but also passively predict negative future events. LFT is only debilitating when experienced to an acute degree, as in the case of severe procrastination.

We ask clients to accept the fact that they can stand to be in tough situations, at least in the short term. We then request them to stop whining, moaning, bitching, or complaining (the word to be chosen from the client's repertoire), and encourage them to develop plans for change, and act immediately on achieving realistic subgoals. It is important that the subgoals are perceived as attainable, which the therapist can determine by checking with the client about the likely outcomes of taking action. Although Ellis prefers to denounce LFT and to disagree strongly with clients who complain of the difficulties involved in change, we like to work within the clients' frame of reference and transform a high degree of unproductive discomfort anxiety into an action-oriented, motivating program of self-help.

A difficulty which commonly occurs when clients claim that something is too hard, too difficult, or too inconvenient, is that they may fail to carry out homework assignments. Most people want to change easily and comfortably. Others fear the discomfort they expect to experience in doing a difficult piece of homework. They desire to feel better *before* changing instead of changing *in order* to feel better. Client problems are then taken "back to the drawing board" in an attempt to uncover what the client fears. In order to accomplish this, imagery and time projection can be employed: imagery to uncover what exactly is seen as fearful, and time projective to help develop mastery and coping skills when facing the actual situation.

A woman gained insight into her personal rules of living which were causing her angry feelings towards father, with whom she lived. "I hate his critical, overbearing manner; he shouldn't talk to me in this way," she recalled when describing a recent argument. She agreed with the opinions of some other group members that "at 71 he is pretty unlikely to change." What she had not accepted previously was the idea that although disapproving of his behavior, she could tolerate it. "How long could you stand his criticism without reacting angrily—10 seconds?" asked the therapist. She laughingly replied that she might manage about 5 minutes and agreed to try. The subsequent corrective experience paid off and she learned to stand being with her father and was thereafter rarely drawn into arguments with him.

In conclusion, RET advocates and CAT actually uses a diverse set of therapeutic mechanisms. In particular, we employ the feedback opportunities the group situation affords, and help clients plan for and carry out new behaviors in order to have corrective experiences. We consider what happens between sessions more important than within sessions.

PRACTICE

Problems

"Can I get help for my problems?" is a question that rests in the consciousness of a new group member. Therapists can provide help when they have the necessary skills and experience, and if their theoretical orientation is appropriate to the problems with which they hope to deal.

Ellis rarely refuses to accept people into his groups. He often refers clients to group therapy following their initial individual consultation with him. His attitude toward individual therapy sessions is laissez-faire; he usually concludes an initial session in which he teaches the *ABC* model, and applies it to the presenting problem, with words to the effect, "You can make another appointment to see me or join one of my groups." He does not develop treatment plans, but rather will discuss whatever problems clients wish to consult with him about. Although he does not make a DSM (Diagnostic and Statistical Manual of Mental Disorders) diagnosis, he has his own system of categories: normal, neurotic, borderline, and psychotic, with pluses and minuses added to create additional points along this diagnostic continuum. Many of his group therapy clients seem psychotic, have severe personality problems, or are "borderline personalities." Since no verbal psychotherapy has been effective with psychotic and neurological disorders, it is not surprising that many individuals remain in RET groups for years without showing much if any improvement.

RET is said to deal with neurotic problems of living, and Ellis sees cognitions as mediating the major emotional disorders. There is no research to support the efficacy of RET with the recognized nosological categories, and no claim that it alters schizophrenia or other thought disorders, for example, those of organic origin. However, one need not be neurotic to have neurotic difficulties. CAT is more conservative in scope, as we confine it to the neurotic problems of living, especially those termed the "moral emotions" (Sommers, 1981), which are characterized by prescriptive statements about living. These contain some form of the word *should* or *ought;* Ellis contends that these are irrational statements, but we disagree that should-, must-, or ought-statements invariably lead to disturbance. Only persons with these problems and for whom group rather than individual therapy is deemed advantageous are appropriate for RET or CAT group therapy.

Other problems call for different tactics, as cognitive appraisals may not be involved in the disturbance. Phobias are an example. Ellis says phobias have a cognitive basis; however, it seems apparent that phobias may have a noncognitive origin, at least in some cases; but cognitions may be crucial to the maintenance of phobias. Here, a cognitive approach integrated with various behavioral tactics is called for, and one might call the result of such a combination Integrated Cognitive Behavior Therapy, or Multimodal Therapy, the term Lazarus (1981) uses to refer to his work.

The following example illustrates an integrated cognitive behavioral approach. A woman told of her severe bird phobia and how it restricted her from enjoying certain activities. She avoided trips to the beach or countryside with her friends. A three-point treatment plan was agreed upon between she and the therapist, which included both cognitive and behavioral modalities: (a) systematic desensitization; (b) information seeking, especially about their flopping wings, the central element in her fear (she decided to study birds), and (c) her cognitive structures concerning the perceived danger of entering situations where birds might be present was defined and modified to overcome the probability that she would continue her well-rehearsed avoidance behavior and not complete her homework assignments. Although the origin of her phobia was never found, the concerted approach to her problem produced satisfactory results.

Flexibility is the byword of the effective therapist. Practicing clinicians can seldom afford the luxury of a "pure" approach. A well-constructed treatment plan can more fully meet the challenges of the client's problems.

Evaluation

It has been difficult to evaluate RET for several reasons. First, it seems not to be a system of psychotherapy but an approach, according to Lazarus (1979). Ellis has incorporated so many techniques into RET that it is nearly impossible to state what most RET practitioners actually do, except that they follow Ellis's speculations about the nature of disturbance. In this chapter, the term RET has been restricted to the procedures Ellis uses most frequently, specifically cognitive disputing of what he has identified as irrational beliefs. However, even this is problematic, since he has defined irrational beliefs in various ways at various times, and his most frequently cited definition—that irrational beliefs lead to inappropriate emotions and goal-defeating behaviors—is circular and imprecise.

This definition is linked with the neologism *musturbation*, to emphasize that absolute *musts* are crucial features of irrational beliefs (Ellis, 1979d). However, this definition itself is absolutistic and at odds with the notion that irrational beliefs lead to inappropriate emotions and self-defeating behaviors. For it does not necessarily follow that a must-statement must always have such consequence, despite Ellis's assertions to the contrary. Ellis has produced well-known lists of irrational beliefs (Ellis, 1962; Ellis & Harper, 1975), but these do not consist exclusively of must-statements, which they should if must-statements are crucial to irrational thinking.

The lists provide the basis of scales or measures of irrationality. Such scales are troublesome in that they assume that irrationality is a unitary dimension, although such an assumption is neither consistent with RET principles (Wessler, 1976) nor supported by data (Woods, 1983). Further, such scales assume that a *statement per se* can be irrational even though Ellis's definition of irrational beliefs clearly indicates the opposite conclusion: beliefs are irrational if they work against the individual's well-being and happiness, that is, they are idiosyncratic. Further, Ellis contends that nonempirical beliefs are also irrational (Eschenroder, 1982). These definitions result in paradox. For example, one might believe wrongly that one is a great writer, feel confident because of this self-delusion, and complete projects one might abandon if one thought one were only average. In other words, a nonempirical belief, which fits one of Ellis's notions about irrational thinking, might have positive consequences for the individual, which contradicts another of Ellis's notions about irrationality.

Because it is difficult to say what constitutes RET as a system of therapy, it seems better to agree with Lazarus that RET is an approach to treatment. An approach to treatment cannot be evaluated. One might attempt to specify what procedures are characteristic of RET and not of other approaches or systems of psychotherapy. Even if these procedures could be specified, their evaluation might be meaningless because there are no guidelines in the RET literature prescribing when to use them. Neither Ellis nor others who have written about RET has stated when to use, say, cognitive disputing and when not to, or when to employ rational–emotive imagery rather than cognitive disputing.

The rationale for explaining why procedures are successful (or should be successful) is open to several interpretations. Cognitive disputing might prove effective because the client wants to think empirically and logically and hence surrenders irrational beliefs, or likes the therapist and wants to think as he does, or has faith in the therapist and aligns his thinking with the therapist's while not understanding what the therapist's arguments mean, or is simply so demoralized that he is willing to try anything to attain relief—and this is only a partial list of possible explanations.

There is a straightforward evaluation study that has not been conducted, that would test Ellis's hypothesis about the pivotal role of irrational thinking and provide some validation for scales of irrationality. (One or two similar studies have been cited by T. W. Smith, 1982.) Ironically, the study would not furnish any information about the effectiveness of RET procedures. The study involves pre- and posttesting of irrational beliefs using any of the available scales developed for this purpose. The independent variable would be some form(s) of therapy or counseling other than RET itself. If Ellis is correct about the necessity of cognitive change, then "successful" cases should show less irrational thinking on the posttest. This design also overcomes one of the main objections to irrationality scales, that they are so transparent that anyone who knows anything about RET can fathom their meaning and easily give rational responses—and RET clients can certainly be expected to get some knowledge of RET principles, basic irrational beliefs, and *ABC* theory in RET treatment.

Evaluation of individual change is another issue. Although it could be attempted with irrationality scales, these are so inadequate as to make it scarcely worth the effort. More importantly, it is not the mediating variable (cognitions) that signals clients' progress, but their moods and patterns of behavior. For this reason we advocate relying on self-reports of mood as evidence that target behaviors have been affected. A direct assessment of progress can be obtained by asking the question, "What do you want to stop doing (i.e., habit modification) that you are now doing, and what do you want to start doing that you are not doing (taps fears)?" While it is flattering to have clients claim to feel better or more satisfied as a result of therapy, probing for concrete evidence is strongly recommended.

Treatment

Perhaps the most prevalent format for RET group treatment is the one Albert Ellis has used for many years. Weekly meetings of personal problem-solving, in which he concentrates on irrational and other cognitions, are followed by an "aftergroup" session conducted by an associate therapist, who often designs the required homework tasks. However, it is possible to work in many different ways and settings.

Although the open-ended, ongoing group session may be typical, more specialized assignments can also be undertaken. Increasingly, there is an interest in closed-ended, short-term groups that are specially structured to deal with the problems of particular client populations. We have found that people who share similar problems and goals can work together on such issues as recent bereavement, parenting, depression, or public speaking and other social anxieties.

Groups of this type are tightly structured and meet for between six to eight sessions. Follow-up sessions are made the responsibility of the group members themselves, and are normally held *without* the therapist. There is large educational input, especially in the first two sessions. Bibliotherapy is encouraged, and reading lists and other information are available at the outset of each session. These groups are especially suited for a task-oriented approach (as opposed, say, to nonspecific self-exploration). Termination is already an expectation and the time limit seems to add to clients' motivation. The art of the therapist here is to keep the group working toward its agreed goals and to prevent members from digressing too far into other problem areas. If other problems are pressing, the person can be referred to another therapist for individual sessions or to a different group.

There are other specialized problem areas which are best treated with an integrated or eclectic approach. Habit control is a good example. Medical treatment is often necessary to help addiction, but a cognitively oriented approach may be useful in helping clients with their low frustration tolerance and other resistances, and with the social anxieties which in some cases precipitate a drug or alcohol problem.

Integration of treatment methods is illustrated by the use of CAT in a specialized drug treatment unit. The authors worked with the staff of the unit in two ways. First, as consultants in regular staff meetings. The staff experienced many personal problems as a result of working in a highly stressful, emotionally charged situation. This often led to burnout, personal stress reactions, and poor communications among staff. The consultants dealt with the staff, using a CAT approach, to alleviate these problems. Second, as a result of their own experience, the directors of the unit decided to include CAT as part of a treatment package for their clientele, to help reformed addicts reenter society and adopt a new life-style, particularly by reducing fears about this transitional period (Comberton, 1982).

It is possible to combine different approaches to psychological therapy and counseling, as well as to combine psychological treatment with other procedures to fashion effective tools for specialized problems. The research literature is full of comparative studies which are unhelpful to therapists who want to improve their skills. Nor are the studies designed to help clients. For example, there is a notable absence of research into the preception of psychological therapy and counseling from clients' viewpoints. Rather, comparative studies attempt to show that one system of therapy is more effective than its rivals. We make no such claims, and urge more effective efforts to provide help for clients and to work from the client's, not the therapist's, frame of reference.

Management

The leader of a therapy group is a therapist who has the task of providing structure for group experiences and problem-solving efforts. The group members are clients who have the task of furnishing content for each session. The leader is not a facilitator who merely creates conditions for positive growth potentials to become fulfilled, nor a member of the group and thus free to probe his own problems or socialize with clients outside the therapy sessions. The therapist is a professional with the ethical responsibilities of a professional in the psychological counseling and therapy field.

The therapist takes an active role each session unless he deliberately chooses to withdraw from the discussion and act as a coach rather than teacher-therapist. The therapist manages each session to insure that no one or two people dominate it, that no one becomes disruptive, and that antitherapeutic statements and actions by group members are not allowed to influence other group members in a detrimental way. The management of the group discussion can be done diplomatically, and the discussion steered into productive areas rather than allowed to wander aimlessly.

When the therapist acts as a coach, the group members are responsible for solving personal problems presented by a focal client, processing a group experience, and applying the therapeutic model in a helpful manner. If the group does not stick with its task or does it poorly, the therapist can intervene. Because group members are likely to propose practical solutions without attempting to work on psychological difficulties or cognitions, the therapist should remain alert and actively involved in this discussion even when silent.

The therapist also has responsibility for emotional-expressive interactions within the group. Although cognitive and rational therapy groups are primarily task oriented, they are not exclusively so. Personal and interpersonal concerns are not uncommon in the course of a discussion, unless the therapist takes a highly didactic, therapist-focused approach to the conduct of group therapy.

Finally, the therapist may also see individuals from the group for private sessions. Individual sessions may supplement group sessions for clients with pressing problems or acute disturbances. Group sessions may also supplement individual sessions for clients with interpersonal and social problems. Clients who initially appear suitable for group therapy but later prove otherwise might be referred for individual sessions, or for medication, and even hospitalization. Clients' acceptance of such referrals can be made a condition for remaining in the group or for rejoining it at a later time.

Group Selection and Composition

Selection and composition of groups depend on their purposes. Ellis's RET groups are general-purpose groups. He uses an exclusion criterion: persons who are thought to be disruptive because of active psychosis or excessive talking (as assessed in an individual screening interview) are referred for individual treatment.

Special-purpose groups might focus on a single diagnostic category, for example, depression, or a special topic, for example, a woman's problems or fear of flying. For the former, clinical assessment by means of interviews and/or psychological tests is recommended. For the latter, self-selection may be sufficient. For some purposes, for example, combined CAT and behavioral training for social skills deficits, it is wise to include members of both sexes, because many problems of interpersonal anxiety involve relations with the opposite sex and unsegregated groups provide more realistic behavioral rehearsal possibilities.

Group Setting

A circular seating arrangement facilitates interactive communications. Sufficient space for role playing and other forms of behavioral rehearsal is also desirable. The space should be private enough to preserve confidentiality.

Group Size

In an ongoing group with a personal problem-solving focus, discussions may lag, become routine and predictable, if there are fewer than six group members and little turnover in membership. On the other hand, if there are more than 12 in a group with a personal problem-solving format, it is difficult to include everyone and there may be low or variable involvement. Ellis's groups have about 13 members, plus one or two associate therapists who are present primarily for the training experience; Ellis provides the charismatic leadership, and group members seek his pronouncements as a respected authority figure, while the associate therapists have the special task of promoting participation by all members.

In some settings, very large numbers of people may participate in certain imagery exercises, for example, the "suitcase and plastic bag" described in this chapter. Large groups, however preclude everyone's participating in individual processing of the exercise.

Therapy Frequency, Length, and Duration

Groups may be either ongoing or time-limited. General-purpose groups are often ongoing; for example, Ellis's groups have continued for many years with several complete turnovers in membership. Special-purpose groups may work better on a time-limited basis, ranging from 6 to 12 weeks depending on the purpose and size of the group. A time-limited group tends to encourage clients to actively work on their problems, to seek corrective experiences rather than additional insights.

The length of session may vary, and can be adapted to the purpose and size of the group. Weekly group meetings are probably typical, but less frequent meetings can be effective, especially when the therapist wants to provide ample time for group members to try out new behaviors and have corrective experiences.

Media Usage

Forms for written homework or for completion within the group session may be employed at the discretion of the therapist. The use of videotape recordings enhances behavioral rehearsals, and are quite valuable for giving feedback to participants about their mannerism and style of self-presentation. Chalkboards and flipcharts can be used, especially if the therapeutic methods are educational, or the therapist wishes to record clients' cognitions (Covi, Roth, & Lipman, 1982; Hollon & Shaw, 1979; Sank & Shaffer, 1984).

Clients seem to benefit from audiotape recordings of portions of personal problem-solving sessions when they are the focal clients. Such tape recordings can be reviewed several times between sessions, and seem especially helpful because clients do not retain in memory everything that has been said to and about them during a discussion. They might also record didactic portions of a therapy session. Tape recordings can readily lead to breaches of confidentiality, and clients should be cautioned not to play tapes for nongroup members that contain revelations made in the group session by anyone but themselves.

Leader Qualifications

A leader should be professionally qualified to practice psychological counseling or therapy in his or her state or country. Further, he or she should be competent to practice the specific procedures selected. The experience of working with an already qualified therapist is the ideal method of attaining such skills, and the qualified leader can validate the neophyte's competence.

Wessler and Ellis (1980) have discussed the general clinical and counseling skills possessed by professionals who most effectively learn to do cognitively oriented psychotherapy. These include skill at assessing clients' problems (including defensive maneuvers that work against change), ability to empathize with clients, knowledge about monitoring the relevant aspects of the interaction between therapist and client, willingness to work actively and directively with clients and to provide structure for sessions, and having the flexibility to vary one's approach in order to fit each client's individuality.

In addition, Ellis (in the foreword to Walen, DiGiuseppe, & Wessler, 1980) lists the following characteristics as highly desirable for a rational–emotive therapist: intelligence, wide knowledge of psychotherapy, persistence, interest in helping others, scientific outlook relatively free of dogmas of overgeneralizations, and personal use of RET by the therapist. Grieger and Boyd (1980) discuss specific skills used in RET and rational behavior training, and Wessler and Wessler (1980) present a self-supervision checklist of competencies used in RET and CAT.

Ethics

A qualified leader is a member of the psychological, counseling, social work, psychiatric, or closely allied professions, for example, nursing, or the clergy. The leader is, therefore, bound by the ethical code of his respective profession, and subject to its discipline. In addition, some professional organizations, for example, Association for the Advancement of Behavior Therapy, accept as members persons from the above-named fields, and have their own codes of ethical conduct. Finally, states that license or certify professionals may specify codes of ethical conduct. Should paraprofessionals or nonprofessionals employ the methods described in this chapter and its references (a practice we do not necessarily recommend), they too should follow generally accepted codes of ethical conduct. In short, leaders should not knowingly harm clients, should keep privileged information confidential, and should avoid such dubious practices as sexual contact with clients.

In addition, the therapist has the responsibility to assure that group members conduct themselves according to ethical standards. The therapist should prevent any harmful actions or statements made by group members, and if harm is done to try to correct it. The confidentiality of group discussions should be stressed; client breaches of confidentiality should be met with warnings followed by expulsion from the group for a repeated violation.

RESEARCH

Studies reviewed by Ellis (1979e) focus on the cognitive hypothesis as a factor in emotional disturbance, not on pure RET. DiGiuseppe, Miller, and Trexler (1979) summarized therapeutic outcome studies, few of which were pure RET and none of which was group therapy *per se*, as Hollon and Shaw (1979) have done for Beck's Cognitive Therapy. T. W. Smith (1982) critically reviewed many of the same studies, plus some new ones. It seems safe to conclude from these reviews that cognitions play an important role in human behavior; that neurotic behavior correlates with unrealistic ideas and illogical thinking; that mood is affected by cognitive content. However, the fundamental postulate of RET—that irrational beliefs determine self-defeating emotions, and that rational beliefs do not—has not been adequately investigated.

Few studies of therapeutic outcomes have used pure RET as an independent variable. DiGiuseppe *et al.* (1979) review about 50 studies and note their limitations. Some used no behavioral outcome measures, and obtained data only for paper-and-pencil measures of irrationality (the inadequacy of these procedures has already been discussed in the evaluation section of this chapter). Some studies were of educational efforts, not psychological counseling or therapy. Others reported outcomes of other cognitively oriented psychotherapies, not pure RET. A few RET analog studies support its effectiveness in reducing public-speaking and test-taking anxiety.

There are several reasons that account for the difficulties in conducting RET studies and for distrusting the results of therapeutic efficacy studies (Wessler, 1983). These are: failure to conduct adequate RET, failure to select an appropriate research design, failure to include relevant therapist and client variables, and failure of RET to present empirically testable hypotheses.

Some investigators misunderstand RET and are therefore unable to reproduce its procedures accurately enough for controlled study. Few studies involve someone expert in RET who can verify that it has been performed accurately. Some persons we have trained assume they are doing RET because they emulate the mannerisms of its founder or assume that the only irrational beliefs are the ones Ellis has compiled. Others confuse an approach or system or psychotherapy with its typical procedures; for example, Herink (1980) indiscriminantly includes specific procedures (e.g., bibliotherapy) used in many approaches along with complex systems of psychotherapy, and labels both procedures and systems "therapies." When research reports omit crucial information about the independent variable, it is impossible to know precisely what was done. Thus, a research report that compares "behavior therapy" with "rational therapy" might in fact have studied thought-stoppage and written homework, but there is no way to know this unless such details are reported *and* one knows that these are two procedures not two approaches to therapy.

Even when the labels are appropriately used, there is no assurance that the procedures have been appropriately selected. For example, one might dispute a fact reported by a client and incorrectly label it "disputing of irrational beliefs." Or, one might dispute the wrong irrational belief (i.e., one not central to the emotional disturbance under investigation).

The model for therapy outcome studies that has been most widely used is that of the drug-outcome study. This model consists of an experimental drug or drugs and a placebo administered to subjects, and the differential effects compared. Ideally, neither the subjects nor the experimenter knows who got the drug and who the placebo until the data are ready for analysis. Although subjects are selected according to diagnostic criteria, it is irrelevant who administers the medication. But, in psychotherapy it is highly relevant who administers the therapeutic procedures and whether the client is cooperative or not. Cooperation depends in part on the client's perceptions of the therapist, which depend in part on the therapist's personal characteristics. Further, therapists are not equal in their competence to perform certain procedures, nor in their belief in their efficacy. A double-blind study is impossible in psychotherapy, and yet it is essential for research using the drug-outcome model.

Psychotherapy resembles surgery more than it resembles medicine. Successful outcomes in surgery depend on both the procedure *and* the practitioner. Just as the skill of the practitioner interacts with the procedures he employs, so the "bedside manner" of the practitioner and the confidence it inspires in the patient interacts with procedures. Few RET studies account for these important interactions among therapist variables, client variables, and procedural variables.

Good research demands control, good therapy flexibility. A skilled RET practitioner will vary the form of cognitive disputing; if a direct "where's the evidence" approach seems to get nowhere, the therapist can quickly switch to anecdotes, analogies, parables, poetry, witty sayings, or other cognitive techniques, not to mention the behavioral and affective-expressive techniques advocated but seldom used in RET.

RET is both a theory of disturbance and a set of procedures for treating disturbance. Ellis (1979e) has proposed 32 hypotheses central to and generated from RET theory and practice. But the research data he presents in support of RET hypotheses are inappropriate because most of the hypotheses cannot be empirically tested. We can add little to Mahoney's (1979) critical analysis of Ellis's hypotheses:

> Many of the hypotheses are never stated, and, when one tries to distill an hypothesis, the result is often disappointing. . . where Ellis does offer relatively clear hypotheses, their parentage is often disputable. Hypothesis 25, for example,—"people tend to focus mainly one thing at a time"—can be traced back as far as William James and is hardly an RET insight. . . . . this is a collection of loosely related and poorly elucidated propositions. (Mahoney, 1979, p. 177)

Ewart and Thoresen (1979) point out that some of Ellis's hypotheses are untestable, some uninformative, that his research review neglects negative evidence, his logic is escaloped, his predictions at times inconsistent, that some hypotheses fail to distinguish RET from other therapies, and that weak evidence is presented for uniquely RET hypotheses.

Even though RET lacks an empirical basis or the kind of conceptual basis that promotes empirical research, the cognitively oriented psychotherapies taken as a whole have begun slowly to accumulate a sounder footing (Schwartz, 1982). Tosi (1979; Tosi & Baisden, 1984) has published several studies of his Rational Stage Directed Therapy. Some outcome studies of Beck's cognitive therapy of depression are impressive (Beck et al., 1979). Mahoney and Arnkoff (1978) have carefully reviewed research and conclude that support for cognitively oriented assumptions and procedures is encouraging but as yet not conclusive. At present, the conservative view such as advocated by Lazarus (1981), that favors selecting procedures with some empirical backing and deferring grand theorizing, seems appropriate.

If one accepts an attitudinal account of neurotic disturbance and treatment, with the indirect support offered by several decades of research in attitude change and persuasion and by contemporary research into emotion, then a different form of research question emerges. Can attitudes and appraisals be influenced in dyads and in larger groups? The answer is yes, and metaanalyses of therapeutic processes, for example that of Strong and Claiborn (1982), furnish a rationale for the cognitively oriented psychotherapies to employ these tactics to bring about evaluative and other cognitive changes.

Group Session Illustration

1 THERAPIST: I noticed, Jane that you had tears in your eyes during this experience.

2 JANE: Yes, I did.

3 THERAPIST: Do you want to talk about it?

4 JANE: I'm thinking about Linda—she's my little girl. Now that her baby days are over, I've decided to go back to college and leave her with a friend during the day. I dread leaving her. She cries when I do and I feel really guilty.

5 DAVID: What made you decide to go back to school?

6 JANE: I've always felt insecure that I'm not really qualified to get a good job. If anything happened to my husband, I don't know how I'd manage to support Linda and myself. It's something I really have to do.

7 THERAPIST: Is the program of study full time?

8 JANE: Yes, it is. And it's just not designed for people like me. There's no evening classes in accounting. I think it's unfair that they don't think about women with children. I don't want to leave her at all.

9 MARGE: Oh, lots of people leave their children these days and go to school. I left my two little boys when they were quite small to go to school and it worked out fine. Why are you feeling so guilty?

10 JANE: Oh, it's just that Linda has always been so close to me. She's our only child. She doesn't like to play with other children very much. She just follows me around the house and likes to be with me. We like to do things together. I'm sure she'd find it very difficult. I know I would. I'm just used to having her there all the time. I'm not happy even being away from her to come to this group.

11 MARGE: Well, you know she may find it difficult at first, but she will get used to it. I still don't know why you feel so guilty about that. It seems like something you want to do very much.

12 JANE: I just get this picture of her face. She always cries when I leave; I must say that she does settle down after a while. I just don't feel good about leaving her. I can't explain it anymore.

13 THERAPIST: I suspect you'd like to go back to college and feel somewhat less guilty. Let's see what we can do about that.

14 JANE: Yes, I feel like crying a bit now. It seems like such a big problem.

15 THERAPIST: I think you have some very strong rules about mothers and children being together, especially when they are so small. Could you tell me some more about that, Jane?

16 JANE: Yes, I don't like the ideas of mothers and children being apart. I think it's quite wrong. I really disapprove of these women who go out to work and leave their babies with other people. I feel sorry for the children. They don't grow up and know what a real mother and father are like.

17 DAVID: Well, you know, most fathers have to leave their children, have to go out and work, and do that all the time. I do that, and I have a very good relationship with my son. I think you're being too hard on yourself.

18 THERAPIST: I think a lot of people would share your ideas, Jane, but I think you hold them very strongly. Do you think that it's terrible for mothers and children to be separated at all? What degree of separation do you think is acceptable?

19 JANE: Well, I think when they're babies they should be together all the time, but I suppose when they get big some degree of separation is inevitable. I just don't think I'm doing my job properly if I let someone else take care of her during the day.

20 MARGE: Do you know this person well? Is she caring?

21 JANE: Oh, yes. Of course. I wouldn't leave her with just anyone. I just don't think she can do as good a job as I can. I think Linda will miss me, and I think she won't forgive me for deserting her.

22 THERAPIST: We don't know about that, do we. That's really a guess. Most children forgive their mothers when they go to school. Do you forgive your mother for leaving you when went to school?

23 JANE: I never thought of that. I never thought of that at all. I guess I must have. I hardly remember really starting school.

24 THERAPIST Let's suppose Linda's a bit older and is looking back on her childhood. What might she say about you if you left her and went back to college?

25 JANE: She'll probably say that I deserted her and that I'm a bad mother. I didn't give her the love she needed. She'll probably grow up to be a difficult teenager, and get back at me for deserting her.

26 DAVID: Don't you think "deserting her" is rather strong language for leaving her with someone while you go back to college during the day? I think you're still being very hard on yourself.

27 JANE: My relationship with Linda is so important to me that I'd hate to have anything upset it. I don't want her to dislike me. I really don't think I could stand it.

28 THERAPIST: Well, Jane, I think you're making some very black predictions about what might happen. Most of us were left by our mothers, and we don't seem angry about it. You don't seem angry at your own mother, either. Let's just stop for a moment and see what's going on here. What sort of things are you saying about yourself because you're planning this course of action?

29 JANE: Oh, I think I'm a bad mother. I don't think I should do that. Mothers shouldn't do that. I never did think so. I'm surprised I decided to do it. It's something I said I'd never do. I'm shirking my responsibilities to

her. I don't think people should have children if they're going to leave
them and go back to work, when they are so small. I really wanted to
stay at home until she was about 11 or 12.

30 MARGE: You sound to me like you're trying to be too good a mother. You
know, that kind of mothering can be bad, too.

31 JANE: I don't know what you mean. I don't see how taking too much care
can mean being a bad mother.

32 THERAPIST: There are lots of different definitions of what a bad mother is.
Your definition seems to be a very hard one. Do you really think you'll
be a bad mother because you are making this decision?

33 JANE: Oh, yes. I really should have had more money before we had Linda. I
should have worked longer so we wouldn't have this problem. I'm a
disorganized person. I'm sick of that and I'm really depressed about it.

34 THERAPIST: How are you depressing yourself, Jane?

35 JANE: Well, I suppose I'm doing that by thinking of what a bad person I am.
How stupid and irresponsible! I'm always getting into scrapes like this!

36 THERAPIST: David's right. You're being very hard on yourself. If I had those
ideas I'd be depressed too. Come on, Jane, how can leaving your child
with a responsible person make you into a stupid person?

37 MARGE: You really do look on the dark side. I mean, you don't really know
that Linda's going to grow up to hate you.

38 JANE: Well, I suppose that's true. When we go around to my friend, Linda
enjoys going there. She might, I suppose, get used to it. She might not
hate me, but I'll hate myself.

39 MARGE: Then, why do it? I don't know why you're putting yourself
through this.

40 JANE: You know, Peter (Jane's husband) and I have had our troubles. We
split up last year for 3 months. I've often wondered if we won't end up
getting a divorce. It happened to my friend, you know. I'd be in a bad
position then. He doesn't have much money—just his job. I'm not
prepared to do anything, and I'd feel better if I had a college degree.

41 THERAPIST: In a perfect world, you'd be able to do all things easily. You'd be
able to stay home with Linda, and get a degree in accounting, the
classes would be exactly at the time you want them. But it isn't that
way, is it?

42 JANE: I wish it was! I get angry that it isn't a better place for mothers with
children.

43 DAVID: I think you think it's worse for you than for anyone else. I don't see
my children much except on weekends, and I'm so tired. I have to work
so hard to make ends meet I hardly get to enjoy them at all. Yet, they
don't hate me and I certainly enjoy the time we do have together.
That's the way the world is, you know.

44 MARGE: I think he's right. Have you thought about it this way: you're really
making the best of the difficulties you face, by getting someone to look
after your child while you go back to school. Why are you being so hard
on yourself?

45 THERAPIST: I'd like to try something, Jane. I'd like you to sit back and relax;

close your eyes and imagine something that's going to take place some time far into the future. Everyone else in the group can join in, too. Try and *be* Jane. Now, here's Jane, a young mother of 24, who's going back to college for the first time in several years. She's going to leave her child, and imagine her home with her child, making pastry, watching television, and talking. Stay with that thought for a minute. (Pause.) I want you to make a magic leap. I want you to go 10 years into the future. Everybody come with us and be Jane. If you want to substitute your own children for Jane's, that's OK. Imagine, Jane, what you'll feel like 10 years in the future if you go on doing what your are doing now. Staying at home with Linda—she'll be 16 then—still doing things together, maybe going shopping, watching TV, and enjoying each other's company. What kind of person will you be if you've been a housewife all these years. What kind of person will your daughter become then? An active 16-year-old with friends of her own? (Pause.) Right, Jane? Now substitute another image for a minute. You go back to college and Linda stays with your friend. Imagine that you do get a degree and become an accountant. Imagine how your life will be different in 10 years time. What sorts of things do you think you will be doing? Some of the dreams and hopes that you must have had when you thought about getting some occupational skills. (Pause.) And, how different will your daughter be? Will she still be the pretty 16-year-old, making friends, going to high school, and dating? What will be different? (Pause.) Which of those scenes gives you the most satisfaction? Stay with that thought for a minute. (Pause.) Now, let's try another magic leap, 10 more years. Your little girl is a big woman now, of 26. She has a career, maybe traveling around the world—people travel so much these days. She'll not be at home with you anymore at 26. What will *you* be doing then? If you've chosen to be a housewife and a mother full time? (Pause.) And again, change the scene: and let's see you as the working accountant. What satisfactions do you get from each of those scenes?

46 JANE: You know, it's really interesting. I've never thought of it like that before. I hadn't thought about it much at all. I hadn't thought of it much beyond going to college. I don't think I'd be satisfied just being a housewife all that time. I certainly always wanted to do something else as well. I like it, but I only have one child and don't plan to have any more. And, gosh, at 16, she's probably not going to want to stay home with me all the time. I'll be entirely different then. I realize now that I certainly do want to go back to college and get a degree, and I don't want to wait any longer. That's interesting. I do wish it were easier.

47 DAVID: I found it interesting, too. I hope I'll be retired in 10 years time. I was thinking, Jane, about you, though for the first time, as you were describing yourself becoming an accountant. I think it means a great deal to you, doesn't it?

48 MARGE: How did you see your little girl being different?

49 JANE: Well it's funny. I only have one image of her, as this bright teenager. I really didn't think she'd be that much different. I can't really imagine that in all those years, she wouldn't get used to it. I think I might have exaggerated the situation.

50 THERAPIST: I've got a suggestion, Jane. I think you gained quite a lot of insight by that imagery exercise. Why don't we actually go out into the field and check out how this sort of relationship is changed—when mothers and daughters don't spend so much time together. Do you know anyone who's gone back to college or gone back to work recently? With little girls or boys the same age as your daughter?

51 JANE: Oh, yes. There's plenty of people in my apartment building. It's a young apartment block. Many of them go out to work.

52 THERAPIST: Well, let me suggest this idea. Why don't you ask them what they think. Have you ever discussed it with them?

53 JANE: No, not really. Because I've always gone around saying that I don't approve of mothers going out to work. I'd be a bit ashamed to say that I've changed my mind.

54 DAVID: So, you don't know what they think!

55 JANE: Well, I see the children. I don't suppose they look any different. I hadn't actually thought about it. I suppose I could ask. People do change their minds, and one or two of them are close friends of mine. I suppose I could ask them.

56 THERAPIST: What kinds of questions could you ask, Jane?

57 JANE: I could ask how difficult it was for them to leave their children. How they got along, and what the children thought about it.

58 THERAPIST: What might you discover?

59 JANE: You know, I really don't know.

60 MARGE: Well, it might be worth finding out. Because I didn't share your view of the situation.

61 JANE: That's true. No one here seemed to agree with me. I guess I'll do it.

62 THERAPIST: How many people will you ask before next week?

63 JANE: Well, I know four people I can think of immediately. Yes, I will ask them. I think I will ask them.

64 DAVID: I'll look forward to hearing what they say. I wonder whether they'll say what you think?

Comments

Following a group exercise, the therapist asks a client Jane to talk about her obvious sadness.

The client presents a problem of leaving her small daughter to return to college. The emotions she is experiencing are guilty anxiety, anger, and possible depression.

Helped by other group members, David (5) and Marge (9), the therapist sets out to gain further factual information to highlight the problem. The following three areas are covered.

1. The relationship between the client Jane and her daughter Linda is briefly explored.
2. Facts about the college course and the involvement required are elicited.
3. The client's predictions about what she anticipates will happen if she leaves her daughter are examined. The therapist (13) then suggests a goal for the work to be undertaken by the group, and Jane agrees (14).

The therapist focuses on the guilt issues although the cognitions leading to anxiety, anger, and suspected depression are hypothesized but not stated at this time. They are:

1. Jane's negative predictions about financial insecurity (40) (marital problems are mentioned later) causing anxiety.
2. Jane's personal rules of living regarding the extreme unfairness of the world to mothers and children (8) leading to anger.
3. Jane's many negative thoughts about herself and the impact of separation from her child (10) which are typical of depression.

The aim is to uncover Jane's cognitive structures which interface with guilt. "I think you have some very strong rules about mothers and children being together (Therapist 15).

Jane supplies some information immediately (16) when she expresses her strong disapproval of women who leave their children in order to study or work.

In response (29), Jane defines herself as a bad mother who is shirking her responsibility. Her depressive ideation about her past failure to have adequate money before having a child and her self-judgmental statement that she is disorganized, are revealed. The therapist (28) begins to raise questions about the client's rules—"I think you are making some very black predictions"—and supplies evidence for this statement.

Other group members supply further evidence to support the therapist's words (Marge 30 and David 43).

In response (45), the therapist embarks on an exercise combining imagery and time projection. The group is invited to join in the hope that they will have a reinforcing impact on Jane's personal rules of living by sharing their own experiences.

A "corrective experience" is the aim. CAT therapists much prefer this approach and it is hypothesized that a straight cognitive disputation format as favored by Albert Ellis could cause Jane to become resistant to change. Corrective experiences are fully discussed elsewhere in this chapter.

The therapist relaxes the group (45) and verbally paints a picture of the client and her daughter in two differing life situations.

1. The client is asked to view herself and her child as they might be in 10

years time if the client chooses to remain as a full time housewife and mother.

2. The second imaginal scene is the same as the above except that Jane is asked to add the role of working accountant and to internally speculate on the effects of this difference on herself and Linda.

The exercise is then repeated, projecting an image 10 years hence, because in 20 years the much feared separation of Jane and Linda will almost inevitably have taken place.

After the exercise, Jane (46) explains to the group the insights which she has gained from this new experience.

1. Jane has reinforced her desire to become qualified and return to work.
2. Jane cannot predict any real differences in her image of her daughter if she does not remain with her full time. Also she sees the separation as happening whichever course of action she might choose.

The therapist (50) suggests a homework assignment designed to build on Jane's experiences. Jane is asked to undertake a small research project to see if other women in a similar situation share her thoughts and feelings. She is asked to report her findings in the next group session.

The therapist is very specific in order that the assignment is actually possible, clearly understood, and obviously relevant to the client's problem. Jane is asked (Therapist 62) to ask several people certain questions in the hope that she will gain a broad spectrum of opinion. She is also asked to outline the kind of questions to be asked (Therapist 56) to check for relevance. Marge (60) and David (64) reinforce Jane in her effort by expressing interest, friendly disagreement, and enthusiasm.

The description of a segment of a typical CAT group session is an attempt to illustrate the focal group member, the therapist, and other group members working together in a collaborative, therapeutic alliance. A wide range of cognitive and behavioral interventions is employed to aid the group process. Jane's problems are by no means solved and there are many other areas she may choose to deal with as illustrated by the therapist's unstated hypotheses cited at the beginning of this annotation. She has provided a wealth of information and it is the job of the therapist and the group to assist her toward her stated goal of reduced emotional disturbance. Other group members may gain by acting as cotherapists and by working covertly on their own related issues.

STRENGTHS AND LIMITATIONS

The cognitively oriented psychotherapies assume that faulty cognitions underlie emotional disturbance and that their correction is the key to successful outcomes. These approaches take the individual, not the group, as the focus. They can treat specific problems, for example, public-speaking anxiety, and thus operate like behavior therapy. They can promote self-exploration and self-awareness, and thus share a goal with psychodynamic and humanistic approaches. The cognitively oriented psychotherapies can utilize specific procedures developed within the context of other approaches to treatment to promote cognitive, emotional, and behavioral change. Versatility in counseling a range of human problems is one of their outstanding strengths.

Like other forms of verbal psychotherapy, the cognitively oriented approaches are most easily employed with clients who want very much to change rather than simply to understand how their personalities developed according to some theory. Since they make no claim that the individual is a victim of parents, society, bungled child-rearing practices, or past passive conditionings, clients who accept responsibility for the creating of their disturbances, and who wish to become less disturbed, benefit most quickly.

The cognitively oriented approaches work well with clients of average or above-average intelligence, but can be used with other people in a somewhat rote manner. Pure RET is inapplicable to persons with strong religious beliefs, but some variant of RET, for example, the authors' CAT, can be used instead. Other cognitively oriented approaches do not ordinarily attend to philosophic content as do RET and CAT.

The approaches discussed in this chapter are limited to the counseling of personal problems of living and neurotic disturbances. Conditions for which verbal psychotherapy in general has not proved effective, for example, psychosis, antisocial personality, fall outside the scope of the cognitively oriented psychotherapies.

Group therapy has additional limitations. Very disturbed clients, those who refuse to participate in group proceedings, and those who require a great deal of personal attention would benefit more from individual therapy sessions. On the other hand, for certain clients group treatment is better than individual treatment. Many problems of living involve relations with other people, and therefore a group is an ideal setting in which to work on such problems.

The group can provide a phasing-out experience for clients who have been in individual therapy. Such clients may have begun to make important changes but require additional practice to complete the process. The group, if it is ongoing, can also be a place for clients to return when faced with new life crises.

The strengths and limitations of the cognitively oriented psychotherapies as approaches to treatment in individual sessions also apply to treatment in group sessions. At present, CBT is an important trend in psychotherapy and counseling. Additional research is needed to validate such enthusiasm, remembering that procedures can be studied but broad approaches to therapy cannot. Pure forms of therapy and counseling applied in a doctrinaire fashion are unlikely to benefit clients; favoring theory and adherence to a school of therapy over service of clients' interests is not only ineffective, it is unethical.

REFERENCES

Arnold, M. B. *Emotion and personality* (Vol. 1.). New York: Columbia University Press, 1960.
Bandura, A. *Social learning theory*. Englewood Cliffs, New Jersey: Prentice-Hall, 1977.

Bard, J. A. *Rational–emotive therapy in practice*. Champaign, Ill.: Research Press, 1980.

Beck, A. T. *Cognitive therapy and the emotional disorders*. New York: International Universities Press, 1976.

Beck, A. T., & Emery, G. *Anxiety disorders and phobias: A cognitive perspective*. New York: Basic Books, 1985.

Beck, A. T., Rush, A. J., Shaw, B. F., & Emery, G. *Cognitive therapy of depression*. New York: Guildford Press, 1979.

Becker, I. M., & Rosenfeld, J. G. Rational Emotive Therapy—a study of initial therapy sessions of Albert Ellis. *Journal of Clinical Psychology*, 1976, *32*, 872–876.

Berkowitz, L. *Roots of aggression*. New York: Atherton, 1969.

Brown, R. *Social psychology*. New York: The Free Press, 1965.

Comberton, J. *Drugs and young people*. Dublin: Ward River Press, 1982.

Corsini, R. J. A medley of current personality theories. In R. J. Corsini (Ed.), *Current personality theories*. Itasca, Ill.: Peacock Publishers, 1977.

Covi, L., Roth, D., & Lipman, R. S. Cognitive group psychotherapy of depression: The close-ended group. *American Journal of Psychotherapy*, 1982, *36*, 459–469.

Davison, G., & Neale, J. *Abnormal psychology: A clinical experimental approach* (3d ed.). New York: John Wiley, 1982.

DiGiuseppe, R. A., Miller, N. J., & Trexler, L. D. A review of rational–emotive therapy outcome studies. In A. Ellis & J. M. Whitely (Eds.), *Theoretical and empirical foundations of rational–emotive therapy*. Monterey, Cal.: Brooks/Cole, 1979.

Dolliver, R. H. The relationship of rational–emotive therapy to other psychotherapies and personality theories. In A. Ellis & J. M. Whiteley (Eds.), *Theoretical and empirical foundations of rational–emotive therapy*. Monterey, Cal.: Brooks/Cole, 1979.

Dryden, W. *Rational–emotive therapy: Fundamentals and innovations*. London: Croom Helm, 1984.

Ellis, A. *Reason and emotion in psycho-therapy*. New York: Lyle Stuart, 1962.

Ellis, A. *Growth through reason*. Palo Alto, Cal.: Science & Behavior Books, 1971.

Ellis, A. Rational–emotive therapy. In R. Corsini (Ed.), *Current psychotherapies*. Itasca, Ill.: Peacock Publishers, 1973.

Ellis, A. Rational–emotive theory. In A. Burton (Ed.), *Operational theories of personality*. New York: Brunner/Mazel, 1974.

Ellis, A. The biological basis of irrational thinking. *Journal of Individual Psychology*, 1976, *32*, 145–168.

Ellis, A. The basic clinical theory of rational–emotive therapy. In A. Ellis & R. Grieger (Eds.), *Handbook of rational–emotive therapy*. New York: Springer, 1977.

Ellis, A. Toward a theory of personality. In R. J. Corsini (Ed.), *Readings in current personality theories*. Itasca, Ill.: Peacock Publishers, 1978.

Ellis, A. On Joseph Wolpe's espousal of cognitive-behavior therapy. *American Pyschologist*, 1979a, *34*, 98–99.

Ellis, A. The issue of force and energy in behavioral change. *Journal of Contemporary Psychotherapy*, 1979b, *10*, 83–97.

Ellis, A. Discomfort anxiety: A new cognitive behavioral construct. *Rational Living*, 1979c, *14*(2), 1–7.

Ellis, A. Toward a new theory of personality. In A. Ellis & J. M. Whitely (Eds.), *Theoretical and empirical foundations of rational–emotive therapy*. Monterey, Cal.: Brooks/Cole, 1979d.

Ellis, A. Rational–emotive therapy: Research data that support the clinical and personality hypotheses of RET and other modes of cognitive-behavior therapy. In A. Ellis & J. M. Whitely (Eds.), *Theoretical and empirical foundations of rational–emotive therapy*. Monterey, Cal.: Brooks/Cole, 1979e.

Ellis, A. Rational–emotive therapy and cognitive behavior therapy: Similarities and differences. *Cognitive Therapy and Research*, 1980, *4*, 325–340.

Ellis, A. Rational–emotive group therapy. In G. M. Gazda (Ed.), *Basic approaches to group therapy and group counseling* (3d. ed.). Springfield, Ill.: Charles C Thomas, 1982.

Ellis, A., & Abrams, E. *Brief psychotherapy in medical and health practice*. New York: Springer, 1978.

Ellis, A., & Harper, R. L. *A new guide to rational living*. Englewood Cliffs, N. J.: Prentice-Hall, 1975.

Eschenroder, C. How rational is Rational–Emotive Therapy? A critical appraisal of its theoretical foundations and therapeutic methods. *Cognitive Therapy and Research*, 1982, *6*, 381–392.

Ewart, C. K., & Thoresen, C. E. The rational–emotive manifesto. In A. Ellis & J. M. Whiteley (Eds.), *Theoretical and empirical foundations of rational–emotive therapy*. Monterey, Cal.: Brooks/Cole, 1979.

Frank, J. D. *Psychotherapy and the human predicament*. New York: Schocken Books, 1978.

Fromm, E. *The anatomy of human destructiveness*. London: Penguin Books, 1977.

Goldfried, M. R. Toward the delineation of therapeutic change principles. *American Psychologist*, 1980, *35*, 991–999.

Greenwald, H. *Direct decision therapy*. San Diego: Edits, 1973.

Grieger, R., & Boyd, J. *Rational–emotive therapy: A skills-based approach*. New York: Van Nostrand, 1980.

Guidano, Y. F., & Liotti, G. *Cognitive processes and emotional disorders*. New York: Guilford Press, 1983.

Hauck, P. A. *Brief counseling with rational–emotive therapy*. Philadelphia: Westminster Press, 1980.

Herink, R. (Ed.). *The psychotherapy handbook*. New York: New American Library, 1980.

Hollon, S. D., & Shaw, B. F. Group cognitive therapy for depressed patients. In A. T. Beck, A. J. Rush, B. F. Shaw, & G. Emery (Eds.), *Cognitive therapy of depression*. New York: Guilford Press, 1979.

Horney, K. *The neurotic personality for our time*. New York: Norton, 1939.

Izard, C. E. *Human emotions*. New York: Plenum, 1977.

Janis, I. L. *Short-term counseling: Guidelines based on recent research*. New Haven: Yale University Press, 1983.

Janis, I. L., & Mann, L. *Decision making: A psychological analysis of conflict, choice, and commitment*. New York: Free Press, 1977.

Kelly, G. A. *The psychology of personal constructs* (Vol. 1). New York: Norton, 1955.

Lazarus, A. *In the mind's eye*. New York: Rawson Publishers, 1977.

Lazarus, A. A. Can RET become a cult? In A. Ellis & J. M. Whiteley (Eds.), *Theoretical and empirical foundations of rational–emotive therapy*. Monterey, Cal.: Brooks/Cole, 1979.

Lazarus, A. A. *The practice of multimodal therapy*. New York: McGraw-Hill, 1981.

Lazarus, R. S. Thoughts on the relations between emotion and cognition. *American Psychologist*, 1982, *37*, 1019–1024.

Lazarus, R. S. & Folkman, S. *Stress, appraisal, and coping*. New York: Springer, 1984.

Mahoney, M. J. *Cognition and behavior modification*. Cambridge, Mass.: Ballinger, 1974.

Mahoney, M. J. Reflection on the cognitive-learning trend in psychotherapy. *American Psychologist*, 1977, *32*, 5–13.

Mahoney, M. J. A critical analysis of rational–emotive theory and therapy. In A. Ellis & J. M. Whiteley (Eds.), *Theoretical and empirical foundations of rational–emotive therapy*. Monterey, Cal.: Brooks/Cole, 1979.

Mahoney, M. J., & Arnkoff, D. Cognitive and self-control therapies. In S. L. Garfield & A. E. Bergin (Eds.), *Handbook of psychotherapy and behavior change: An empirical analysis* (2nd ed.). New York: John Wiley, 1978.

Maultsby, M. C. *Help yourself to happiness*. New York: Institute for Rational Living, 1975.

McGuire, W. M. The nature of attitudes and attitude change. In G. L. Lindzey & E. Aronson (Eds.), *The handbook of social psychology* (Vol 2). Reading, Mass.: Addison-Wesley, 1969.

Meichenbaum, D. H. *Cognitive-behavior modification*. New York: Plenum Press, 1977.

Moore, R. H. Defining the cognitive components of "A" and "B" in RET. *Rational Living*, 1983, *18*(1), 25–28.

Neisser, U. *Cognition and reality*. San Francisco: Freeman, 1976.

Nelson-Jones, R. *The theory and practice of counselling psychology*. London: Holt, Rinehart & Winston, 1982.

Petty, R. E., & Cacioppo. J. T. *Attitudes and persuasion: Classic and contemporary approaches*. Dubuque, Ia.: Brown Publishers, 1981.

Plutchick, R. *Emotion: A psychoevolutionary synthesis*. New York: Harper & Row, 1980.

Raimy, V. *Misunderstandings of the self*. San Francisco: Jossey-Bass, 1975.

Rotter, J. B. *Social learning and clinical psychology*. Englewood Cliifs, N.J.: Prentice-Hall, 1954.

Sank, L. I., & Shaffer, C. S. *A therapist's manual for cognitive behavior therapy in groups*. New York: Plenum Press, 1984.

Schwartz, R. M. Cognitive-behavior modification: A conceptual review. *Clinical Psychology Review*, 1982, *2*, 267–283.

Smith, D. Trends in counseling and psychotherapy. *American Psychologist*, 1982, *37*, 802–809.

Smith, T. W. Irrational beliefs in the cause and treatment of emotional distress: A critical review of the rational–emotive model. *Clinical Psychology Review*, 1982, *2*, 502–522.

Sommers, S. Emotionality reconsidered: The role of cognition in emotional responsiveness. *Journal of Personality and Social Psychology*, 1981, *41*, 553–651.

Strong, S. R., & Claiborn, C. D. *Change through interaction*. New York: Wiley-Interscience, 1982.

Tosi, D. J. Personal reactions with some emphasis on new directions, application, and research. In A. Ellis & J. M. Whiteley (Eds.), *Theoretical and empirical foundations of rational–emotive therapy*. Monterey, Cal.: Brooks/Cole, 1979.

Tosi, D. J., & Baisden, B. Cognitive experiential therapy and hypnosis. In W. Wester & J. Smith (Eds.), *Clinical hypnosis: A multidisciplinary approach*. New York: Lippincott, 1984.

Walen, S. R., DiGiuseppe, R., & Wessler, R. L. *A practitioner's guide to rational–emotive therapy*. New York: Oxford University Press, 1980.

Wessler, R. A., & Wessler, R. L. *The principles and practice of rational–emotive therapy*. San Francisco: Jossey-Bass, 1980.

Wessler, R. L. On measuring rationality. *Rational Living*, 1977, *12*(2), 25–30.

Wessler, R. L. Varieties of cognitions in the cognitively oriented psychotherapies. *Rational Living*, 1982, *17*(1), 3–10.

Wessler, R. L. A critical appraisal of therapeutic outcome studies. *British Journal of Cognitive Psychotherapy*, 1983, *1*, 39–46.

Wessler, R. L. Alternative conceptions of rational–emotive therapy: Toward a philosophically neutral psychotherapy. In M. Reda & M. J. Mahoney (Eds.), *Cognitive psychotherapies: Recent developments in theory, research, and practice*. Cambridge: Ballinger, 1984a.

Wessler, R. L. A bridge too far: Incompatibilities of rational–emotive therapy and pastoral counseling. *The Personnel and Guidance Journal* 1984b, *63*, 264–266.

Wessler, R. L. & Ellis, A. Supervision in rational–emotive therapy. In A. K. Hess (Ed.), *Psychotherapy supervision*. New York: Wiley-Interscience, 1980.

Wessler, R. L., & Hankin, S. W. R. (1986). Cognitive appraisal therapy. In W. Dryden & W. Golden (Eds.), *Cognitive-behavioral approaches to psychotherapy*. London: Harper & Row.

Woods, P. J. A taxonomy of instrumental conditioning. *American Psychologist*, 1974, *29*, 584–597.

Woods, P. J. On the relative independence of irrational beliefs. *Rational Living*, 1983, *18*(1), 23–24.

Woods, P. J. Learning paradigms, expectancies, and behavioural control: An expanded classification for learned behaviour. *British Journal of Cognitive Psychotherapy* 1985, *3*, 43–58.

Zimbardo, P., & Ebbesen, E. G. *Influencing attitudes and changing behavior*. Reading, Mass.: Addison-Wesley, 1969.

GLOSSARY

ABC **Theory or Model.** Ellis's term for his theory of personality and of disturbance. *A* variously stands for activating event, experience, or thought; *B* for beliefs or belief system; *C* for emotional and behavioral consequences.

Active-Directive Therapy. Any form of therapy in which the therapist actively participates, usually by asking questions and offering comments, as opposed to passive listening and/or reflecting whatever the client says. Directive refers to the therapist's structuring the session according to some hypotheses or theory of disturbance.

Anxiety, Ego versus Discomfort. In Ellis's RET, ego anxiety is any anxiety resulting from threats to ego or self-esteem; a fear of demonstrating one's worthlessness or inadequacy to self and/or others. Discomfort anxiety is simply fear of discomfort, either physical or psychological, or of inconvenience, emotional experiences, or difficult tasks.

Appraisal. A mental or cognitive evaluation or rating of an event or experience; appraisals are crucial processes in several theories of emotion.

Cognition. A thought, especially of what one has conscious knowledge; more generally, any idea, image, meaning, or other symbolic representation in one's mind. A "cold" cognition refers to what one knows; a "hot" cognition to an appraisal.

Cognitive Appraisal Therapy. The authors' term for their cognitively oriented therapy derived from Ellis's RET but employing many different philosophical and theoretical assumptions and treatment procedures.

Cognitive Behavior Modification. Meichenbaum's term for his treatment approach that uses silent and aloud statements to direct one's behaviors, especially new behaviors.

Cognitive Behavior Therapy. A generic term that refers to any of several approaches to treatment that are basically behavioral but with additional cognitive dimensions.

Cognitive Disputing. Ellis's term for challenging the logical or empirical basis for one's beliefs.

Cognitively Oriented Psychotherapies. Any form of therapy in which cognitions are assumed to be central in emotional and behavioral processes; these include some approaches, for example, Kelly's, which are not primarily behavior therapy with cognitions added to the account of disturbance or its treatment.

Constructs, Personal. Kelly's theoretical notion about the implicit categories or dimensions which each person develops and employs to construe reality and make sense of one's experiences.

Corrective Experiences. Experiences which lead to modifications of maladaptive thoughts, emotions, and patterns of behavior.

Diathesis. A genetic predisposition to certain diseases.

Direct Feedback. Comments from therapist, group members, or others about a person's behavior, including emotional expressions and verbalizations.

Double-Blind. An experimental design used in drug outcome studies in which neither patients nor drug administrators know what medication the patients receive.

Elegant Solution. Ellis's term for pervasive philosophical restructuring of one's belief system. Ideally, it involves full self-acceptance, nonglobal ratings of other people, and a stoic acceptance of reality. Inelegant solutions to emotional problems consist of either attitude changes about specific events or more accurate perceiving of reality.

Emotional Episode (Cognitive-Emotive-Behavioral Episode). A term introduced by Wessler and Wessler to replace Ellis's *ABC* theory, to account for the interrelations of cognition, emotion, and behavior in a specific situation.

Humanistic Philosophy. Humanism in philosophy rejects notions of divinely given rules for humans to live by, and states that humans are capable of generating their own codes of ethical conduct through their powers to reason. It differs from humanistic psychology, the so-called third force in psychology, which rejects psychoanalysis and behaviorism, and embraces everything human as its proper subject matter.

Iatrogenic. The causation of a new disorder or the worsening of a disorder by the process of treatment itself.

Internal Dialogue. Conversations, usually silent, with oneself.

Low Frustration Tolerance (LFT). In RET, a set of beliefs about one's inability or unwillingness to withstand discomfort, inconvenience, or frustration, or the behavioral consequences of such beliefs, for example, procrastination or other forms of withdrawal or avoidance.

Multimodal Therapy. A. A. Lazarus's term for his approach to treatment, featuring assessment and intervention in seven basic modalities (behavior, affect, sensation, imagery, cognition, interpersonal behavior, and psychological processes); a systematic form of technical eclecticism.

Must-Statement. Any statement that contains an absolutistic must, should, ought, or other unqualified imperative. In RET, must-statements are hypothesized to be central to most emotional disturbance. Ellis occasionally distinguishes between absolute musts and preferential musts, but in practice condemns all musts as the bases of irrational thinking.

Musturbation. A term coined by Ellis to refer to irrational thinking.

Personal Rules of Living (PRL). In CAT, statements of personal values and ideas about the ways people should act and the ways they typically act.

Placebo. In drug outcome studies, an inert substance administered to patients to test the effects of the taking of medication and to differentiate them from the chemical effects of the drug. More generally, any intervention that produces results, due to patients' expectations that they are getting help, whether or not the interventions have proved effective.

Rational Belief versus Irrational Belief. Ellis has provided several sometimes contradictory definitions of rational and irrational beliefs. In general, rational beliefs are either accurate representations of reality or nonexaggerated evaluations, and lead to emotions that appear appropriate to the situation. Irrational beliefs fall along a separate dimension, and consist of distortions of reality, exaggerated evaluations, must-statements, and all other cognitions that theoretically lead to disruptive, inappropriate emotions.

Rational–Emotive Therapy (RET). Ellis's approach to therapy. He distinguishes between general or unpreferential RET, which he claims is synonymous with CBT, and elegant or preferential RET, which has a humanistic philosophical emphasis.

Self-Acceptance. In RET, this term refers to nonrating of self, unlike self-esteem, which implies a positive rating of the self. Self-acceptance rather than self-rating is a goal in RET.

Social Learning Theory. Identified with the work of Bandura and of Rotter, it is a cognitively oriented theory in which people develop expectations or anticipations of their behavior and its outcomes, especially its reinforcing consequences; behavior is understood in terms of expectations about reinforcement rather than a history of reinforcement.

5

Gestalt Group Therapy

ROBERT L. HARMAN

INTRODUCTION

Gestalt therapy needs no introduction to serious students of psychotherapy. Along with the several good books that have been published recently, almost every theory of psychotherapy textbook contains a chapter about Gestalt therapy. Rapidly increasing is the number of journal articles about Gestalt therapy and its use in a wide range of settings with different patient problems. All of this does not mean that Gestalt therapy is well understood. In fact, I find just the opposite; though widely talked about and "used" by psychotherapist, the conceptual understanding of Gestalt therapy is pretty much superficial.

Gestalt Therapy Verbatim by Fritz Perls (1969a) has been widely read and a lot of people confuse this book with the whole of Gestalt therapy. It is far from that. The main theoretical exposition of Gestalt therapy continues to be *Gestalt Therapy: Excitement and Growth in the Human Personality* by Perls, Hefferline, and Goodman (1951).

Yalom's (1975) statement that Gestalt groups are not examples of group psychotherapy indicates a basic misunderstanding of Gestalt group therapy and a lack of awareness of the way Gestalt therapy is practiced. I imagine Yalom to be describing a Fritz Perls's workshop or demonstration and not Gestalt group psychotherapy as I and many others practice it. Several authors (Kepner, 1980; Melnick, 1980; Simkin, 1976a; and Zinker, 1977, 1980) devote all or portions of their books or articles to Gestalt group work. Still, misconceptions persist. My purpose in this chapter is to provide a clear statement about Gestalt group psychotherapy and the ways groups can be led and are led by Gestalt therapists.

DEFINITION

Gestalt therapy is a term used to describe a particular type of psychotherapy, the essence of which is "I and thou, here and now" (Simkin, 1976b, p.

Throughout this chapter I use "we" when writing about something that I believe most Gestalt therapists would agree with; I use "I" when voicing my own opinions and beliefs.

Robert L. Harman • Counseling and Testing Center, University of Central Florida, Orlando, Florida 32816.

226). With the focus of attention on the present ongoing situation, the therapist is an active participant, applying himself in and to the situation in a style that does not violate the integrity of the patient. According to Laura Perls (Rosenfeld, 1978a, p. 26) "Gestalt therapy is existential, experimental, and experiential."

HISTORY

Frederick S. (Fritz) Perls, usually considered the founder of Gestalt therapy, was born in Germany in 1893. He received his medical degree and became a trained psychoanalyst, working with Karen Horney, Clara Happel, and was especially influenced by Wilhelm Reich. The story as Fritz has told it is that Karen Horney referred him to Reich because "he is the only one who might get through to you" (F. Perls, 1969b). In 1929, after completion of his training in psychoanalysis though still a patient, he married Laura Posner, who had received her doctorate from the University of Frankfurt where she majored in Gestalt psychology. The Perls escaped from Nazi Germany in 1933 and, after brief stopovers in Holland and England, settled in South Africa where they established a successful psychoanalytic practice. It was in South Africa that the ideas which gave birth to Gestalt therapy and the break from psychoanalysis were generated by Fritz and Laura Perls. His book, *Ego, Hunger, and Aggression* (F. Perls, 1947), was published while they were still living in South Africa, and although the American edition of this book did not mention it, Laura Perls (Rosenfeld, 1978a) claims to have written the chapters on the "dummy complex" and "the meaning of insomnia." My hunch is that intellectually she made an even larger contribution than those two chapters.

Shortly after World War II the Perls moved to New York City and set up a private practice. In 1951 with Hefferline and Goodman, Fritz Perls published *Gestalt Therapy: Excitement and Growth in the Human Personality*, which remains the primary theoretical statement about Gestalt therapy. The book's first half reports results of some Gestalt experiments developed by Fritz Perls and done by Hefferline's students at Columbia University; the second half, the real meat of the book and *the* theoretical statement about Gestalt therapy, was written by Perls and Goodman. Supposedly, Fritz Perls wrote the original manuscript and it was not very readable, so Paul Goodman was brought in to clear it up. While speaking on this topic in a recent interview (Rosenfeld, 1978a), Laura Perls said that in the published version, Fritz Perls contributed intellectually and Goodman did the actual writing.

At about the same time *Gestalt Therapy* (Perls et al., 1951) was published, the New York Institute for Gestalt Therapy was organized, the "original" fellows of the Institute being Fritz and Laura Perls, Paul Weisz, Paul Goodman, Elliot Shapiro, Sylvester Eastman, and Isadore From (Rosenfeld, 1978b). The Institute began to offer workshops for the training of Gestalt therapists. James S. Simkin, one of the first trainees, worked with Fritz Perls and others at the New York Institute from 1952 to 1955. Later, Simkin was the first Gestalt therapist to settle on the West Coast, where he was in private practice in Los Angeles for many years before moving to Big Sur in the early 1970s. Simkin's practice, now, is devoted exclusively to the training of other psychotherapists in Gestalt therapy. Fritz Perls laid the initial groundwork by giving some workshops in Cleveland and, in 1952, Isadore From started going to Cleveland on a regular basis to train five or six psychologists in Gestalt therapy (Rosenfeld, 1978b). Later, these people organized the Gestalt Institute of Cleveland, which remains today one of the leading training institutes.

The real boost to the popularization of Gestalt therapy is attributable to several factors. *Gestalt Therapy Verbatim* (1969a) and *In and Out of the Garbage Pail* (1969b), two of Fritz Perls's books, became widely read. But even before the publication of these books the popularity of Fritz Perls had spread and become legend while he was at the Esalen Institute in Big Sur, California. Perls, James Simkin, and Walter Kempler led the first Gestalt therapy training workshop at Esalen in 1963. From this, Gestalt therapy has burgeoned to the point where there are now nearly 80 training centers listed in the *Gestalt Directory 1977*, as well as several hundred Gestalt therapists.

GOALS

Awareness and contact stand out as the paramount goals of Gestalt therapy and both of these concepts are discussed in detail in the theory section of this chapter. Several other lesser goals can be enumerated. For example, I published an article on the goals of Gestalt therapy (Harman, 1974) in which I listed the following goals: (1) awareness, (2) integration, (3) maturation, (4) responsibility, (5) authenticity, (6) self-regulation, and (7) behavior change.

Zinker (1977, pp. 96–97) states "Gestalt therapy does not seek to fit people into molds, to deny that goals are implicit in the therapy would be unrealistic." Zinker goes on to say that through involvement in the Gestalt process, it is his hope that a person:

> (1) Moves toward a greater awareness of self—body, feelings, environment; (2) learns to take ownership of experiences, rather than projecting them onto others; (3) learns to be aware of needs and to develop skills to satisfy her or himself without violating others; (4) moves toward a fuller contact with sensations, learning to smell, taste, touch, hear and see—to savor all aspects of his or her self; (5) moves toward the experience of personal power and the ability to be self-supporting, rather than rely on whining, blaming, or guilt making in order to mobilize support from the environment; (6) becomes sensitive to surroundings, yet at the same time wears a coat of armor for situations which are potentially destructive or poisonous; (7) learns to take responsibility for his or her actions and their consequences; and (8) feels comfortable with the expression of his or her fantasy life and its expression. (Zinker, 1977, 96–97)

Although the goals listed by Harman (1974) and Zinker (1977) are certainly appropriate, and few Gestalt therapists would disagree with them, they can all be subsumed under the terms *awareness* and *contact*. In other words, it is through awareness that one knows if one is responsible or authentic, or if one is in contact with sensations, and so forth. Without awareness and contact we are lulled into believing that we are doing what we think we are doing.

The goals discussed here are applicable to therapy done individually or in groups. Gestalt therapists are interested in individuals in the group and not the group *per se*. The integrity of an individual would never be violated in order to achieve some group developmental stage.

THEORY

Basic Concepts

Necessary to the understanding of Gestalt therapy are a number of basic concepts. Foremost and underlying our theoretical approach and much of our practice is the concept of awareness, defined by Perls *et al.* (1951) as "the spontaneous sensing of what arises in you, of what you are doing, feeling, planning." When people are aware they know what they are doing. This is not as simple as it sounds. For example, it is possible to "feel" one's facial expression and know that sadness is being expressed; or, to be aware that one is strutting and preening in order to impress another person.

Several levels of awareness are possible. First of all, we can be aware of our emotional state; that is, we can feel sad, joyous, loving, and so forth. Second, we can be aware of our physical state. At this level of physical awareness we might be in touch with such feelings as tension, tightness, tingling, posture, breathing, physical discomfort, or pleasurable sensations. Third, we can be aware of what is "out there" in the environment, utilizing the sensory system, seeing, hearing, touching, smelling, and tasting. Sometimes guesses and interpretations are confused with this third level of awareness. I have heard people say, "I'm aware that you are sad"; this is not awareness, instead it is a guess, hunch, or interpretation. A more accurate response based on awareness might be, "I notice that your eyes are teary and your lips are trembly," or "I'm aware of thinking that you are sad."

In a broad sense, then, awareness means knowing what we are doing, which includes knowing about one's motives and intentions. When we have full awareness we can take over our own lives, for this permits us to rely on our own organism to tell us what to do, to make our own decision, to be self-sufficient. When we are totally aware we know what is necessary to satisfy ourselves, and we do not need some external source to guide our lives. Awareness is helpful in making decisions; it helps us pick and choose that which is nourishing for us. Without this awareness, decisions might be based on what someone else thinks is good for us.

Gestalt therapists frequently speak of "contact." Perls *et al.* defined it as "the awareness of, and behavior toward, the assimilable; and the rejection of the unassimilable novelty" (1951, p. 230). Seeing, hearing, touching, talking, moving, smelling, and tasting are sensory motor components involved singularly, or in some combination during contact. Acknowledging, recognizing, and coping with the "other" in our existence constitutes contact. While contacting this "other," we have an awareness of what is "me and not me." When we are able to maintain our awareness of this boundary that separates "me and not me," then excitement and growth are possible.

As Gestalt therapists we are interested in how our patients contact other people, or we are concerned with how they avoid contact. Our patients' intellectualization is a way of talking about and not talking to. Gestalt therapy has no inherent opposition to intellectualization as long as patients do not drain off energy and excitement and prevent a contactful encounter. We must remember that, from a Gestalt point of view, it is at the contact boundary that the possibility for excitement and growth resides.

Zinker (1977), describing the awareness–excitement–contact cycle, indicates the various stages a person goes through from withdrawal to contact to be: (1) withdrawal, (2) sensation, (3) awareness, (4) mobilization of energy, (5) action, (6) contact, and (7) withdrawal. (p. 97). One male member of the group might be working with the therapist on a problem of relating to the coldness of his mother. Another female participant, looking on, may become aware of a warmth in her chest and a tingling in her arms. She then associates the sensation of warmth and tingling with a desire to mother and contact the other patient in some way. Feeling fully expressed, she then can go on in her role as participant in the work of the patient and therapy can resume. When this awareness–contact cycle is not interrupted, a person becomes aware of a need and fulfills it through one of the contact functions. In other words, when the contact–withdrawal cycle is functioning properly, a person is able to pay attention to, to concentrate on what is novel and assimilable in the environment; a clear figure emerges and the person does what is necessary in order to fulfill that need. The figure then fades into the background and the person is in a state of withdrawal or stasis until this whole process starts over again. At times Perls (1969a) referred to this as the process of "destroying gestalts," or "destructuring gestalts"; when this takes place the emerging gestalt becomes a need and either is destroyed through assimilation or is rejected. In either case, the person returns to a state of withdrawal on the contact–withdrawal cycle.

We can now begin to understand how Gestalt therapy is grounded in Gestalt psychology; the awareness–contact cycle is another way of describing the formation and destruction of gestalts, and the figure–ground relationship. Out of the ground of all the possibilities in our environment a gestalt begins to emerge. This gestalt or figure may be experienced as a need to express ourselves to others, the awareness of a bodily need, the intention to gain knowledge; the figure or gestalt then stands out from the background until we have satisfied our need in some way, in which case it then is destroyed or destructured and fades into the background. For example, a male participant in a group might become aware of certain sensations in his body; let us say his arms and upper body begin to tighten and he feels heat rising to his face. He knows that for him this is resentment and it is his response to what has been said to him by another group member. These feelings and the need to express them then become foreground (figure) for him; he can then decide to express himself in some contactful way, such as "I don't like what you said to me," "I resent that," or "when you say that I become tense and feel hot." When he does so, that gestalt fades into background so that another clear figure can emerge. If, on the other hand, this person interrupts his expression in some way, the gestalt might become fixed and interfere with this healthy process of gestalt formation and destruction. In Gestalt-therapy jargon, this becomes "unfinished business" (Perls, 1969a).

"Every healthy contact involves awareness (perceptual figure/ground) and excitement (increased energy mobilization)" (Perls et al., 1951, p. 118). To assimilate or reject that which is novel, there must be some excitement, some manifested energy by way of interest and attention. That is, contact cannot be made unless in some way one is drawn toward the figure. Contact, then, is a natural result of experiencing novelty, of following up on interests, and of satisfying needs. The natural experience of true contact is enlivening, as opposed to the dullness, staleness, or draining that results from a forced making of contact.

As I have already stated, the basic concepts of Gestalt therapy have a *strong* theoretical foundation. Serious students of Gestalt therapy know this. Psychotherapists who use a "little Gestalt," "combine TA and Gestalt," or whatever, violate the essence of Gestalt therapy, a holistic approach in which the therapist is dedicated to restoring the awareness continuum and expanding the contact boundaries.

Assumptions about Human Nature

A basic assumption in Gestalt therapy is that of organismic self-regulation. We all have the innate capacity to take care of ourselves. More specifically, we have the ability to meet our own needs through picking and choosing from the environment that which benefits us. This, of course, does not mean that we always choose correctly, that there are no mistakes; it does mean that we can recover from poor choices and not be incapacitated, but through organismic self-regulation we can then make a more nourishing choice.

F. Perls et al. (1951, p. 247) wrote that "it is not necessary deliberately to encourage, to schedule, or to inhibit the prompting of appetite, sensuality, and so forth, in the interests of health and morals. If these things are let be, they will spontaneously right themselves, and if they have been deranged, they will tend to right themselves." For this kind of self-regulation to work we need to trust the wisdom of the organism. We, as individuals, know what is best for us through the awareness continuum. "Awareness," as Zinker states, "is a blessing because it enables me to understand what is going on inside, and what I can do to make me feel better" (1977, p. 90).

I do not want to give the mistaken implication that organismic self-regulation is appropriate for physiological needs only. I have learned to use organismic self-regulation, for example, when I am approached about giving a speech, teaching a class, or presenting a paper. Before responding to the request for services I focus my awareness on my stomach. If I am feeling nothing in my stomach, I say "yes" to the request; if I experience "butterflies" and a whirling sensation, I say "no." I have rarely made a "bad" choice in these matters since I have learned to trust my organism. In this same vein, Simkin (1976b, p. 228) wrote:

> Recently a patient was describing a conflict between continuing a project on his own that he had begun with a partner or dropping the project. His truth button was a hard, rocklike feeling in the pit of his stomach. He worked through his conflict by imagining first he would continue the project without his partner and would see it through the acquiring of property, erecting a building, and manufacturing the article in the new plant. As he fantasized these various steps, he experienced increasing discomfort in his stomach; his "rock" was getting more and more unbearable. He then proceeded to fantasize dropping the project, abandoning the plans that had already been made plus his investment of time and money. At this point, he reported feeling more relaxed and comfortable, especially in the pit of his stomach. Experimenting several times (reversing so that at times he fantasized giving up the project first and at other times continuing the project first) brought the same results. The patient became convinced that he knew via his truth button which was the appropriate decision for him.

As organismic self-regulating people or individuals, we use our intellect as well as our senses and emotions, in a balance of all three modes of experiencing.

Most people who come for therapy experience a disturbance in this capacity to be organismically self-regulating. The work of the therapist, therefore, is to help patients regain this capacity to take care of themselves. Disturbances usually are the result of the familiar mechanisms of projection, introjection, retroflection, and deflection.

Personality Theory

Gestalt therapists are not primarily concerned with the development of a theory of personality. However, this does not mean that we lack assumptions about the motivational and emotional traits that distinguish people from each other. We also have some ideas about the drives or inner forces that influence the way we interact with our environment. Fritz Perls's first book, *Ego, Hunger, and Aggression* (1947), grew from his ideas about "oral resistance." From this early work we have come to recognize oral aggression, or dental aggression as some prefer to call it, as the basic drive to preserve the individual, as contrasted to the sexual drive which preserves the species. The infant is first a suckling, that is, all he needs to do is to suck and swallow. Little aggression is required at this point, and according to Perls *et al.* (1951) this amounts to total introjection, because the material, food, is swallowed whole. This is healthy behavior at this stage for it is the only way that infants can nourish themselves. The infant goes from being a suckling to a biteling. During this stage infants become more active, more aggressive in the process of taking in food; they bite and chew. And, as all parents know, they learn to reject what they do not like. As a biter and chewer a person is actively involved in the destruction of food. Destruction is necessary for the food to be digested, to be assimilated; when this is done properly, the nutrients literally are transformed and become the person. This process of destruction and transformation is essential for physical growth. Perls, *et al.* (1951) went on to say that

> instead of accepting what is given and uncritically introjecting it, the "chewling" works over what is provided by the environment so as to insure his assimilation of it. It is on the basis of such competence, combined with almost complete development of sensory discrimination and perception of objects, that the child begins to speak and bring to a head the process of forming his "I". (pp. 224–225)

This stage is not without trauma. When the nursing baby cuts teeth the confluent relationship between mother and child is altered. What once was a pleasurable time for the mother can now be filled with pain and the baby can discover that the nipple is offered conditionally, or that he is punished for biting. Improper weaning can result in forcing solid food on the child and in the child's consequently learning to "swallow whole" without much chewing or tasting.

Consider some analogous adult behavior. We describe gullible people as "swallowing anything." Some adults are not very adept at chewing and assimilating new "material"; they take it in chunks without it really becoming a part of them. Some therapists even swallow therapeutic material in chunks; they take in *all* Gestalt therapy, for instance, in one gulp, and employ a "Gestalt technique" without using much aggression in studying and digesting the theory; instead, they introject the techniques. On the other hand, there are those who resist taking in much that is new. Sometimes they literally have their jaws "locked" in grim determination to prevent anything being forced on them. In their efforts to prevent having something shoved down their throats, they resist a lot of nourishment. It is during this "suckling to biteling to chewling" stage that the early groundwork for discrimination and differentation is laid. The first experiences of "I," or the "self," or "what is me and not me" also occur during this crucial stage of development.

Homeostasis, a governing force within humans, is a way of maintaining balance, equilibrium. Physiologically, this process of homeostasis is easily understood. For example, when our body liquids are low we experience certain sensations that we label as thirst; we then drink, our physiological balance is restored, and the sensations disappear. Psychologically, the homeostatic process is more difficult to describe. At any given time, the most paramount need will stand out as foreground and the other needs will recede into the background. To attend to whatever figure becomes foreground is a way of restoring our balance, our equilibrium. That figure then fades and another one begins to emerge. Right now, what I am writing is foreground for me, everything else is background. Last night, as I wrote, I began to distract myself about the whereabouts of my son; I created some mental pictures of him until finally, I phoned him. There was no answer, but the need to contact my son receded into the background and my writing again became figural. This is the homeostatic process at work.

For individuals to be self-regulating, to satisfy their needs, they must be able to sense their most important need, to do what is necessary in closing the gestalt; then the whole process repeats itself. One way that we become neurotic is to lose the ability to sense our most important need at any given time. We might interfere with our process of homeostasis through socialization, by doing what we think we should do, by accumulating "unfinished business," incomplete gestalts. Thus we do not know what is foreground, or by "hanging on" we thereby prohibit the formation of new gestalts.

Finally, and very importantly, Gestalt therapists take a holistic view of man. "A holistic understanding of man," according to Latner (1973, p. 6),

> brings the functioning of his physical body, his emotions, his thoughts, his culture, and his social expressions into a unified picture. They are all aspects of the same client—man. The mind does not cause the body to operate, nor the body the mind; to conceive of things in that way is to emphasize their separateness. Instead, the pounding of our heart, our excitement, and the concurrent anxiety are manifestations of the same occurrence, like the heat and the light from the sun. Holistically, we cannot understand ourselves by summing our understanding of our heart, our brain, our nervous system, our limbs, our circulatory system. We are not simply an accumulation of functions. The ordinary language expression for this is: The whole is greater than the sum of its parts. "Greater" means difference in quality from; it also refers to the entirety of the object or event. Therefore, the whole is a new event, as water is greater than two parts of hydrogen and one part of oxygen, and the hand is greater than four fingers and a thumb.

This holistic approach, adhered to by Gestalt therapists, espouses the belief that normal, healthy man reacts as a whole, not as a disorganized organism. This approach empahsizes the unity and integration of the "normal" personality. Any fragmentation is objected to. Some systems of therapy tend to deal only with the cognitive aspects and ignore the sensory and emotional modes of experiencing. The statement by Straus (1963), "Man thinks, not the brain," appropriately reflects the Gestalt therapy point of view.

Comparisons with Related Theories

The differences between Gestalt therapy and other therapeutic approaches are quite noticeable. Rational–Emotive Therapy (RET) espouses the belief that what we say to ourselves influences what we feel. I do not particularly disagree with this; I just think it is incomplete. Try the reverse: What we feel influences what we say to ourselves.

The RET assumption seems to be that all people are internally auditory. I do not think that is true. Recent work by Grinder and Bandler (1976) has exquisitely demonstrated that people represent their experiences visually and kinesthetically as well as auditorially. From watching the famous film series of Perls, Ellis, and Rogers, all working with the same client, Gloria, it becomes apparent that the RET therapist, as exemplified by Ellis, tries to argue the patient out of some belief. This "persuading," on the part of the therapist aims to convince the patient of the "irrationality" of the belief. I disagree with this approach and contend that it violates the basic Gestalt principle of working with the patient "where she is."

Whenever I work with someone who has been to a Transactional Analysis (TA) therapist before coming to me, I hear statements like, "That's my child saying that," or "I have a really powerful parent." Patients speak as if it is not even them who has said or done something, but rather their "parent" or "child." This practice reinforces splits, disowning, and fragmentation. I believe that implicit in TA therapy is the belief that "one should be in their adult." This runs counter to the Gestalt beliefs of integration and freedom from "shoulds."

Some popular schools of therapy (Carkhuff, 1969; Egan, 1975) emphasize empathy. In fact, empathic responses are rated and said to fall into various levels. Counselors and therapists are taught to give the highest level response they can. From my observations of therapists who adhere to these systems I notice that they spend a lot of time "trying" to give a level-5 response. That is, much of the time they are withdrawn into their own heads trying to figure out what a level-5 response would be. I think this reinforces two things: therapist incongruity and lack of authenticity.

The emphasis of psychoanalysis is on the past, on explanations, and on interpretations; Gestalt therapy differs greatly. We consider these three areas by-products of our therapy instead of the central focus, as they are with some psychoanalysts. In other words, patients might understand themselves better as a result of Gestalt therapy, but this would come out of their experience in therapy and would seldom be accepted as a working goal by most Gestalt therapists. Regarding interpretation, Applebaum (1976, pp. 756) stated:

> Gestalt therapists minimize and some no doubt abstain completely from explicitly interpretive or "explaining" remarks. Thus, they try not to tell the patient in so many words about himself (although I *have* seen this done by some esteemed Gestalt therapists along with hortatory, educative, inspirational, and summing up comments). They do make highly educated guesses about what to emphasize, what roles to play out in dialogue, what should be repeated louder, what elements in a dream should be attended to—all under a guiding clinical sophistication, reflecting *their* insight or awareness and encouraging the same in the patient.

Gestalt therapists regard highly the integrity of the individual. Therefore, we resist offering interpretations or explanations that would invade that integrity. We do not assume to know more about patients than do the patients themselves.

THERAPY

Theory

Just as it is not enough to use techniques without theory, it is not enough to be well-grounded in theory and unskilled in applying the knowledge to groups. In the next three sections on therapy, practice, and application I will attack the problem of synthesizing these parts into the process which is Gestalt therapy.

Because we believe that awareness alone can be curative and furthermore that awareness at all times is necessary to start the curative process, Gestalt therapists spend a great deal of time facilitating group members' awareness. Awareness gets at the "hows" and "whats" in a patient's existence. The "hows" and "whats" tend to reinforce the present-centeredness of Gestalt therapy. "Whys," on the other hand, are deemphasized and are viewed as fostering excuses and rationalizations; "whys" frequently lead to a focus on the past.

Gestalt therapists believe that awareness and contact, among other things, make behavior change possible. It is by being aware that one can "contact" with other group members and therapists. Therefore, the therapist works with the group in a variety of ways to develop awareness and contact, and to help participants discover their ways of blocking and avoiding these naturally curative processes.

Critics frequently criticize Gestalt therapy groups because there is no interaction, saying they are really doing individual work in the presence of others. At times this is true, but often it is nonsense. Simkin (1976a, p. 16) stated: "In Gestalt therapy it is not necessary to emphasize the group dynamics, although some Gestalt therapists do. All Gestalt therapists focus at one time or another on the interactive process between the therapist and the group member in the here and now and/or the interactive process between group members as it is ongoing." For a Gestalt therapist to be disinterested in group dynamics is acceptable, but to deny their existence belies his or her expertise. A critic who states that Gestalt therapists are unaware of and do not utilize group dynamics and processes is limited in his understanding of the scope of Gestalt group psychotherapy. So the matter appears to be up to the therapist's individual preference and individual style. The continuum appears to consist, on the one hand, of doing individual work within a group and, on the other, of focusing on Gestalt group process.

After running ongoing Gestalt groups since 1972, my experience is that I could not stop interaction if I wanted to. I definitely pay attention to group dynamics and occasionally make "process comments" (Yalom notwithstanding). Anyone who keeps up with Gestalt literature, for example Polster and Polster (1973), Zinker (1977), and Rosenblatt (1975), would know that it is incorrect to assume that there is no group interaction and that therapists pay no attention to dynamics in Gestalt groups. Zinker (1977, p. 161) stated: "Gestalt group process, as it has been developed at our institute in Cleveland, operates according to four basic principles: (1) the primacy of present ongoing group experiences; (2) the process of developing group awareness; (3) the importance of active contact between participants; and (4) the use of interactional experiments stimulated by an actively involved leader." Polster and Polster (1973, p. 28) wrote about Gestalt groups. "Going beyond the hot seat and including the spontaneous participation of the rest of the group broadens the dimensions of interaction—well *within the range* of Gestalt methodology."

Furthermore, Rosenblatt's (1975) vivid description of one of his groups pointed out the interactional and participatory spirit of his group. Interaction, then, certainly occurs in many Gestalt groups and many Gestalt therapists pay attention to group dynamics.

We do not want to throw out the baby with the bath water! Gestalt therapy offers a powerful way for individuals to change their behavior and that style of working in groups ought to be preserved along with the more recent emphasis on group process. One-to-one work, that is, the therapist working with one individual within the group, may occur in any group and has a number of advantages over private sessions. First, the working client is usually energized by the process of becoming the center of attention; working in front of a group can be singularly exciting. Second, the client who agrees to work in front of others is learning to take responsibility for his or her own behavior, is learning assertive behavior, and is learning to deal with acceptance or rejection by others. Third, by observing group interaction, the therapist can see how an individual patient interacts and can consequently direct awareness and group experience appropriately. Fourth, the nonworking group members are given the opportunity to extract and assimilate personal meaning from the work being done. Finally, the group can be used experimentally in ways not possible in private sessions (Polster & Polster, 1973).

It is nearly impossible for 6 to 10 people to gather weekly over a period of time and not have anything to say to each other. How participants affect each other and what impact they exert on the group are grist for the therapeutic mill. At times when group members want to interact with each other, the therapist will become more background and become a facilitator rather than work directly with one of the group members. The therapist facilitates awareness and contact by making sure that participants are not "laying trips" on each other, pushing someone around, or in some other way violating the privacy and integrity of other group members. If group members are communicating in a contactful way, that is, with awareness, there is no need for therapist intervention. The therapist can then become an active observer while the interaction continues to a natural conclusion.

Becoming an "active observer" involves several options. One possibility is to pay attention to the entire group. Who is participating in the interaction and who is not? How are group members reacting? Do they look interested, "turned off," angry, energized, agitated? The therapist, in addition, might focus awareness on any themes that are re-emerging; that is, if the interaction involves/concerns a specific topic, say the expression of anger, are the same persons involved and the same ones withdrawn as happened the last time? As an "active observer" the therapist should constantly remain alert to the need to intervene in case one person is pushing another around, or in case a participant is not capable of taking care of her or himself and is being overwhelmed.

Generally, our theory of putting people together in Gestalt groups is that the activity in a group creates the possibilities for behavior change. More specifically, we believe that awareness and contact, as developed in Gestalt groups, allow participants to make nourishing decisions about their lives.

Process and Mechanisms

Process and mechanism in Gestalt therapy are intertwined and difficult to separate. Mechanisms seem to be the same as "techniques" and I admit to a bias against techniques (Harman, 1977). I agree with Laura Perls (1978, p. 32) when she says, "A good therapist does not use techniques, he applies himself in and to a situation with whatever knowledge, skills, and total life experience have become integrated into his own background and whatever awareness he has at any given moment. Thus I speak of styles of therapy rather than techniques." However, I am not inflexible, and for the sake of clarity will include in this section what might be called mechanisms or techniques.

The term process can have several meanings in Gestalt therapy. First of all, it can refer to the dynamics of the group, that is, what is actually said and experienced by members of the group as well as a sort of "collective process" reflected in statements like, "The group was sad today." Second, process can refer to the mechanisms, techniques, experiments, or interventions employed by the therapist as he works with the group. Third, from a strictly Gestalt point of view, process could be considered as the awareness and contact functions within a group. Finally, we can consider the process of what goes on within the therapist as he or she leads a group; how the therapist combines style, artistry, techniques, skill, and theoretical knowledge in order to accomplish the group's goals.

A Gestalt group, with its "here and now" emphasis, is a lively, exciting, energizing place to spend some time. This does not imply fun and games. Experiences range from joy and hilarity to pain and suffering, and even to grief. The experience and expression of these feelings becomes possible when participants permit themselves to be aware and to express and share this awareness with the therapist and the group. Gestalt therapists promote this process by directly asking from time to time for participants to contact and report what they are experiencing. The therapist may ask, "What are you aware of now?" "What's happening?" "What are you doing?" "Where are you?" and so on. These statements by therapists reinforce awareness and help to establish a sharing and interacting climate within the group. The message that group members can talk about what is happening to them remains both explicit and implicit. It is apparent then that Gestalt therapy is more direct than are most schools of therapy in attempting to establish a "here and now" focus in the group interaction.

Development of awareness may occur when an individual has asked "to work on" a specific problem. If the therapist agrees, the rest of the group may become background as he or she focuses awareness and attention solely on the "working" patient for a while. Although at these times the work is concentrated on the one patient, this does not mean that the "nonworking" group members withdraw. They may be very actively involved and closely identify with what is going on; some may be stimulated by what the other person is working on and start to internally articulate problems of a similar nature; some may become aware of their disgust and revulsion at the nature of the work;

others might be completely uninterested and withdraw into their own unrelated fantasies.

In the flux of such group energies, Gestalt therapists have their individual styles for working with the group. Some might do nothing overt, allowing participants to decide for themselves about what they want to do; patients can then discover when they can interact in the group process or when they prefer to remain withdrawn from it. Other Gestalt therapists prefer to be more active, inquiring directly of "nonworking" patients. At other times, the group-oriented Gestalt therapist might respond to nonverbal expressions of clients. He or she may notice one client's physically "drawing away" or sitting back from the group at the onset of working with another client on a given subject. Thus the inquiry: "Bill, I'm wondering if you have anything to say?" or "June, you always seem to look away when René works." Such process-oriented statements, based on the perceptions of the therapist and put out by the therapist without any preconceived ideas about what will happen, draw responses which run the gamut from, "Yeah, so what?" to "Yes, and I would like to work on that."

Interaction is further promoted in Gestalt group therapy by encouraging and reinforcing feedback. Authentic sharing and self-disclosing helps develop a spirit of trust and mutuality, even if it is noncomplimentary. Patients are encouraged to talk or share with others their own inner experience. It is not unusual to hear: "I really identify with you," "I feel warm and tender toward you," or "I don't like what you were doing, I am turned off."

"Dual focus" Gestalt group therapy is a phrase coined by my colleague, Ken Tarleton, to describe the kind of Gestalt group work that I do and about which I am writing here. The dual focus blends group process with the power of individual work within a group. In focusing thus, therapists do not have to choose one or the other directions, but can integrate group process and dynamics into a Gestalt therapy mode.

When giving feedback, patients are discouraged from advising, instructing or questioning. This is to discourage noncontactful ways of interacting. "Why did you do that?" frequently is just a disguise for "I don't approve of what you did." This noncontactful interaction distances group members. In light of such interaction Gestalt therapists can and do make much therapeutic "hay" with group dynamics and process.

Using the group experimentally, as part of one patient's work, transforms groups into a laboratory for trying out and developing new behaviors. Suppose, for example, that a male group member says he cannot talk to women and wants to work on that. One possibility is to ask him to say something to each female group member and to be aware of himself as he does so. Or, on the other hand, he could be asked to say something to every group member, both male and female, and to be aware of differences within himself as he does. During or after such an experiment, some group members may want to give feedback to the "worker." This can be a powerful learning experience, especially when it is discovered that "talking to women" is possible and that the dreaded consequences of talking to women did not occur.

Experiments do not necessarily include other group members. Whether they do or not depends on the style and creativity of the therapist. Experiments are used as ways of involving the patient and group experientially and avoiding the dullness that comes from "talking about" a problem. Patients are "invited," never coerced, to participate in an experiment, which if accepted in good faith and openness, without predictions, will lead to new learning about themselves. Experiments are always based on the phenomenology of the individual or group and are never preplanned or "packaged," and, according to Zinker (1977, pp. 123–124), "can involve every sphere of human functioning; however, most experiments have one quality in common—they ask the client to express something behaviorally, rather than to merely cognize an experience internally."

Polster and Polster (1973) have categorized experiments into five modes: (1) enactment, (2) directed behavior, (3) fantasy, (4) dreams, and (5) homework. Enactment, which aids in working through unfinished situations from a person's life, permits the patient to gain a new perspective while antiquated ways of behaving give way to invigorating new behavioral possibilities. Enactment may be used in dealing with polarities, such as strength and weakness. For example, patients may enact dialogues in which they play both their perceived strengths and weaknesses. Directed behaviors may be employed to exaggerate and accentuate certain behaviors; for example, we might ask a patient who is a monotonous speaker to speak with more monotone. Fantasy can be used as an alternative in the session when it is impractical to experience something directly. I once asked a patient who complained of "never having fun" to fantasize having fun and to put me in the fantasy with her. She launched into a fantasy of the two of us preparing a gourmet meal together, while I reported my fantasy of attending a Willie Nelson concert with her. This seemed to loosen up both of us and added zest to our therapy.

Gestalt dreamwork is fairly well known due largely to the numerous demonstrations, books, and films of Fritz Perls. Dr. Perls believed the dream was projection, everything in a dream being a part of the dreamer. Following this lead, the therapeutic task, then, consists of guiding the dreamer into "becoming" the various parts of the dream so that disowned, alienated parts of the self are embraced. The dream may contain, for example, a tree whose aspects (rootedness, straightness, broadness, etc.) can be owned as psychological aspects of the dreamer. Certainly an accepted way of working on a dream both in a group and individually, this is, however, not the only way. Recently Isadore From (Rosenfeld, 1978b) wrote about treating the dream as a retroflection, especially if it occurred the day before or the day after a therapy session. If the patient dreams of murder or violence, hostility or anger toward the therapist could be explored. Zinker (1971) uses dreamwork as theatre, where in a psychodramatic fashion group members play out parts of a dream.

Finally, homework may be assigned to a patient. Like other experiments, homework must be based on the phenomenology of the patient and on particular problem areas that emerge in the group. One of my patients once seemed compelled to be "open," wanting to disclose to the group every detail of his life. He went on to say that liveliness in his relationships was diminished and he imagined people to be avoiding him. I suggested that during the ensuing week, that he experiment with "keeping a secret," and that he might even want to tell a few friends that he "has a secret." At the next group meeting he reported a new effervescence to his life; just having a secret had made him livelier.

Experiments are based on the belief that learning requires action. Besides being involved in a cognitive way, the patient may be honing his awareness, having contact with other members of the group, or utilizing some sensorimotor aspect of himself. The goals of Gestalt experiments according to Zinker (1977, p. 126) are: (1) to expand the person's repertoire of behaviors; (2) to create conditions under which the person can see life as his or her *own creation*; (3) to stimulate the person's experiential learning and the evolution of new self-concepts from behavioral creations; (4) to complete unfinished situations and overcome blockages in the awareness–excitement–contact cycle; (5) to integrate cortical understandings with motoric expressions; (6) to discover polarizations which are not in awareness; (7) to stimulate the integration of conflictual forces in the personality; (8) to dislodge and reintegrate introjects and generally place "misplaced" feelings, ideas, and actions where they belong in the personality; and (9) to stimulate circumstances under which the person can feel and act stronger, more competent, more self-supported, more explorative and actively responsible to him or herself.

By now it should be obvious that Gestalt therapists spend time and energy developing the awareness of group members. Perhaps not so obvious is the meaning of contact. Remember that contact is the acknowledgment of the other while maintaining a sense of self. "Through contact, each person has a chance to meet the world outside himself nourishingly. . . . In contacting you, I wager my independent existence, but only through the contact function can the realization of our identities fully develop" (Polster & Polster, 1973, p. 99). Consistent with the Gestalt paradoxical theory of change (Beisser, 1970) is our belief that through contact one need not strive for change, because change is absolutely unavoidable. After a contactful encounter I am no longer the same person; if I have assimilated something new I must change. The same male group member who complained that he "couldn't talk to women" was asked if he would be willing to say that to each woman in the group; he did. After the first encounter he turned to me and said he was shaking. I suggested he allow himself to shake and continue with the experiment. With the second woman he became more talkative, verbally acknowledging that even though he felt shaky, he *was* talking to her. By the time he reached the last woman in the group he felt and acted like a different man; his shaking had changed to excitement, he looked alive and solid, his voice resonated. Women in the group began to respond to him, engaging him in contactful ways. After a time, still flushed with excitement, he said to me: "Well Bob, I can talk to women when I want to." After he had destroyed his myth, experientially learning from contact with others, he was no longer the same.

Patients interfere with contact in myriad ways, with projection, deflection, introjection, retroflection, and confluence leading the way. *Projection* is a common behavior in groups because projectors attribute to others their own feelings and thoughts. No matter what was said to Colleen by Jim and Cathy, she "knew" they did not like her. When I asked how she knew that, Colleen became confused, finally stating she just knew. I suggested she "try on" the reverse, that she state to Jim and Cathy, "I don't like you." With that she perked up, and after saying my sentence, spontaneously went into what she did not like about Jim and Cathy. Invigorated by her contact with Jim and Cathy, Colleen was willing, when asked, to role play, saying all the things to herself that she had said to the other two. This produced a surprised, "yes, yes, yes! Those are all the things I can't stand in me." Reowning what she had projected onto Jim and Cathy increased Colleen's self-identity and permitted her to have contact in a nourishing way.

In *deflection*, another way of interfering with contact, the person turns aside or in some way defuses possible contact. Words from others seem to have little effect, they bounce off as if from invisible shields. Deflections serve to "water down" feelings; not only do they weaken the impact others have on us, they also sap the vitality of our own responses. In group, the deflectors' responses will often seem inappropriate or out of context, or they may seem confused and "off the mark." A recently divorced man was disclosing to group the agony he experienced each time he said goodbye after visiting his children. One group member asked him how many children he had, another asked how often he visited them, and the therapist-in-training asked how old they were. These statements helped to get away from whatever feelings were being aroused in the group members and in the therapist. The divorced man may also have been led from his feelings to a "talking about" interaction.

I believe that in the early developmental stages of a group, projection and deflection will be particularly evident. This necessitates an especially keen awareness during early group sessions so that we can intervene when necessary, facilitating the reowning of feelings and establishing contact between patients. This is not to say that projection and deflection do not occur throughout the stages of a group; they do. It is just that these two ways of interfering with contact surface early and must be worked with effectively if the group is to progress.

Through the process of *introjection* people take in beliefs, values, and feelings from others. The material taken in is not assimilated and remains as an unintegrated part of the person's personality. Introjectors report experiencing themselves as phony, superficial, automatic, and not feeling close to people; and it is not unusual for others to have similar impressions of them. Introjectors make poor contact, as they have difficulty developing a sense of "me and not me." They have taken in so much from others that they literally have no self-identity.

The astute Gestalt therapist will recognize introjectors by their compliance. Introjectors experiment willingly and appear to get little from it, or, they get what they think they "should" get, parroting the good patient. Introjectors tend to "swallow whole," without chewing or evaluating to see if the material suits them. Because introjectors are so solicitous, Gestalt therapists must be particularly careful to avoid giving advice to them.

Of primary importance when working with introjectors is establishing a firm sense of boundary, or what is "me and not me." Working with Mike, I began to suspect he was taking in everything I said without discriminating, so I suggested that he stand up, then sit down, stand up, sit down, and so on. This went on for several minutes, by now the rest of the group had caught on. Finally Mike said, "No, I won't do this anymore." This experiment permitted Mike to make a choice and to experience a sense of self-identity. Any kind of interaction in which the introjector makes "I" statements may help to undo the introjection.

Doing to ourselves that which we want to do to others is what Gestalt therapists refer to as retroflection. A literal definition of a *retroflection* is a turning back on ourselves what is rightly meant for someone ele, or doing to ourselves that which we would like someone else to do to us. Naturally, contact is impeded through retroflection; at best, retroflectors will be in contact with themselves. What they miss is the enlivenment that occurs from good contact with others.

So much is held in by retroflectors that somatic complaints are frequent; they may complain of headaches, stiffness, an upset stomach, and/or other body ailments. Awareness is essential in order to undo retroflection; with awareness retroflectors know what is going on inside them and then their energy can be mobilized outward in some form of action. They first need to become aware that they want to squeeze, to make tense, to stifle, to soothe or cuddle themselves or someone else in the group. Once this is discovered, the retroflection can be undone by directing the energy outward.

In Gestalt therapy, *confluence* means to come together with or to become one with. Confluence is used by people to reduce differences. Again, no sense of boundary exists. Confluent people seldom disagree. According to Polster and Polster (1973, p. 93), "Confluence is a three-legged race between two people who agree not to disagree." Confluent people see to it that nothing new happens, while at the same time they experience little interest or excitement in their relationships. They are clingers, wanting others to make all the effort. I see a lot of confluence in "leaderless" and "consciousness-raising" groups. Upon hearing one group member discuss the injustice she received at her place of employment, other group members began to feel as if it were happening to them and to feel similarly. A situation like this is easily remedied by electing a leader for each group meeting; the leader could keep some distance from the confluent process, point it out to the group, and work with it in whatever way seemed appropriate.

Guilt and resentment are often clues to disturbed confluent relationships. If Larry and Linda are in a confluent marriage and the confluence is interrupted by Larry, he may feel guilty and attempt to restore the confluence by making restitution. If, on the other hand, Larry believes Linda guilty, he will feel resentful; perhaps demanding that Linda feel guilty, apologize, or accept some punishment. What is needed is actual contact with each other in which they learn to accept and appreciate their differences. This can be done adroitly in a group by helping patients to figure out how they are different from others, and to articulate their differences within the group. Questions like, "What are you doing now? and "Can you express what you are doing?" will help the confluent person have contact.

The quality of the Gestalt therapist's own awareness in group enhances the effectiveness of the work. Therapists need to be aware of the behavior of group members. Who is sitting by whom? Who is looking at the therapist and who is not? Who articulates "I want to work?" When one group member is working, what does the rest of the group do? Being aware is necessary if Gestalt therapists are to focus on the group process; this demands a cognitive awareness of what is going on. Our own self-awareness is essential as we work with a group. How much energy do we have? Whom are we interested in working with? How do we feel about the absent member?

For Gestalt therapists, awareness and style go hand in hand. Awareness improves focus and prevents the pitfalls of "making things happen" and of interfering with the group's natural evolution. Sometimes therapists might decide to disclose their awareness to the group in some way, while at other times, because they think it would be counterproductive, they opt against sharing their awareness. Polster and Polster (1973) apply the term *bracketing off* to the therapist's setting an issue aside, perhaps planning to return to it later. Sometimes therapists "bracket" their personal awareness, realizing that the group's purpose is not to provide a ground for them to express themselves. At other times, they bracket off their expression when there is good contact in the group and for them to say something would be interruptive. Without awareness, their bracketing off would be impossible and they would be interruptive, interfering, and ill-timed.

At times it is helpful to consider patients' original goals for joining a group. This could be done privately by reviewing notes from screening interviews, or notes from the first group meeting where typically group members state their reasons for being there and what they hope to accomplish. My preference is to bring up the matter of goals after the group has had 6 to 10 meetings, asking the group members directly, "How do you feel about the goals you stated when the group started? Are you getting what you want?" Because a lot of my work is in a university setting, my colleagues and I jokingly refer to this as our "midterm" evaluations. We might be more goal conscious than some Gestalt therapists, because our groups are somewhat time limited; to have a member more than one or two semesters is the exception rather than the rule.

Suppose that we discover when we ask our group patients to evaluate their goals that some say they are disappointed, that they believe they are getting nowhere, or in some other way communicate that they are not achieving their goals for being in group. We can then review with those patients what they have been doing in the group. I recently went through this process in a group I am leading. One man reported that no, he was not getting what he came for, which was to learn to be more expressive, hoping that this would help him develop a more intimate relationship with his wife. I remembered that he had hardly opened his mouth, let alone asking to work on anything. He replied that he felt there had not been any appropriate times for him to speak. I speculated that one way he might be blocking his expressivity was by waiting to be appropriate and I went on to suggest that he experiment during the rest of the group with expressing himself at inappropriate times. Starting somewhat tentatively he soon began to comment in an engaging way to others in the group, enlivening himself and the rest of us in the process.

Some Gestalt therapists may consider what, if anything, they have contributed to their patients not working on or achieving their goals for being in group. Aware therapists sometimes discover that they have blocks to working with certain types of patients or certain problems, or that they have other ways of not doing good work. Consulting with colleagues or supervisors is a beneficial way to discover how we might be blocking ourselves with some patients. In a supervisory session four of us were discussing a patient with whom the therapist was having difficulty. The patient complained that he was not getting much from group. As we discussed the situation and offered suggestions, the therapist's usual response was, "If I did that it wouldn't work because the patient would do such and such." It then became apparent that the therapist was predicting what the patient would do and was preventing himself from working well because of this restricted view of the patient.

Patients' originally stated goals should not be viewed as binding or restrictive. This would violate the Gestalt principle of working with what is most important at the moment. Patients and therapists can decide to renew or renegotiate goals at any time. Because patients' lives go on, it is not unusual for something unrelated to the original goal to emerge and for the patient and therapist to contract to work on that. Temporarily, the original goal is "put on the shelf" although it might be discovered later to be related to the more immediate problem.

Most Gestalt therapists, in one form or another, establish agreed upon contracts for what they are willing to do with their groups. I like to differentiate goals from contracts. As previously stated, *goals* are what patients hope to get for themselves from attending group. *Contracts,* on the other hand, are the specific problems I agree to work on with a patient at any particular time. A restatement of the original goal might be an acceptable contract; or, the contract might be unrelated to the original goal. A contract might be stated in one of these ways: "I want to work on how I hold myself back from participating in this group." "I want to work on what happened between me and my husband last night." If the therapist agrees, then the work begins.

There are times when it is necessary to negotiate with the patient before agreeing upon a contract. One time we negotiate is when the patient requests to work on something vague like feeling better or achieving happiness. Negotiating is helpful if therapists feel drained from already having worked on similar problems during that group. For example, Jeff was the third person to ask to work on a dream in one particular group. The therapist replied to Jeff that he was willing to work with him but not on a dream; perhaps they could agree on something else. Occasionally there are groups in which no one contracts to work; this is most likely to occur in a group where there is a lot of interaction. As long as the group members are talking to each other in a contactful way, or are content to sit silently, there is no need to insist on a contract.

Occasionally, either at the start of a group session, as a follow-up to some provocative work, or during a lull in the session, Gestalt therapists will "make rounds." Patients are asked if they are willing to share what they are aware of. When this occurs at the start of a session several patients might say they have something to work on, while others might say something that merely discloses their awareness at that moment. Sometimes while "making rounds" patients want to give feedback to others, share with them something that has happened to themselves, or complete some "unfinished" business for them. Feedback is usually appropriate as long as it is not interruptive. For group members to make statements to others that disclose how they feel toward them or how they were affected by something they did is a relevant type of group interaction. While making rounds, the Gestalt therapist will normally say something to the group about his or her own existence.

Gestalt therapists seldom have a programmed idea about what they want to happen in a group. Instead they prefer to stay with the emerging gestalt, whether it be something an individual is working on, or some group theme: "This capacity to follow the theme and development of a session is called tracking. The therapist is like a complex radar machine, able to consolidate material, see its direction, and keep moving with it until the person is able to surprise himself with an insightful experience" (Zinker, 1977, p. 47). This kind of "tracking" and staying with the patient or the group helps assure that the work is based on the phenomenology of the patient or group as opposed to its being based on interpretation or advice-giving and suggestions.

Gestalt therapists often colead. For ongoing groups it is wasteful and inefficient to have coleaders whose styles are "carbon copies" of one another. It is preferable that the two therapists differ somewhat, that the best use is made of existing polarities. If one leader tends toward being abrasive, the other may be chosen for his or her gentleness. If one is keen on picking up nonverbal auditory cues, the other might be chosen for his or her ability to notice the visual nonverbal. Some Gestalt coleaders prefer a style where one is foreground and the other is background and they change positions based on their needs or the needs of the group. Another style of coleading has both leaders active, intervening and withdrawing in accordance with their interest and focus. Both can be concentrated on the patient, though possibly on different aspects, or one may be paying attention to other group members, which could lead to bringing them into the work. My preference, when working with a coleader, is to negotiate with him or her at the beginning of the group meeting, so that both leaders and group members have a clear idea of the style for that day.

Practice

Problems

A Gestalt group offers a novel approach to solving problems, since the work of the group, directed toward patients' discovering what they are doing to themselves and how they are doing it, presents a new frame of reference. Patients typically expect to be told what they are doing "wrong" and how to correct it. Gestalt therapists do not offer that. We offer, instead, group therapy with an emphasis on experiencing instead of problem solving.

Problems can arise with patients who are determined to have an expert tell them the "right" thing to do. Our experience with some patients is that after hearing a description of a Gestalt group, they decide not to attend, or they attend but go "underground" with their attempted manipulations to get answers as to how to live their lives. Simply put, some people, wanting their problems solved for them and too impatient to discover the answers and solutions within themselves, remain rigid and will not get much from being in a Gestalt group. Ideally, patients will discover the futility of looking to others for answers as to "why" they do what they do. When other group members discover they are being manipulated to give advice, they frequently refuse to cooperate and the patient is left to work on how it feels when manipulation for advice fails.

Some people join Gestalt groups with the mistaken idea that group is a place to gather and emotionalize, a place where they can dump all "bad" feelings onto someone else. True, Gestalt groups can produce a lot of emotion, but effective Gestalt therapy works to tie the emotional expression into making contact or increasing awareness. Seldom will a patient be encouraged to express just for the sake of emotionalizing, which leads only to release or relief and not much else. Gestalt therapists do not strive for a high emotional tenor in group; they might, though, ask the patient who is speaking about a normally "charged" issue in a flat, lifeless tone, to repeat himself with "appropriate" affect.

After stating their initial goals, if patients draw back and wait for the therapist to tell them what to do, patients will probably never make the changes they desire. Patients must be able to take initiative or be aggressive in order to contact and "come out" with whatever it is they want to work on. I usually tell my patients during their screening interviews, and periodically after group starts, that they will not be forced to do or say anything they do not want to, but that they have a better chance of getting what they want if they ask for it. On the other hand, it is possible to benefit from group work and not "come out" and initiate work. Identification with the subject matter of someone else's work tends to be powerfully effective for some. I have had patients tell me that they "got a lot," actually resolved some problems for themselves, by attending closely and privately to another member's work.

Some patients make up a "ticket of admission" for getting into groups while their real intention is just to meet people and fulfill some affiliation needs. If patients are straight about this I see no need to exclude them from group. I do expect, though, that they be willing to work on finding out how they keep themselves from meeting people and learning ways to meet their social needs. This problem of lack of initiative or aggression is sometimes dealt with through techniques like our "midterm" evaluation, which gives patients an opportunity to determine if they are getting from group what they came for. Finally, we have discovered that some patients hold themselves back because they believe their "problem" is not serious enough or because they cannot articulate it. The Gestalt mode encourages working with such patients to alleviate their confusion and enable them to explicitly state their wants.

Patients with "serious" problems may tend to monopolize the group's time and frequently the majority believe their problems to be trivial in comparison with the momentous problems of one or two others. Therapists can unwittingly reinforce this monopolizing by actually giving more time and energy to these patients and, in general, by acting as if they need more than others. Experienced therapists of all theoretical persuasions know that some patients can present a crisis at every group meeting, yet they manage fairly well on their own during the rest of the week. If the monopolizer's problem is, in fact, too serious and time-consuming to handle in group with fairness to the others, the therapist may ask him or her to drop out of the group and may offer individual therapy in its place. He or she may, on the other hand, negotiate with the group to set time limits on each participant's work, or may even opt to "work" on the monopolizing of the patient, perhaps helping him or her "get at" whatever it is that the patient does to create a crisis and "hog" time. The result might be that the patient merely wants attention and can learn more nourishing ways to get it.

Referrals from other therapists can be a problem if not handled appropriately. It is best to have a screening interview before accepting referred patients into a group. Whenever possible a consultation with the referring therapist is helpful. My colleagues and I have been amazed at the number of times therapists refer patients to groups because they are tired of working with them, feel stuck with them, are not getting anywhere, or have given up, believing that they cannot "help" the patient. A joint interview with the patient and the referring therapist has been known to turn into a profitable supervisory session in which the referring therapist becomes aware of how he or she is blocking progress and decides to continue seeing the patient.

I believe it is important to educate our referral sources about Gestalt group therapy, to eliminate such gross misrepresentations of Gestalt therapy as the incident of the psychiatrist who told his referral that we spend most of our time beating on pillows. In order to prevent such misconceptions we need to inform our colleagues in other branches of psychotherapy about how we work, the types of patients we will and will not work with, and what kinds of activities we engage in the group.

Groups establish ground rules, regardless of the theoretical orientation of the leader. Gestalt groups are no exception. Some Gestalt group therapists are explicit about stating rules to group members at the beginning, while others prefer to wait until the need arises. According to Rosenblatt (1975, p. 78) the rules can of course be broken: "To be as honest as possible in what you are feeling and thinking. To come regularly, on time. To be willing to 'work,' to be willing to risk, to try new things. To pay your bill. These are, to my knowledge, the rules, and from here we are on our own."

I favor Rosenblatt's style and prefer not to encumber my group with legislation. With my rules I try to avoid creating a "list of how to behave" in group.

> If we are to do justice at all to the spirit and essence of Gestalt therapy, we must recognize clearly the difference between rules and commandments. The philosophy of rules is to provide us with effective means of unifying thought with feeling. They are designed to help us dig out resistances, promote heightened awareness—to facilitate the maturation process. They are definitely *not* intended as a dogmatic list of *do's and don'ts:* rather, they are offered in the spirit of experiments that the patient may perform. (Levitsky & Perls, 1970, p. 140)

One ground rule that I am willing to be explicit about is confidentiality. I ask group members not to talk about what goes on in groups with *anyone.* Even without giving names I consider it a breach of confidentiality to talk about "what someone is doing in my group."

Owing to the nature of my style, I frequently have to deal with what group members interpret as an implied ground rule: when one member is working the others should not interrupt. Because no such verbalized "ruling" exists, I usually ask the patient who alludes to it, "How did you stop yourself from interrupting?" Being interrupted is okay with me. In fact, I want patients to interrupt when they have something to say; that does not mean I will always "like" it.

Evaluation

Most Gestalt therapists do not find the traditional diagnostic labels that are given to patients useful for doing therapy. Kempler (1973, p. 275) sums up our position quite succinctly by saying: "Diagnostic labels are dangerous. They are like glue, they flow on readily and must be peeled off slowly, bit by bit. They confuse the patient, if he hears them, and they can astigmatize the vision of the next therapist who sees the chart before he sees the patient. And worst of all they impair the vision of the therapist who makes them."

Seldom is a diagnosis helpful to a group leader, so we spend little time making them.

> A diagnosis is a limited way of reducing a person to a concept. To call a person a schizophrenic, an obsessive or a character disorder tells me little more than if you were to call him a father, an uncle, a worker or a friend. Less, as a matter of fact, for one clinician's schizophrenic is another man's hysteric; one clinician's obsessive is another man's blocked habit pattern; one clinician's character disorder is another man's perversion, which is simply another man's pleasure. (Rosenblatt, 1975, p. 16.)

Most Gestalt therapists would agree upon process-oriented evaluation, by which we scrutinize and assess the quality of the contact that group members are having. Where are their boundaries? Are they willing to meet another and risk being rejected or taken in, thereby losing their own identity? When do they withdraw from contact and where do they go? Gestalt therapists do this kind of evaluation consistently, because it helps assist in directing the group's activities as well as develop the experiments that we propose.

I take assessment in another direction and examine the progress of each patient in the group. This can be done by periodically reviewing each participant's goals and by following each patient's work with questions about what was learned. Are they satisfied with what they got? Are they ready to stop, to withdraw from their working? Evaluating in this style insures that we have done more than simply emote.

Treatment

I do not like the word treatment; it implies a medical model. It suggests that we will provide "treatment" for our "patients" (a term, incidentally, which despite its common usage is far from satisfactory) and make them well. It puts therapists in a "one-up" position and increases patients' tendency to look outside for support instead of taking care of themselves. The Gestalt emphasis on contact and awareness insists on an approach that is very different from "treating" someone for an illness. In Gestalt therapy, therapists and patients meet on an equal basis. Granted, therapists do have some expertise not usually possessed by patients; still, we do not offer pat solutions, advice, or answers to problems. To "treat" a problem as a symptom would violate the holistic doctrine of Gestalt therapy. The approaches are diametrically opposed.

We do "treat" people, if I may be permitted a play on words, by treating them as equals, as people who are capable of taking care of themselves. Instead of "solutions" we may offer frustration, so that our patients mobilize their energy and aggression to take some initiative and action in their lives. Through frustrating their attempts to manipulate us for support, our patients learn to support themselves. They learn to solve their own problems and not to depend on some expert or guru or doctor to do it for them.

Management

Sheldon Kopp (1977, p. 49) asserted, "I'm in charge of the therapy, while the patient is responsible for running his or her own life." This strongly and correctly implies two responsibilities: Therapists must be skilled professional people who know how to do Gestalt group psychotherapy; patients must choose for themselves what to do in their lives. Freed from the burdensome responsibility of telling patients how to live, Gestalt therapists create an atmosphere in which patients must take responsibility for what they do from moment to moment. Success in this endeavor means that patients must grapple with, "If I can do this in our session, how do I stop myself from being responsible in life?"

Therapists' related duties include the juggling of schedules and setting the time for the group to meet. Provided the therapists' schedules are flexible, we may survey our potential group members to find out what time is best for them, but as a practical matter I have found it a disagreeable experience to attempt to coordinate the schedules for 8 to 10 people. Therefore, I decide when my group will meet and then let my patients and colleagues know. They do the maneuvering and I have no trouble filling groups this way.

Therapists need to make explicit to their groups their policy on confidentiality. I make a point of stating the definition and gravity of confidentiality, in the initial meeting. Frequently patients will want to discuss this. Of course we cannot enforce any policy, but we need to be "on the record" as having established the policy. A group must necessarily be regarded as different from individual work in the matter of confidentiality. In individual work, we usually assure our patients that we will keep our sessions confidential and what they do with the content of our sessions is their own business. In group we are concerned that members respect the privacy of what others do and say. Therapists working in agencies need to assure the patients that their files are secure and that supervision and discussion of groups and patients be held in private.

Some therapists give their home telephone numbers to patients and tell them to call if they are "hurting" or "need" anything. I prefer not to do this, because I believe people are capable of deciding on their own whether or not they need to call me. Although I have on occasion spent an hour or more on the telephone, in the middle of the night, with a patient, it is the exception rather than a common occurrence with me. We will instead discuss a time when I can see them during working hours.

Most Gestalt therapists do not hospitalize or medicate patients. If my patients insist that they want drug therapy, they must move on to some other therapist who will provide them with what they think they need. I am willing to refer them to a physician. I have worked with patients who terminate with me in order to be hospitalized and then choose to resume with me later. In this case, I must know if my patient is on any medication. It is important for me, in practicing Gestalt therapy with patients taking medication, to acquire sufficient knowledge about the effects of the prescribed drugs.

Application

Group Selection and Composition

In order for patients to benefit from being in a Gestalt group they should be willing to do "work," to risk honesty in their working, and to articulate what they want. Whenever possible this information should be provided to the potential group member in the screening interview. Certain questions help: What do you think you would "work" on in the group? What difficulties do you have being open and honest in what you say? Thus the screening interview can be more than just a sterile gathering of information; it can proceed much like the group meetings will. This way the prospective patients have experiential data to aid them in their decision to join the group or not. One patient of mine, for example, had an appointment with me to discuss his entering a group. When I asked him what he would want to work on he responded first by saying that he did not think he would need to work on his marriage, his relationship with his children, his parents, or his boss. When he mentioned his boss, his voice sounded strained to me and he tightened his jaws and lips. I asked him if he was aware that he had noticeably tightened when he mentioned his boss. Similarly strained, he expressed an interest in finding out more about his tightening at the suggestion of working on his relationship with his boss. So, we worked a few minutes, discovering that he had a lot of stored up anger and resentment toward being treated like an inferior. This sudden awareness of subject matter for working provided him with first hand experience of the kind of activity and surfacing of material for work that occurs in a group.

Some Gestalt therapists prefer to balance their groups by gender. This has certain advantages since in the real world most patients find it necessary to relate to both sexes. An equal number of, say, four men and four women may not be necessary. It generally behooves a group to have members of both sexes to achieve some balance; if a man, for example, is working on his difficulty relating to women, the women in the group can participate in exploring this difficulty. On the other hand, some therapists are finding the sexually "segregated" groups to be effective. Because there are not many "real" situations where people can isolate themselves from the opposite sex, these groups may seem somewhat "staged." A distinction should be made between psychotherapy groups and groups convened for a special purpose such as men's or women's "consciousness-raising" groups, assertive training groups, and so on, all of which apparently offer a valuable service.

Generally, I prefer not to see patients for individual therapy if they are in one of my groups. Even if they are having "trouble" with group, I think it is best to work on that in the group session. Sometimes I have people in group who are receiving individual therapy from other therapists. Because what they do on their own time is their business, I have no objections to them receiving individual therapy from other therapists.

Patients who have had previous group experience or have worked individually with a Gestalt therapist can serve as useful models to the novice on how to work in a group. Without a skilled therapist leading the group though, the experienced patients tend to monopolize the working time while the beginners remain observers of the group activities.

As a part of the screening and selection of patients for groups we have developed a videotape that shows segments of actual groups. We show this to patients before or after interviewing them so that they will have accurate expectations about what will go on in the group. We selected for the tape segments of groups that we thought were fairly typical; that is, about 10 minutes of interaction and feedback, 10 minutes of a patient working on a "problem," and 10 minutes of "dreamwork." Patients report that the videotape helped them to be prepared for any emotional intensity that may occur early in the group meeting.

No selection process is perfect, and there are times when it is appropriate to consider transferring a patient from group to individual therapy. Patients who, in some fashion, continue to disrupt the ongoing activities may be harmful to the total group and could be recommended to be seen individually to work out their disruptive behavior. Sometimes, despite the assurance in the screening interviews that they are willing to work and will ask for what they want, patients remain passive; in this case likewise, a switch to individual therapy might be more appropriate, if other modes of changing fail.

Group Setting

Except in the case of a workshop or demonstration that has been arranged by someone else, therapists usually are responsible for choosing the site where the group will meet. The group room ideally should afford privacy in an informal setting. Because Gestalt therapy frequently and actively involves more than one member, and sometimes the entire group, the room should provide adequate space. The conference room style, with chairs set around a table, offers the least desirable setting.

Group Size

The size of the group may vary depending on many factors. Gestalt therapists are comfortable working with eight persons. Some work, in ongoing groups, with as few as 5 or as many as 10. The Gestalt workshop, in which the group meets all day for several consecutive days, can easily handle more than can the ongoing groups which meet on a weekly basis.

Therapy Frequency, Length, and Duration

Once a week for 2 hours tends to be the usual practice for Gestalt groups. This may vary according to therapists' preference and agency's need and demands. Some therapists prefer to meet twice a week; some prefer more than 2 hours. An agency such as a halfway house may schedule a 1-hour group each evening. A group in a university setting typically meets weekly during a semester or term lasting 15 to 18 weeks, vacation weeks, of course, being excluded. Many of these students in groups, knowing the limitations on their time and predicting future schedule conflicts and class demands that may require their dropping out, will be motivated to move faster toward accomplishing goals and getting the most out of their group experience. A group in a university setting would typically not meet when students are on vacation. Often, scheduling a day-long meeting for a group which normally meets once a week offers a break from the routine, and usually it accelerates the working through of some problems.

The duration of a group's existence depends on several factors. Its termination may be arbitrarily determined by such factors as a semester ending, therapist's schedules, fund cuts in an agency, and so forth. Patients could decide to terminate when their goal for attending has been achieved. Some productive therapy can result from working in group with patients who are considering terminating. Ordinarily, strong feelings have developed toward the therapist and members of the group. Learning to say good-bye and not hanging on beyond the point of nourishingly relating in a group can teach a lot about contact and withdrawal.

Media Usage

The use of audio and video equipment can enhance and facilitate group progress, but audiotaping or videotaping of Gestalt groups should be done *only* with permission of group members. Members should be fully informed about the purpose of taping, who will view or hear the tapes, how long tapes will be preserved, and if they have veto rights after taping. After a thorough discussion of the issue and after permission is given by all group members, taping can serve several purposes. Tapes can be used for supervisory purposes. Supervisors understand better what is going on in a group by seeing and hearing it than they do by getting a "report" from the leaders. Some leaders, upon viewing their own group, become belatedly aware of what they are missing at the moment of group interaction. Tapes can also be employed to facilitate patients' awareness of themselves. A time can be arranged for the interested group members to listen to or watch themselves. Patients report this to be very helpful and sometimes say things like, "Now I know what you were seeing," "How do you put up with me?"

Filming or videotaping can be cumbersome and distracting. Bearing this in mind, and in order to cut down on the interference, it is best not to bring in a "camera operator" who is not known to a group. Instead, group members can take turns running the equipment. The different styles of operating the camera are an interesting group phenomenon. Whom and what group members focus on when operating the camera has been known to stimulate much discussion.

Leader Qualifications

Gestalt therapists should meet required licensing criteria in order to practice psychotherapy in their state. Usually these standards require an advanced degree in psychology or social work, or a residency in psychiatry. Most Gestalt therapists receive their training after they have completed their degrees, either at one of the Gestalt institutes or from an experienced Gestalt therapist. Training time varies depending on the program. Generally, training programs combine theory, practice, supervision, and the opportunity for the trainee to participate in therapy. The necessary qualifications, therefore, are advanced degrees in the appropriate disciplines and completion of a training program.

Because no certification requirements are needed in order for therapists to call themselves Gestalt therapists, it is difficult for patients to tell beforehand about therapists' qualifications. Some information can be gleaned by asking about the training therapists have received. "Who trained you?" or "How long were you in training?" Still, this may not say much about how a therapist will work with a particular patient. The advice I give is for people to have a few sessions and then decide if they are getting the kind of therapy they want. Frequently I initiate this discussion with my patients. This helps to clarify expectations and they can decide to continue with me or not.

Ethics

Gestalt therapists are no different from any other therapeutic school when it comes to ethical conduct. The national association for psychologists, psychiatrists, and social workers all have codes of ethics for their membership that serve as guidelines for ethical behavior. Naturally there are different interpretations on ethical matters.

RESEARCH

There has not been a lot of research in Gestalt therapy in recent years, but this does not mean that there is not a need for more. Questions remain to be tackled: What are the most important effects of Gestalt therapy on patients? What kinds of patients are best suited for Gestalt therapy? Are there any personality styles best suited for Gestalt therapists? In other words, there are some important questions yet to be answered.

Research in following up the effects of Gestalt weekend marathons and ongoing weekly groups by Guinan and Foulds (1970) suggests that Gestalt-oriented groups foster increased levels of self-actualization in normal growth-seeking college students. Foulds and Hannigan (1976) followed up Gestalt marathon participants 6 months later and discovered that achieved gains in self-actualization persisted over time. Greenberg, Seeman, and Cassius (1978) studied participants in a 45-hour marathon experience, in which the therapists worked generally from a Transactional Analysis and Gestalt framework. Using the Tennessee Self-Concept Scale, the Semantic Differential, and the Bach Helpfulness Scale, they found significant positive changes on all measures for the treatment groups. A 2-week post marathon follow-up with the TSCS showed some shrinkage toward baseline, but with continued significant gains on some of the TSCS variables.

Ramig and Frey (1974) applied content analysis and cluster analysis to the ideas of Fritz Perls in order to develop a taxonomy of Gestalt processes and goals. By using these techniques they found that Perls's Gestalt therapy can be defined as a process in which the therapist seeks to skillfully frustrate the client in the here and now so as to facilitate organic contact with the environment, self-awareness, and maturation and autonomy. Most Gestalt therapists believed this anyway. It is nice to find some beliefs statistically validated!

Smith and Glass (1977) "meta-analyzed" nearly 400 controlled evaluations of psychotherapy and counseling. They found, on the average, the typical therapy client to be better off than 75% of untreated individuals. Their analysis included many different kinds of psychotherapy, but there was an inadequate number of studies for them to make firm statements about Gestalt therapy's effectiveness. This points out the absence in the literature of controlled studies involving Gestalt therapy.

In a study of the effects of encounter groups, Lieberman, Yalom, and Miles (1973) compared the effects of 10 different kinds of encounter groups, including Gestalt therapy. Among many findings, they found one Gestalt group to be among the lowest in producing positive change and one Gestalt group to be among the highest in producing positive changes. Equivocal findings like this need to be replicated.

Leslie S. Greenberg and his associates (Greenberg & Clarke, 1979; Greenberg & Dompierre, 1981; Greenberg & Higgins, 1980; Greenberg & Rice, 1981) have published some interesting research in which they have investigated a specific Gestalt therapy technique, the two-chair technique of dealing with splits, conflicts, or polarities. In a series of studies Greenberg and his associates found that the Gestalt two-chair technique led to a greater depth of experiencing than did empathic reflection. Greenberg and Dompierre (1981) substantiated the previous findings on depth of experiencing; they also discovered shifts in awareness, reported conflict resolution, and reported behavior change were greater following the Gestalt interventions than the empathic reflection of feelings. The findings of Greenberg and his associates support the contention of Gestalt therapists that we provide an intense experience in many of our sessions.

Fagan and Shepherd (1970, p. 241) commented on the difficulties of doing research in Gestalt therapy.

> Most often hard data are difficult to obtain: the important variables resist quantification; the complexity and multiplicity of variables in therapists, patient, and the interactional processes are almost impossible to unravel; and the crudeness and restrictiveness of the measuring devices available cannot adequately reflect the sublety of the process. However, the fact that the task is difficult does not reduce its importance, and the need for many questions to be asked and answered by the more formal procedure available to researchers.

Gestalt therapists are seldom found in academic positions, because they would generally rather *do* therapy than theorize about it. More typically they are in private practice or in service agencies where research takes a back seat to practice. Most Gestalt therapists are not academicians and most academicians are not adequately trained in the practice of Gestalt therapy. Yet academicians, whose training is generally superficial at best, are responsible for most research in the field. I contend that their knowledge of Gestalt therapy is only peripheral and they consequently are unable to properly measure its intricasies. One way around this problem is for Gestalt therapists and research-minded academicians to join forces, to set up controlled studies under joint supervision.

STRENGTHS AND LIMITATIONS

Practiced in groups, Gestalt therapy draws some strength from the "collective energy" of the group, with the expectation that something vigorous, something quickening might happen at any time, in any session. Time and again, patients in Gestalt groups relate how their energy builds by watching others work, experiment, or struggle, thereby contributing to their own courage to jump into their own problems. This "collective energy" grows from the present-centeredness and action orientation of Gestalt therapy. Passively "talking about" a problem occurs infrequently; instead, patients are encouraged to "get into" what they are "talking about." If a female patient says she wants to work on her problem with authority figures, not much can be accomplished by her merely "talking about" it. A Gestalt therapist would probably prefer to explore the problem with her. One possibility for exploration is to have her dialogue "empty chair fashion" with some authority figures in her life. Playing both herself and authority figures the possibility exists that she will discover how she causes her own problem. Another possibility is to explore the relationship with the therapist, who is probably perceived as an authority figure.

Another strength is in "coattailing," or vicarious therapy. Some patients resolve problems or make decisions without working directly or overtly with the therapist or group. In the preceding example, others who have similar problems will be working simultaneously without being directly involved. At times "coattailing" initiates a theme, and an entire session's working will follow the theme stimulated by the first "worker."

Gestalt therapy offers a way of getting into therapy rapidly. The first session, whether a group or individual session, is a working session, as opposed to a history gathering or a passive listening by the therapist for the purpose of formulating ideas about what the group or individual patient "needs." Personally, I prefer to "do therapy" from the start. This furnishes the patients with a sample of how I work and they can then decide whether or not to continue on the basis of some experiential data about what group will be like.

It must be noted that, "Gestalt therapy offers powerful techniques for intervention into neurotic and self-defeating behaviors, and for mobilizing and redirecting human energy into self-supporting and creative development" (Shepherd, 1970, p. 234). Herein is a major strength of Gestalt therapy when practiced by a well-trained, skilled Gestalt therapist. On the other hand, when practiced by a poorly-trained therapist it can constitute a serious limitation. Gestalt therapy does get people into their feelings, into emotionality. Therapists not grounded in theory, especially in the concepts of closure–finishing and contact–support, tend to render the patients vulnerable and to abandon them there. At other times, poorly trained therapists will facilitate a powerful process then interrupt it before the patient has a chance to finish, thereby reinforcing "unfinished business" in the patient.

Patients who insist on taking a causality approach to their problems, who persist in eliciting advice from their therapists about how to live, will probably not benefit from Gestalt therapy. Although most Gestalt therapists would agree that this is not a limitation, we could better articulate our position and supply a rationale for our opposition to "whys" and *advice* giving.

Both Shepherd (1970) and Simkin (1976a) caution against using Gestalt therapy with patients who have "acting out" tendencies. Because "acting out" patients experience some problems with impulse control, the expressive techniques of Gestalt therapy may be experienced as tacit approval of their actions. In extreme cases, some patients believe they are being encouraged to leave therapy sessions and act on the "outside" as they did during the session, Shepherd states: "A skillful Gestalt therapist will design experiments to facilitate the patient's working within the therapy session, thus reducing his need to act outside. However, work with acting-out individuals, as with psychotics, cannot be considered without commitment to a longer and often slower process than many Gestalt therapists are willing to undertake" (Shepherd, 1970, p. 236). It is clear that some peril exists, that care should be taken, and that techniques which facilitate expression are not useful with some patients. Skilled Gestalt therapists would work with "acting-out" patients in some alternative mode, maybe by teaching them some suppressive skills so that they are not always on the verge of an explosion. Working with contact boundaries is beneficial, because these patients typically skip the contact phase in the awareness–contact cycle. The impulsive "acting-out" person usually goes from awareness to action and does not contact the other person.

The inherent paradox of Gestalt therapy is one of its limitations. True, Gestalt therapy is lively and invigorating, often dramatic. On the other hand, there are no instant cures; bringing about real change can be a lengthy process. The lure of a quick cure has attracted many patients and pseudotherapists who, because of impatience or greed, are unwilling to spend the time necessary for authentic integration and assimilation.

GROUP SESSION ILLUSTRATION

Members begin to trickle into the group room about a quarter to two for our eighth weekly session, and situate themselves on the cushions: one consciously chooses the Mediterranean blue, to "suit her disposition" she kids; others, not particularly concerned with color, opt for the puce or the fuchsia or the orchid, until the periphery of the room is peopled. One woman sits barefooted, cross-legged; one is perched on the cushion, tensely seated, on her heels; one fellow is "at attention" on his seat; another is "laid back," propped on pillows, casing the place with a relaxed gaze. I position myself, quite aware of my choice, at a vacancy between Martha and Becky, with my back to the windows.

Two o'clock. I push the door shut with my foot, and group officially commences. Arms folded, I check everybody out, taking note of who is doing what: who seems to be memorizing the pattern on the rug; who is staring off into the great beyond; who seems to be mentally "whistlin' Dixie"; who is looking determinedly *back* at me.

Kate is looking me right in the eye and she announces, "I really feel good today." I am a bit surprised, although I keep it to myself, as I remember that for the past 4 weeks she has been feeling bad, physically, and has been depressed. I am pleased, and tell her that I am pleased.

"Thanks," she responds, "I have lots of energy and would like to get closer to people."

"Would you be willing to experiment with that?"

"Here?" "Now?" She is confused and I decide to let her stay in her confusion. I do not answer. A moment more of struggling and then she catches on and starts moving about the room, approaching one member, with noticeable hesitation, speaking to him, moving on, speaking to another, stopping to touch another. With Rich she verbalizes her feelings of "being cautious."

"I feel afraid—to get too close—to you."

Rich looks away, not responding, and I inquire of Kate, "What do you imagine there is to fear in getting close to Rich?"

"Well, I think it's happening right now, He'll reject me, look away, pretend I don't exist."

Rich asserts that he is neither rejecting her nor pretending that she does not exist; he is "not wanting to be invaded" and is wary of looking at her for fear she will take his looking as an invitation to move closer. That he does not want.

I suggest that he *could* say that to her, that they *could* have contact with some definite limitations on closeness. Both seem to accept the possibility and they begin to experiment by moving together and apart, until they discover the satisfying "distance," the acceptable "space," exchanging comments about what causes them discomfort about each other. They are contacting; I see no need to intervene. The interaction evolves to a natural closure and Kate proceeds, finishing making rounds in the group and eventually sitting between Holly and Martha, across the room from her original position.

The group attention had been focused on Kate for about 20 minutes; several members have actively participated in what she was doing. By now I am curious about what is "going on" with the other group members so I ask, "Who is willing to say what you are doing, what you are aware of at this moment?" Mary Ann responds that she feels "laid back" and tired. "I want to observe, and I don't want to be very involved." Her posture, consistent with what she says, is restful. Several pillows which she has fluffed are behind her and at her side and she is convincingly "laid back" into them. Becky interjects that she is "alert," "not introspective," that she is interested and wanting, somehow, to be involved. Ken adds, "I'm glad to be here and feel very energetic, for a change." Bill has said nothing so far; I notice he is leaning forward on his seat.

Rich, agitated, is tapping both feet, wringing his hands and I ask him what is going on. He responds that he feels "so cooped up," and he goes on talking, with what seems to me to be forced humor, telling of all the "things he has to do." Gradually his voice takes on a dull monotone. I consider saying to him that one way for him to coop himself up is to think of all the "things he has to do"; resisting this, I propose an experiment. Would he be willing, I ask, to give a voice to the part of him responsible for "cooping up" and let it speak to the rest of him? He agrees. His voice picks up energy as he says to this part of himself, "Look Buddy, I'm in control! Don't try to slide away from me; you know you wouldn't be able to get rid of me." I ask him to move to another seat and to give the other part a voice, the part that feels "cooped up." He moves, and in a whine, begs the other part to lighten up. As he continues to move from place to place, from voice to voice, in this enactment he asks the "cooping up" part what it is trying to do for him. He switches places and says, "To keep you from getting hurt." At this point he starts to sob. This is quite new behavior for Rich, who is a "big bear" of a man and has alternated between looking foreboding and making superficial jokes.

I check to see the impact he is having on others. Most appear to be paying close attention and Becky looks as if she wants to reach out to him or say something to him. She does not do so. I do not want to interfere or in any way cut off what Rich is getting into; I am thinking of what I could do to facilitate his becoming more involved with his experiencing so that he will be able to "finish" with it. His sobbing peaks and he begins to take a few deep breaths. I ask him what is going on. He starts sobbing again and says, "I really hurt."

"Can you tell me how you hurt?"

"I am keeping in so much from the woman I live with," he replies.

I consider asking him to put the woman here and express some of what he keeps from her. I decide not to do this since I am concerned with how much he can assimilate and since, by now, we have been working about 15 minutes. He no longer appears to feel "cooped up" and has ceased crying, so I ask him to experiment by coming back to the part that "coops up" and ask it what it is trying to do.

Emphatically, "I am keeping you from getting hurt, as long as I keep you cooped up you don't get hurt."

Again I am concerned about overloading him, yet to stop here seems premature. So I ask him to talk to me about some other ways he could keep from getting hurt besides being cooped up. He comes up with two or three alternatives, acceptable to him.

Becky can contain herself no longer and tells Rich that she likes him and that his work has "moved" her. He seems uneasy and does not know what to say.

"Rich, are you cooping up at this moment?" I ask.

"Yes!" he sighs heavily, then turns to Becky and gives her a solid, "Thank you."

Bill chimes in that he is moved and feels very warm toward the group. "Could you express this directly?" I want to know. He turns to several members, expressing whatever warmth he feels for each, sometimes hugging, sometimes clutching a hand, finally saying to Martha that he "likes her" *and* that he wants to "keep some distance" because he does not know her well, Martha is okay with this and he goes back to his seat.

I am touched by Bill's work. I remember him in individual therapy, how uptight and nonexpressive he was; I remember how skeptical he was that joining group would help him. I share my feelings of pleasure with him and he tells me he is likewise pleased with himself. He is learning to be expressive in group and finding he can do the same outside of group, when he chooses to do so.

Martha contributes that the work of Rich and Bill has made her feel closer to both of them; she is energized by getting to know them in new ways. Impressed with Bill's ability to articulate his feelings, she believes she can learn from him. He responds that he could probably learn a lot from her also, because she represents the antithesis of him, free-spirited, expressive of all her emotions, at times impulsive.

I suggest an experiment evolving from this in which Martha teaches Bill something about being lively and expressive and he teaches her something about being considerate and thoughtful. True to form, Martha gets into it immediately, teaching Bill how to flirt. She tells him, "When you see someone you think is attractive, you approach her to talk to her, to let her know you think she is attractive and that you are interested in her." Self-consciously, he responds that he could not do that.

"How do you know?" I ask.

"Well, I just don't think I can."

"Would you like to find out?"

"Yes."

If there is any woman in the group that he is attracted to, I proffer an experiment to see if he can express it. He goes to Mary Ann and tells her that he "likes her looks," is attracted to her, and at the same time, is afraid of her strength, afraid that she might "overwhelm" him. This surprises her as she is not aware that in earlier interactions she came across as overwhelming. Bill takes some time to tell her what it is that she does that scares him, seeming solid and expressive in his interaction. He ends by turning to me and saying, "By golly, I'm amazing myself."

Five minutes to 4 o'clock. Our time is almost up, so I make rounds and check to see if there is any "finishing" anyone needs to do before we stop. Several want to say something to Rich or Bill—some new appreciation of them. I wonder, privately, at all the "sweetness and light," all the "liking," "complimenting," and "feeling good," bracketing it off until another time. I remember that at the start of our session Kate claimed to be energetic, so I ask her what has become of her energy. She says, "That is the story of my life, to know that I am excited and to wait for someone else to do something and my energy just dies."

"You must frequently feel that you do not get what you want," I comment. She agrees. We are now a couple of minutes over time. If she is interested, I tell her, we could work on that next week.

Summary

This chapter describes Gestalt therapy as practiced by those Gestalt therapists interested in group therapy. Emphasis is placed on strong theoretical knowledge of Gestalt therapy theory and personality development. Awareness and contact are the Gestalt concepts therapists draw upon continuously, so these two concepts are believed to be the primary curative factors and the focus upon awareness and contact leads to a therapy grounded in the present and ongoing activity of the group techniques *per se* are de-emphasized. Gestalt therapists believe that a reliance on technique places barriers between therapists and patients, as well as diminishing the contact function. This does not mean that some experimenting might not be done by some Gestalt therapists, but the best experiments are those which sharpen awareness and improve contact. Some Gestalt therapists pay little attention to group dynamics, while others view group interaction as important, leading in a style that facilitates interaction. An implicit message throughout this chapter is that there are very few "shoulds" in Gestalt therapy. In other words, Gestalt therapists are not expected to behave in canned or programmed ways. Most, however, would agree upon one commandment—awareness—because from this the excitement and energy will mobilize in novel ways to create change.

Acknowledgments

I owe a debt of gratitude to four people who helped in preparing this chapter. They are Martha Gehringer, Charles O'Neill, Richard Franklin, and Martha Herrick; without them I would still be struggling.

References

Appelbaum, S. A psychoanalyst looks at Gestalt therapy. In C. Hatcher & P. Himelstein (Eds.), *The handbook of Gestalt therapy*. New York: Jason Aronson, 1976, 753–778.

Carkhuff, R. *Helping and human relations: A primer for lay and professional helpers* (Vol. I). New York: Holt, Rinehart & Winston, 1969.

Egan, G. *The skilled helper: A model for systematic helping and interpersonal relating*. Monterey, Cal.: Brooks/Cole, 1975.

Fagan, J., & Shepherd, I. *Gestalt therapy now*. Palo Alto, Cal.: Science & Behavior Books, 1970.

Foulds, M., & Hannigan, P. Effects of Gestalt marathon workshops on measured self-actualization: A replication and follow-up study. *Journal of Counseling Psychology*, 1976, *23*, 60–65.

Greenberg, H., Seeman, J., & Cassius, J. Personality changes in marathon groups. *Psychotherapy: Theory, Research and Practice*, 1978, *15*, 61–67.

Greenberg, L., & Clarke, K. Differential effects of the two–chair experiment and empathic reflections at a conflict maker. *Journal of Counseling Psychology*, 1979, *26*, 1–9.

Greenberg, L., & Dompierre, L. Specific effects of Gestalt two-chair dialogue on intrapsychic conflict in counseling. *Journal of Counseling Psychology*, 1981, *28*, 288–295.

Greenberg, L., & Higgins, H. Effects of two-chair dialogue and focusing on conflict resolution. *Journal of Counseling Psychology*, 1980, *27*, 221–225.

Greenberg, L., & Rice, L. The specific effects of a Gestalt intervention. *Psychotherapy: Theory, Research and Practice*, 1981, *18*, 31–38.

Grinder, J. & Bandler, R. *The structure of magic II*. Palo Alto, Cal.: Science & Behavior Books, 1976.

Guinan, J., & Foulds, M. Marathon groups: Facilitator of personal growth? *Journal of Counseling Psychology*, 1970, *17*, 145–149.

Harman, R. Beyond techniques. *Counselor Education and Supervision* 1977, *17*, 157–158.

Harman, R. The goals of Gestalt therapy. *Professional Psychology*, 1974, *5*, 178–185.

Kempler, W. Gestalt therapy. In R. Corsini (Ed.), *Current psychotherapies*. Itasca, Ill.: F. E. Peacock Publishers, 251–286, 1973.

Kepner, E. Gestalt group process. In B. Feder & R. Ronall (Eds.), *Beyond the hot seat: Gestalt approaches to group*. New York: Brunner/Mazel, 1980.

Kopp, S. *Back to one: A practical guide for psychotherapists*. Palo Alto, Cal.: Science & Behavior Books, 1977.

Latner, J. *The Gestalt therapy book*. New York: Julian Press, 1973.

Levitsky, A., & Perls, F. The rules and games of Gestalt therapy. In J. Fagan & I. Shepherd (Eds.), *Gestalt therapy now*. Palo Alto, Cal.: Science & Behavior Books, 1970, 140–149.

Lieberman, M., Yalon, I., & Miles, M. *Encounter groups: First facts*. New York: Basic Books, 1973.

Melnick, J. Gestalt group process therapy. *Gestalt Journal*, 1980, *3* (2), 86–96.

Perls, F. *Ego, hunger and aggression*. New York: Vintage Books, 1947.

Perls, F. *Gestalt therapy verbatim*. Lafayette, Cal.: Real People Press, 1969a.

Perls, F. *In and out of the garbage pail*. Lafayette, Cal.: Real People Press, 1969b.

Perls, F., Hefferline, R., & Goodman, P. *Gestalt therapy: Excitement and growth in the human personality*. New York: Julian Press, 1951.

Perls, L. Concepts and misconceptions of Gestalt therapy. *Voices*, 1978, *14*, 31–35.

Polster, E., & Polster, M. *Gestalt therapy integrated*. New York: Brunner/Mazel, 1973.

Ramig, H., & Frey, D. A taxonomic approach to the Gestalt theory of Perls. *Journal of Counseling Psychology*, 1974, *21*, 129–184.

Rosenblatt, D. *Opening doors: What happens in Gestalt therapy*. New York: Harper & Row, 1975.

Rosenfeld, E. An oral history of Gestalt therapy: Part 1. A conversation with Laura Perls. *Gestalt Journal*, 1978a, *1*, 8–31.

Rosenfeld, E. An oral history of Gestalt therapy: Part 2. A conversation with Isadore From. *Gestalt Journal*, 1978b, *1*, 7–27.

Shepherd, I. Limitations and cautions in the Gestalt approach. In J. Fagan & I. Shepherd (Eds.), *Gestalt therapy now*. Palo Alto, Calif.: Science & Behavior Books, 1970, 234–238.

Simkin, J. *Gestalt therapy mini-lectures*. Millbrae, Cal.: Celestial Arts, 1976a.

Simkin, J. The development of Gestalt therapy. In C. Hatcher & P. Himelstein (Eds.), *The handbook of Gestalt therapy*. New York: Jason Aronson, 1976b, 225–233.

Smith, M., & Glass, G. Meta-analysis of psychotherapy outcome studies. *American Psychologist, 32*, 752–760, 1977.

Straus, E. *The primary world of senses: A vindication of sensory experience*. Glencoe, Ill.: Free Press, 1963.

Yalom, I. *The theory and practice of group psychotherapy* (2nd ed.). New York: Basic Books, 1975.

Zinker, J. Dreamwork as theatre. *Voices*, 1971, *7*, 18–21.

Zinker, J. *Creative process in Gestalt therapy*. New York: Brunner/Mazel, 1977.

Zinker, J. The developmental process of a Gestalt therapy group. In B. Feder & R. Ronall (Eds.), *Beyond the hot seat: Gestalt approaches to group*. New York: Brunner/Mazel, 1980.

GLOSSARY

Awareness. Spontaneously sensing or knowing what one is doing, planning, or feeling.

Contact. The sensory-motor way that a person encounters the environment. Through contact, one acknowledges others while at the same time, maintaining a sense of self.

Empty Chair. Refers to a technique developed by Fritz Perls, in which patients are asked to fantasize other people or various parts of their personalities in the empty chair and develop a dialogue with them.

Experiment. "A creative happening which grows out of the group's experience" (Zinker, p. 167, 1977).

Hot Seat. A term used to designate "the worker" in a Gestalt group.

Organismic Self-Regulation. A psychophysiological cycle that maintains equilibrium through the meeting of needs.

Worker. The person in a Gestalt group who is the center of attention and actively involved in doing something of his or her choosing.

6

Behavior Therapy Groups

MELVYN HOLLANDER and KATSUSHIGE KAZAOKA

INTRODUCTION

In any behavioral approach to change, major emphasis is placed upon the clear delineation of the goals as conceived of by the change agents. Following this emphasis, the authors wish to begin this chapter by stating the goals which they had in mind as they wrote for the reader. The goals for the chapter are:

1. To describe behavioral group therapy as a legitimate form of group therapy which, as with other forms of group therapy, has its unique advantages. These advantages enable it to meet the goals of individual change, as in individual therapy, while at the same time augmenting the change process in ways which are not possible in a one-to-one context.
2. To describe the similarities and differences between behavioral group therapy and the other group therapies.
3. To provide the reader with a new classification system which would allow for a coherent view of the varieties of behavior therapy groups.

Behavioral group therapy represents the amalgamation of two trends in the history of treatment approaches developed to deal with the multitude of problems experienced by man: group therapy and behavior therapy. Group therapy has a long history as a treatment approach, with its beginnings dating as far back as the early 1900s. However, group therapy did not begin to have major impact as a treatment alternative until World War II, with the work of S. H. Foulkes and others in England (Kaplan & Sadock, 1972a). These early pioneers were analytically oriented and were attempting to modify and extend the principles of individually oriented psychoanalysis to the treatment of individuals in groups. This extension of individual treatment to groups occurred in

Melvyn Hollander • Department of Psychology, Queens College, City University of New York, Flushing, New York 11367 and the Center for Behavioral Psychotherapy, White Plains, New York 10605.   **Kasushige Kazaoka** • Late of the Greer-Woodycrest Children Services, Pomona, New York 10703 and the Center for Behavioral Psychotherapy, White Plains, New York 10605.

response to the increasing awareness of mental health professionals that they were failing to reach the large numbers of persons who were in need of help.

Behavior therapy, unlike group therapy, represents a historical trend which owes its origin to forces outside of the traditional mental health mainstream. In fact, it developed in response to the increasing dissatisfaction of some professionals with the traditional views of and approaches to changing disordered behavior. Thus, where group therapy had its origin in the traditional therapies, with their acceptance of the intrapsychic and medical models, behavior therapy had its origin in the behavioral model, with its acceptance of situationism (Bowers, 1973).

It is of interest to note that the historical forces which led to the development of group therapy share much in common with the forces which led to the development of behavioral group therapy; namely, those forces which led to the increasing awareness by mental health professionals of the apparent inadequacies of the existing approaches in attempting to meet the demands for dealing with the problems faced by the consuming public. In addition, like the earlier workers, behavioral clinicians did not fail to appreciate the unique features of the group as providing a context which enabled them to deal with interpersonal issues which would be difficult or impossible to focus upon in a one-to-one relationship.

DEFINITION

Behavioral group therapy, as noted above, represents an attempt to wed the virtues of group therapy with those of behavior therapy. The most general definition would thus include such characteristics as the presence of two or more persons who are seeking help; one or more persons who by virtue of training and inclination function as providers of help; and the helping process as focusing on the issues of change in the behavioral, cognitive, and affective domains. However, these characteristics are insufficient to distinguish the behavioral group from any other group. Before we can suggest a meaningful definition of behavioral group therapy, it becomes necessary to deal with several common myths regarding behavior therapy which characterize the views of many mental health professionals.

Myth 1. Behavior therapy focuses on changes in behavior and not on changes in cognition and affect. Contrary to this widely held belief, current behavior therapy holds that changes will invariably occur in the cognitive and affective domains. The therapeutic issues have to do with the emphasis and timing in dealing with these domains as they relate to behavior. In general, the assumption is made that it is easier to effect changes in behavior, with subsequent changes occurring in relevant cognitions and affect, than to effect changes in cognitions and/or affects, with subsequent changes occurring in behavior. Clearly, this is not always the case, and it is the task of the behavioral clinician to ascertain the most effective focus of intervention for a particular individual, his or her particular problem, at that particular time, given the resources of the individual and the clinician.

Myth 2. Behavior therapy takes its theory and methods from learning theory and the psychological laboratory. To some extent this myth is accurate, but fails to provide an adequate picture of the extent to which contemporary behavior therapy has borrowed from other sources, as well as its emphasis on the development of methods on purely empirical rather than theoretical grounds. We believe that it is more accurate to characterize behavior therapy as an empirical approach to behavior change which is characterized by a neo-behaviorist model of humanity. More specifically, the model of human behavior which represents most accurately the state of the art is that espoused by Bandura (1977, 1978) and Mischel (1973).

Myth 3. Behavior therapy is incapable of dealing with the wide range of complex issues which are of concern to modern humanity; rather, it deals only with discrete behaviors which are symptomatic of more important and far-reaching problems. In answer to this myth, we agree with the point made by Ullman (1973) in an early paper where he provides a rationale for the ability of a behavioral approach to deal with the most complex of human issues. Ullman argued that even the most complex and ambiguous human issues arise in response to specific antecedent and consequent variables, and that their very complexity and ambiguity simply presents a problem capable of empirical analysis. The example he used was that of existential issues, and the behavioral clinician's task in these cases would be the same as in the case of any other problem area: namely, to pinpoint the relevant behaviors, define them, and identify the antecedent and consequent events related to them. Once a functional analysis is completed, then the clinician's task would be to implement the appropriate interventions in order to obtain the desired changes.

These myths are widespread and are held by clinicians of practically all persuasions, including some behavioral clinicians. The latter point is important, because it implies that the term behavior therapy and its referents are still somewhat unclear. Indeed, this lack of clarity is emphasized by the fact that there are a number of terms currently used in describing the activities of behavioral clinicians, for example, functional analysis of behavior, multimodal therapy, behavioral psychotherapy, behavior management, and so forth. In spite of the proliferation of terms and the differences which they attempt to stress, it is the belief of the present authors that a generally acceptable definition applicable to the activities and content of behavior clinicians is possible as well as desirable.

First, in terms of the content which might legitimately be identified as comprising the domain of interest of behavioral clinicians, it would be safe to state that it must encompass all of those phenomena which are thought to be of interest and importance both to helpers and to those seeking help. This then would include all behaviors, whether occurring in the external or internal environments. Whether these behaviors are to be addressed within a clinical context depends upon at least two things: (a) whether or not such behaviors are capable of translation (given the current state of the art) into the language of empirical psychology, and (b) whether or not there are available (given the current state of the art) empirically determined procedures for manipulating these behaviors in ways which are susceptible to empirical evaluation. If the phenomena of interest to clinicians meet at least these two stipulations, then they are capable of systematic and verifiable change. In effect, it is our contention that the behavioral clinican would deal with all the phenomena of interest to other clinicians regardless of their theoretical persuasion. The difference lies not in the phenomena addressed, but rather in the approach to those phenomena.

Second, in terms of the methodology employed in bringing about change, the behavioral clinician has no allegiance to any particular method or methods. Rather, his allegiance is to data within the context of an empirical psychology. Thus, we believe that the only restriction applicable to the methods used by the behavioral clinician to bring about desired change is that a particular method should have been demonstrated to be effective on the basis of empirical vaidation, rather than of clinical belief. We appreciate the fact that in the heat of operating in the front lines of the mental health battle, it is the rare clinician who has the luxury of relying solely upon methods which have been empirically validated as appropriate to the persons and/or situations which are of concern at any particular moment. With this in mind, we believe that what is important is that regardless of the specific intervention to be implemented, the clinician proceed with full awareness of the problems and pitfalls related to the intervention of choice. Equally important is that the clinician also proceed with the intervention in the context of an empirical framework which would allow for the evaluation of the impact of such intervention on the basis of data, rather than clinical intuition. This latter demand may appear to be irrelevant and/or impossible to many clinicians but, to our mind, it constitutes the core of a behavioral approach. Indeed, it is this experimental model with its emphasis on data which uniquely distinguishes the behavioral clinician and his or her activity from the activities of clinicians of other persuasions.

In light of the foregoing discussion, the formal definition of *behavioral group therapy* is as follows: any attempt by a person or persons to modify the behaviors of at least two or more other persons, meeting as a group, through the systematic application of empirically validated procedures within a framework which allows for the collection of data relevant to the assessment of the impact of these procedures upon the members of the group as individuals, and upon the group as a whole. It is our intent that this definition be clearly distinguished from other definitions which identify behavior therapy with a particular theory or approach limiting its definition to a naive behaviorism. Indeed, it is our intent to confine our definition to a methodological framework, and to exclude any reference to a particular theory or set of theoretical constructs. This is not to say that we, as teachers and clinicians, do not subscribe to a theoretical framework, but rather, that we wish to emphasize the possibility of many theoretical viewpoints existing under the roof of an experimental clinical model (Browning & Stover, 1971).

HISTORY

The application of behavioral principles and techniques to the behavior of individuals in groups appears to have occurred as a function of three different orientations. The first orientation is to extend, to a group setting, interventions which had been developed for the modifications of the behavior of individuals. In one of the first applications of a behavioral procedure in the context of a group, Lazarus (1961) extended the use of systematic desensitization to a group of phobic individuals. This trend of extending particular interventions to groups of persons can be seen in the extension to groups of such interventions as assertion training, stress management training, skill training, and so forth. The second orientation is to provide specific skill training in a group context in the interest of economy. Thus, in order to save time and effort, Patterson and his colleagues (Patterson, Ray, & Shaw, 1968) were among the first to train parents in parenting skills in the context of a group. Finally, the third orientation is to see the group as providing a unique context for modifying behaviors which would not occur, or would be difficult to modify, in the context of a one-to-one relationship. Liberman (1970) was one of the first to apply this approach when he attempted to systematically modify the dynamics of a group by means of a series of behavioral interventions.

In the almost two decades since Lazarus first applied systematic desensitization in a group context, there has been a slow expansion of behavioral group therapy. This expansion has been based primarily on the application of behavioral procedures to groups, as simple extensions of those developed for use with individuals, as well as on the use of skill-training programs in the context of a group. Such extensions require practically no change in the basic interventions and, indeed, need not require a group for their application.

On the other hand, the intervention procedures designed to modify those behaviors which are unique to the group setting, such as group dynamics, have to be developed specifically for that purpose. Such interventions thus are more than a simple extension of procedures developed previously for use with individuals. Unfortunately, there is a dearth of such procedures, and very few investigations have reported work with interventions which are designed to operate upon the unique characteristics of the functions and content of groups. Recently, however, there have been attempts to address issues such as a model for group therapy (Flowers, 1979), the role of the group in behavioral group therapy (Sansbury, 1979), process analysis in group therapy (Piper, Montvila, & McGihon, 1979), and group interaction (Rose, 1977). Other than these volumes, there are a few isolated reports of relevant works in the literature of the last two decades (Aiken, 1965; Bavelas, Hastorg, Gross & Kite, 1965; Bennett & Maley, 1973; Dinoff, Horner, Kuppiewski, Richard, & Timmons, 1960; Heckel, Wiggins, & Salzberg, 1962; Lieberman, 1975; Oakes, 1962; Oakes, Droge, & August, 1961; Shapiro, 1963; Shapiro & Birk, 1967) which focus on issues unique to the behavioral group. The lack of such work is particularly problematic in light of the professed and actual increase in interest in behavioral group therapy, particularly as witnessed by the text edited by Upper and Ross cited previously, as well as two currently available texts by Rose (1972, 1977), and a number of chapters or sections of other texts devoted to behavioral group therapy (Gazda, 1975; Hardy & Cull, 1974; Kaplan & Sadock, 1972a,b).

One might ask why there has been such a scarcity of investigations relevant to phenomena unique to the behavioral group therapy approach. In our judgment, this scarcity can be attributed to a number of factors. First, although there has been some interest in group behavior therapy for the last two decades, as noted earlier, it is only recently that this approach entered the mainstream of behavior therapy. Second, the historical emphasis of theorists in the areas of personality, psychopathology, and treatment has been upon the individual, and there is a marked lack of earlier work dealing with phenomena unique to groups. Third, this historical emphasis is in part related to the Western emphasis upon the individual as it is reflected in the sphere of Western psychology. Fourth, there is the empirical fact that group phenomena present the theorist with a degree of complexity greater than that evident in the psychology of the individual. Thus, the task of developing theoretical models and clinical interventions unique to behavioral group therapy requires a degree of theoretical and clinical sophistication not generally available in the field today. Fifth, and finally, empirical investigations and their theoretical products face the practical difficulties inherent in the implementation of programs which require large groups of people. It is, in fact, more difficult to obtain sufficient numbers of individuals for a group program, and this poses a significant obstacle for the initiation and implementation of appropriate research programs.

GOALS OF THE BEHAVIORAL THERAPY GROUP

The goals of the behavioral therapy group may be grouped within three distinct areas: the practical, the clinical, and the theoretical/conceptual. The practical goals are those related to nonclinical issues such as economy of time, money, and energy. Among them are such goals as: (a) achieving therapeutic contact with the greatest possible number of persons in need of change; (b) the use of the behavioral clinicians's time and effort in the most economical fashion; (c) the use of the group format to provide individuals with a learning set appropriate to a teaching/learning model of behavior change; and (d) providing a context which maximizes the probability that group members will develop the skills necessary to generate change in themselves and others; this is done by encouraging mutual information exchange. As can be seen, the assumption is made that the group provides a context of change which is qualitatively different from that found in one-to-one therapy, a context which makes it possible for the clinician to achieve goals precluded in the case of individual approaches to change.

The clinical goals of the behavioral therapy group are related to those issues which have to do with the specifics of change as agreed upon by the clinician and the clients. That is, the characteristics of the situation which directly influence the nature and quantity of change possible within the group setting, and which may or may not occur in a one-to-one context. They include such factors as: (a) that the group context makes possible the assessment of individuals and their behaviors in a situation which allows for the sampling of behaviors, which is not possible in a one-to-one situation; (b) that the group provides a context for change, which makes it possible for individual members of the group to learn and practice new behaviors in a setting where they can receive maximal support, feedback, and reinforcement; (c) that the group provides a context for change which makes it possible for individual members to learn the flexibility of response style necessary to cope with the idiosyncratic styles of those about them; (d) that the group provides a unique context for learning the social and interpersonal skills which are so important to successful living, by providing an immediate arena for change and practice; (e) related to this last point is the fact that the group provides a context for change which allows the individual to try out new behaviors in a setting which is appropriate to the spontaneous emission of such behaviors, but where the behavioral cost of errors or misjudgments are minimized and the payoff for success is maximized; and (f) that the group provides the clinician with the flexibility to choose between a context where members share a homogeneous set of issues or one where they face issues which are heterogeneous in nature. In addition, the members of a group may be chosen for their homogeneity or heterogeneity in relation to a large number of characteristics such as age, ethnicity, sex, income level, educational level, degree of impairment, and so forth.

It is also possible to view clinical goals as falling into two types: personal or individual goals and interactional goals (Thorensen & Potter, 1975). The individual goals would be those relevant to each of the group members. Individual goals may be shared in common by some or all of the members of the group, or they may be idiosyncratic to one member. In terms of these individual goals, the group simply provides the context for change and, in theory, these changes may be possible as well in a one-to-one context. The interactional goals, on the other hand, are unique to a group context, and refer to the quality and quantity of behavioral interactions which are made possible by the presence of a group of individuals, as opposed to the dyad of clinician and client. Thus, these interactional goals refer to such phenomena as group cohesiveness, level of activity of a group, group style, and so forth (Rose, 1977). These interactional goals may or may not be directly related to the members' individual goals, but rather are the goals set by the clinician for the group as a whole, with the purpose of providing the most salutary context for change. Thus, such things as group cohesiveness would likely influence the reinforcing characteristics of individual group members for others in the group, and by enhancing their reinforcing effectiveness, increase their impact upon those other members of the group.

Finally, there are the theoretical/conceptual goals of the behavioral group. These goals are related to the continuing need for a meaningful theoretical/conceptual framework which would make it possible for behavioral clinicians to understand and predict the nature of behavioral change as it occurs in the context of a behavioral group. Thus, there is a continuing need for behavioral clinicians to evolve the necessary theories or concepts which would lead to greater understanding of behavioral group therapy and its relationship to such phenomena as group norms, group cohesiveness, group control, and social reality (Lieberman, 1975).

In the next section, which will discuss the basic concepts applicable to the process of behavioral group therapy, it will be apparent to the informed reader that these concepts are also applicable to behavior therapy in general. That is to say, the basic concepts applicable to behavioral group therapy are those which were established in behavior therapy in general, and as yet no set of concepts unique to the group has emerged from the work of behaviorally oriented clinicians.

THEORY

Basic Concepts

Unlike the great majority of conventional diagnostic systems, the behavioral orientation asserts that there is little fundamental difference between behavior labeled normal and that labeled abnormal. Behavioral theoreticians suggest that the same learning processes which account for the development and maintenance of desirable, functional behavior are also sufficient to explain behavior labeled as maladaptive.

From a behavioral perspective, the only discernible difference between acceptable and problem human behavior is related to the content of what has been learned rather than to the process. As an example, any two individuals who have been raised in separate family environments are very likely to have been subjected to the same parent influencing procedures—rewarding child behavior, punishing child behavior, and modeling adult behavior that the child is expected to adopt. Yet, through these same procedures, one individual may have been taught by his or her parents to be confident and assertive in dealings with people and the other may have been trained to mistrust people and respond to their demands with anxiety or anger. Regardless of diagnostic labels, behavioral theorists see most forms of abnormal behavior as nothing more than the failure to have learned select coping skills, or as the unfortunate and sometimes accidental learning of inappropriate and self-defeating behavior.

The major aspect of a behavioral assessment is the repertoire inadequacy evaluation (Hollander, 1975). An individual has repertoire inadequacies when select aspects of behavior are viewed as discrepant by the individual or by others. These inadequacies are viewed as discrepant whenever the individual is not performing the way he or she would like to perform or the way others expect him or her to perform (Gottman & Leiblum, 1974). Most often the individual's performance is being unfavorably compared to his past performance, to group performance norms (the acceptable performance level of fellow workers, students, housewives, etc.), or to future performance self-expectations.

Problem behaviors may also be further classified as behavioral excesses, behavioral deficits, or behavior under inappropriate stimulus control (Kanfer & Saslow, 1965). Problem behaviors that occur at a rate in excess of cultural standards are called behavior excesses. Compulsive rituals, exhibitionism, assaultiveness, and hallucinations are examples of behavior patterns that have become exaggerated in frequency, intensity, or duration parameters. It should be noted that every person evidences some forms of problematic behavior but at too low a frequency to necessitate professional intervention. Commonplace examples are unusual or depressive thoughts, anxiety reactions, fears, and antisocial acts.

Thus, behavioral excesses are not intrinsically abnormal, but only become defined as problems when they are engaged in to an abnormal degree. Due to the disruptive nature of most behavioral excesses, these responses are easily recognized as problem behaviors. They interrupt the routine of the individual, create threat or discomfort in others, and sometimes require the involvement of social and legal agencies. In public schools, the child demonstrating behavioral excesses (classroom disruptions, threats directed to teachers, and truancy) is the most likely candidate for special school programs or outside therapy referrals. Similarly, adults with a chronic or psychotic adjustment pattern are usually institutionalized only after their interactions become excessive and incapacitate others (Langner & Michael, 1963).

Whenever a person is found to have gaps in his or her social, educational, or vocational repertoires large enough to obstruct effective actions, behavioral deficits are evident. Of course, factors such as age, social status, past performance, and setting must be considered in deciding whether an absent or low-frequency behavior serves a deficit function in the individual's current repertoire. In children, lack of success in mastering such essential developmental tasks as self-feeding, proper toilet habits, speech acquisition, cooperative play, and attending school are viewed as deficit behaviors. In adults, forms of sexual dysfunction such as impotence and frigidity, lack of assertiveness, social withdrawal reactions, and ineptness in responding to such changes as living independently, getting married or divorced, and losing one's job are similarly viewed as behavior deficits.

The third form of problem behavior is termed behavior under inappropriate stimulus control. Here the label "problematic" is based on the observation that the behavior in question occurs under undesirable, unrealistic, illegal, or dangerous circumstances. The behavior itself is not considered discrepant in frequency, intensity, or duration.

There is nothing clinically striking about the comment that an individual changes his clothing once or twice per day until the added fact is introduced that he makes these clothing changes in the middle of public meeting places. Similarly, engaging in active conversation is acceptable behavior unless no one else is present during this "conversation." A more subtle example can be illustrated by the situation where a person exclusively seeks love, support, or admiration from people who lack the capacity or interest to provide for the requested needs. Changing clothing, engaging in conversation, and seeking emotional support are adaptive behaviors until they occur outside of appropriate situational limits.

All human behaviors (problematic and nonproblematic) appear in the context of environmental antecedents and consequences. Thus, any behavior is subject to two distinct environmental forces—antecedents and consequences. Antecedents set the occasion for the occurrence of certain responses. On the other hand, consequences serve to strengthen, weaken or maintain responses already performed.

The identification of antecedent variables related to problem behaviors requires careful study of what factors are continually pesent each time the behaviors occur. In one of our cases, a male client complained that he experienced anxiety and social inhibition while attending parties. Further office assessments and some self-observation assignments revealed that he was relatively confident at work, at home, on vacation, and in most other typical settings. Parties seemed to be the only setting where social anxiety and subassertion reliably reached clinical levels.

A further antecedent appraisal indicated that such factors as the number of people present at the party, the degree of familiarity with others and the setting, and the purpose of the party exercised no antecedent control over his problem behavior. Only the factor of being alone at a party with an attractive female appeared to be significantly related. In all other settings this client arranged his life carefully so that he would not be alone in an informal social context with appealing women. Continued assessment efforts led to the conclusion that he was specifically afraid of being asked to dance (he did not know how), that he did not know how to handle anticipated sexual overtures from women, and that he was hypersensitive that someone might distort the meaning of his social contact with women at parties. Treatment involved systematic desensitization for his fears and assertion training to help him cope with shyness and negative self-evaluations.

Perhaps what is more important in clinical assessment than the identification of antecedents is the evaluation of consequences (Hollander & Plutchik, 1972). One such example, the direct–indirect control loop (Hollander, 1974) is a dysfunctional form of family interaction that becomes clear when one studies behavior consequences. Originally, this pattern was observed from a videotape playback of a family session conducted by one of the authors. Three family members were present: a mother, a father, and the indexed patient—a 12-year-old son diagnosed as schizophrenic. On the tape the family interacted normally until the father began disagreeing with the mother over financial expenditures and announced in a belligerent tone that she would have to make many extra sacrifices. Her weak protestations that he would not make similar sacrifices went unnoticed. Then the son began to exhibit bizarre speech and ritualistic movements. Both parents stopped arguing and the mother comforted the son.

In future sessions, this pattern was recorded whenever family arguments ensued. As to the maintaining consequences of this faulty interaction pattern, the mother's attention and concern appear to have reinforced her son's psychotic behavior. In turn, the son's psychotic behavior may have been reinforcing to the mother in that it terminated marital arguments, which she could not do through her own efforts. In other words, the mother directly controlled (reinforced) the son's psychotic behavior so as to indirectly control (punish) the husband's offensive actions.

Analysis of consequences is critical to the practice of behavior therapy when one considers how rapidly behavioral and emotional problems can be treated. If a behavior therapist fails to gain a thorough understanding of what reinforcements the symptoms provide, resistance or other untoward reactions could easily result from direct symptom modification (Lazarus, 1971).

Let us look at the problem of agoraphobia and the interplay with consequences. We treated a woman who had previously consulted another behavior therapist. The therapist had immediately attempted to desensitize her to leaving the house, but the therapy failed and she contacted one of the authors. Through a behavioral assessment it became most apparent that powerful reinforcements maintained her agoraphobia. For one, her husband pampered her only after she had become phobic, at which time he began to center his life around her. Also as a result of the agoraphobia, the husband arranged for a live-in maid who relieved the client of distasteful household chores. Systematic desensitization proved to be an effective procedure, but only after it was used in conjunction with training the husband to withdraw his reinforcement from the phobia and to direct his encouragement exclusively toward her attempts to be more independent. Furthermore, the live-in maid was released, although she continued to maintain a long friendship with the client.

Assumptions about Human Nature

In our judgment, several prevalent misconceptions exist about the behavioral view of human nature. Many people believe that behavioral theory reduces human behavior to a set of isolated, externally conditioned responses that do not reflect the essence of human nature.

Contrary to this popular belief, human beings are not automatically conditioned to behave in select ways by the external forces of stimulus antecedents and consequences. The capacity to learn in humans partially reflects the ability to think and process information about external and internal experiences. This capacity allows people to assess the potential benefits and costs of performing certain behaviors in future circumstances. It insures that we are not solely motivated by the short-term profit of immediate consequences (Mischel, 1974). Instead we can defer engaging in actions that produce immediate rewards if it becomes apparent that such practice will result in long-term aversive consequences. In fact, this capacity to defer action based on a cognitive appraisal of short- and long-term consequences is a form of insightful behavior.

In social learning theory, there is recognition of the importance of awareness and self-produced consequences in learning. Bandura (1969) cites evidence that rewarding consequences do not automatically strengthen human actions. He asserts that it is the person's capacities to value the incentives, the agent(s) dispensing the incentive, and the behavior to be performed, that determines responses to rewarding consequences. Thus, human conduct is not merely a by-product of consequences; people respond to self-evaluation reactions, as well as external outcomes. People do more than react to their environment; they act on it to promote changes which serve them. As humans, we can inform ourselves, symbolically enact what we observe in others, and reinforce ourselves for accomplishments. We can influence the world as well as be influenced by it in lawful ways.

It has long been held that determinism is a key concept in behavioral theory. All discernible events are elicited or caused by prior events and so forth in an infinite regression of causes. Although behavioral theory embraces determinism as a conceptual underpinning, it does not negate the existence of freedom as a force in human behavior.

Both concepts can be embraced in a perspective on human nature if the notion that freedom and determinism are antithetical is reconsidered. Bandura (1974) proposed that freedom can be conceived in terms of prerequisite skills available and the exercise of self-influence over decisions to act. Even if prerequisite skills and self-influences are themselves determined by prior events, the individual has partial freedom insofar as he or she can control future events by managing his or her own behavior. Hence, freedom is not the absence of controls or external constraints; it is now defined by the existence of self-controlling features in human behavior. People have certain degrees of freedom to act even if the self-controlling features are themselves determined by prior external conditions.

It follows that acceptance of this dual position implies a generally positive view of human nature in which people can partially transcend environmental influences and controls. Further extrapolations of behavioral therapy characterize human nature in terms of the concepts of uniqueness and striving for competence. Although humanistic theory sees uniqueness in terms of totally individual perceptions of the world, current behavioral theory sees people as unique in terms of their particular learning history and the resultant repertoire of skills available to master life situations. Because no two people experience the same learning history (even if they were identical twins who resided in the same home), it is not expected that people will respond identically to divergent situational demands in the home, office, school, and so forth.

Another essential feature of the behavioral view of human nature is the concept of striving for competence. In some respects there is an overlap with the ego psychology view of competence as advanced by White (1959). However, the behavioral view differs in that it specifically identifies the varying coping behaviors and enumerates at least three kinds of environmental challenges and demands (Goodstein & Lanyon, 1979). For example, with respect to environmental challenges there are: (a) direct challenges from the physical environment; (b) challenges involving people's reactions to their own physical and intellectual limitations; and (c) challenges posed by the interpersonal environment. It is primarily, but not exclusively, problems in the area of interpersonal challenges that bring people to seek counseling and psychotherapy. Often they express an inability to relate to others in ways that clearly satisfy their personal needs and find difficulty in coping with demands made by others.

Even when people falter with interpersonal challenges and develop neurotic symptoms, they still attempt to achieve some modest level of social competency and control. Usually people get minimal rewards from securing attention and recognition, even at the price of experiencing uncomfortable symptoms. Thus, problem behavior may lead to some achievement in interpersonal strivings. In essence, a basic force of human nature is the achievement of some social reinforcement, regardless of the means by which it is achieved.

Personality Theory

In behavioral terms personality is an abstraction that is based on inferences drawn from observed samples of behavior in various life situations. An individual's personality cannot be understood apart from his or her response patterns. In this sense, the study of personality is synonomous with the study of behavior patterns, and particularly with the interaction between these patterns and environmental consequences. Personality can be satisfactorily accounted for in terms of concurrent interpersonal skills and environmental influences, as well as previous social learning history. It is not necessary to postulate underlying dynamics—defenses, drives, or traits—to achieve a full and rich understanding of personality.

In contrast, most traditional personality theorists rely heavily on the concept of underlying dynamics to afford them a working picture of human personality. They consider that all significant behavior (personality) is a product of nonobservable, intrapsychic phenomena such as traits or personality structures, which are enduring entities and reside within the individual. Accordingly, it is only through a careful appraisal of intrapsychic phenomena that human behavior can be understood and predicted. This view is consonant with a centralist orientation, where the focus is on the individual and his or her characteristics.

At the other end of the continuum is the radical behavioral view. It is most consonant with a peripheralistic orientation: the study of human behavior should focus entirely on environmental influences. We subscribe to a more moderate behavioral view of personality and maintain an interactional orientation. Personality, in our view, is the sum total of the reciprocal interactions between the individual's responses and his or her internal and external environments. Furthermore, we assert personality is not what one has, but what one does and the specific conditions under which one does it.

The interactionist behavioral view (Goldfried & Kent, 1972; Mischel, 1968, 1973) states that behavior referred to as personality is highly situation specific.

One could argue, however, that what we learn in terms of one situation does transfer to new, relatively similar situations. How are these statements reconciled? Behavioral theorists would point out that, although transfer does occur, it is much less prevalent than suggested by traditional personality theories. These latter theorists have assumed that people acquire internal personality traits that produce similar reactions across a variety of different situations.

If behavior is situation-specific, we would not expect to find children who are labeled as aggressive behaving in an aggressive fashion in most situations. Children are usually aggressive when the aggression is elicited by others (verbal challenges, taunts, lack of affectionate displays) and/or when it works for the child (attention, submission by others, withdrawal by others). It should be obvious that all situations are not characterized by these antecedents and consequences; as a result the child would not be expected to show a generalized trait of aggression. Surprisingly, a child may be found to defer to the father, be affectionate to the grandparents, verbally abusive to the mother, and physically abusive to siblings and schoolmates. He or she may act out whenever anyone denies a meal but not necessarily when people fail to play with him or her. He or she may even laugh a great deal and care tenderly for animals. Does it make sense to give this child a generalized trait label—aggressive? We think not.

In the same vein, depressed persons do not always act depressed, psychotic persons do not always evidence psychotic symptoms, happy people are not always cheerful, and so forth. A careful behavioral assessment, including observation, interviews, and paper-and-pencil questionnaires may lead to a determination of precise circumstances under which these characteristics of personality (behavior) occur and do not occur. For example, Ullman and Krasner (1969) and Braginsky and Braginsky (1967) showed that hospitalized mental patients were very aware of the social rules in their institutional environment. Patients were found to present themselves as more or less disturbed, depending upon which type of behavior would offer greater rewards at any point in time. These research conclusions not only suggested that personality behavior is situation-specific, but also support the interaction orientation (reciprocal interaction between an individual's behavior and the environment).

The aforementioned discussion does not negate the existence of behavioral consistencies. Rather, such consistencies are to be viewed as the product of specific learning histories (Baer, Wolf, & Risley, 1968; Karoly & Steffen, 1980). Those of us who practice psychotherapy find ourselves dealing with individuals whose typical behavior happens to be problematic in the home, school, work, and related contexts. A fairly stable pattern of maladaptive interpersonal behaviors has been learned and it is by way of these behaviors that a person comes to be characterized by others as troubled.

There have been few attempts among behavioral theorists to develop a comprehensive theory of personality. Instead, research and theorizing has tended to be limited to select topics in personality such as conflict, dependency, social responsiveness, and aggression, as well as the learning principles that account for their development. There are several learning theorists whose contribution to personality research and theory are noteworthy. Among them are Dollard and Miller, Wallace, Wolpe, Bandura, Krasner and Ullman, Rotter, and Mischel. A brief synopsis of their theories follows:

Dollard and Miller (1950) took on the difficult task of unifying learning theory and psychoanalytic theory in their book *Personality and Psychotherapy*. Essentially they adhered to Freud's basic concepts, such as psychosexual stages of development, innate drives, and defense mechanisms, to name a few. Their interpretation of these phenomena, however, relied heavily on the learning theory concepts of stimulus and response associations.

For example, anxiety was viewed as a learned or conditioned drive, and any response that reduced the stimuli associated with this drive was strengthened. As to the defenses, repression was described as an active response of avoiding the thinking of anxiety-arousing thoughts by use of cognitive distraction and mislabeling strategies. Transference was proposed to be a special case of response generalization which occurs when one responds alike to a current person and a previous similar person. Attitudes and responses toward parents may generalize later to teachers, friends, and spouse because of similar stimulus characteristics. Dollard and Miller, unlike Freud, thought it was superfluous to postulate a symbolic connection between parents and say, teachers. They felt that similarity in overt stimulus features between these two groups, as well as the social status accorded them by society, was sufficient to explain the transference phenomenon.

Another contribution made by Dollard and Miller was to the study of conflict. Rather than accepting the psychoanalytic notion of conflict as a battleground between id, ego, and superego structures, they offered a learning explanation. In their explanation, conflict was a result of pursuing mutually exclusive goals of equal or nearly equal strength, and having to make a forced choice. Conflict was divided into specific types according to whether the goals elicited approach or avoidance tendencies.

The view of personality developed by Wallace (1966) emphasized the individual's physical and interpersonal competencies for coping with varying life circumstances. Wallace introduced the term "response capability" to refer to the measurement and prediction of human response probabilities which are thought to be determined by early socialization experiences. Response capability is any learned proficiency within the person's repertoire. These proficiencies are arranged in a hierarchial order of occurrence in situations.

Wolpe (1958, 1969) devoted his attention to the study of neurotic personality. Wolpe assumed that a neurosis was a persistent learned habit of responding with irritational anxiety to situations that do not present any actual threat or danger. This learning comes about through a classical conditioning paradigm. An initially neutral stimulus occurs in close temporal association with an extreme anxiety situation. Through pairing or association learning, the neutral stimulus comes to acquire fear arousing properties, the result being called conditioned fear. Characteristically, avoidance learning takes place next. Here attempts are made to avoid the physical, and sometimes imaginal, presence of the learned fear stimulus. Avoidance learning prohibits the opportunity to face the learned fear and thus become desensitized to it. In clinical practice the authors have treated numerous clients whose phobias are a function of conditioned fear. Previously neutral or pleasurable stimuli such as water, bridges, the dark, home, sleeping, and audiences have, through temporal association with traumatic events, come to precipitate phobic neuroses.

Krasner and Ullman (1973) developed an approach to personality they called behavior influence. To them, the concept of personality is an intellectual creation used to explain acts that have uncertain origins. They also proposed a rather different point of reference for personality investigations, urging that such investigations include historical, economic, contextual, sociological, ecological, and organizational variables. Krasner and Ullman diverge further from conventional practice by including the investigation of the personality of the personality theorists. "Personality theory is human activity; hence, we can and should study personality theorists" (p. 23).

Bandura, Rotter, and Mischel have given considerable attention to the area of behavioral cognitions in their study of personality. At the same time all have accorded the concept of reinforcement a slightly lesser role in their theory. Bandura adopted the view that personality was largely the product of modeling and imitation. People tend to be influenced by what they observe in select ways. Bandura's extensive research investigated and studied, among other variables, the characteristics and perception of the model and the consequences experienced by the model under different performance conditions. In summary, models who possessed high status and were perceived as nurturant were likely candidates to be imitated. What behaviors got modeled depended largely on the observed consequences to the model.

As an example, if a child observes an older and respected classmate engaging in boisterous classroom antics and then getting severely reprimanded, there is little chance that the model's conduct would be imitated. Besides overt behavior tendencies, Bandura found that attitudes, expectancies, and even emotional responses, can be vicariously learned without the observer experiencing any direct consequences. Thus, it becomes easier to understand how children whose parents are phobic develop the identical phobia without ever experiencing the uptoward consequences themselves.

Rotter (1954) discussed meaningful environments as a key concept in his exposition of personality theory. To Rotter, what affects the individual is not the environment *per se*, but the environment as it is uniquely perceived. Furthermore, he postulated that the occurrence of a behavior is not only the function of the nature of reinforcement, but also the expected probability of a successful outcome. For example, whether an employee asks for a raise depends as much on his or her expectation of success in getting the request approved as on the desire for reinforcement. If the goal of securing a raise is very important while the expectation of reaching it is very low, the employee will likely decide against making the effort to make a request.

According to Mischel, individuals have differing capacities to absorb information from various sources. Once information is absorbed, it is encoded, and the event observed now has meaning. Other personality variables studied by

Mischel are the perceived value of the goal, the outcome expectancy, and self-regulatory capacities.

Comparisons with Related Theories

For many years, behavior therapy has been strongly contrasted with counseling and psychotherapy, as if it embodied a set of assumptions and treatment procedures foreign to customary clinical practice. Behavior therapists themselves have added to this schism by dissociating their research and theoretical endeavors, as well as treatment efforts, from other therapeutic orientations. Early behaviorists denied the importance of such parameters as subjective experiences, the influence of the past, the therapeutic relationship, and other cherished ideas of psychodynamic theory.

The winds are changing now. More and more, practitioners and theoreticians of a behavioral persuasion are seeing the value of traditional clinical concepts and at the same time expanding behavioral technology. We believe, along with others (Kendall, 1982), that the time has already come for a serious rapprochement between behavioral and other pragmatic approaches. Furthermore, we feel that behavior therapy as currently practiced by ourselves and other colleagues is a form of psychotherapy. In fact, we have introduced the term "behavioral psychotherapy" to describe the philosophy of the postdoctoral training programs at our center. However, we will adhere in this chapter to common practice by retaining the term behavior therapy throughout.

Regardless of theoretical orientation, all systems of psychotherapy (including behavior therapy) share some common practices and hold many of the same fundamental assumptions. The classic oft-quoted studies of Fiedler (1950, 1951) compared the therapeutic relationship as established by psychoanalysts, nondirective therapists, and Adlerian therapists. Fiedler found that the therapeutic relationships established by experts from different schools of thought were more like one another than those established by experts and novices of the same school. An assumption of these studies, still widely held, is that experienced clinicians of varying persuasions are more similar than different in treatment practices.

All forms of psychotherapy begin with an assumption that human behavior can be changed. Psychotherapy provides the conditions whereby psychological problems can be treated through unlearning and relearning. The actual form that this learning process takes is dependent on the type of therapy practiced. Learning takes place in the context of a professional therapeutic relationship. Experienced therapists all work toward establishing the kind of therapeutic relationship that will optimize learning experiences for clients. The specific nature of the relationship established depends on many variables, including the nature of the client's problems and the form of learning experiences undertaken (e.g., insight, behavior change, emotional catharsis, awareness).

There is some evidence that the effectiveness of the psychotherapies is largely dependent upon the client's motivation for change and expectations that he or she will be functioning better as a result of the treatment (Coe, 1980; Garfield, 1978). The degree of congruence between the client's expectations of what will transpire in therapy and the actual process of therapy is another important parameter in treatment outcome. In our behavioral practices, we have noted that client motivation, faith, and positive congruence expectations are crucial to our successes. In fact, the initial phase of every behavioral program we provide, whether it be for individuals, groups, families, or institutional residents, involves strategies to foster motivation and realistic treatment expectations. Strategies we have used to create these conditions are social reinforcement for change efforts, use of pretherapy videotapes of ideal therapy sessions, shaping and reinforcement for successive approximations of the goal, verbal persuasion, and giving prior examples of similar successful cases.

Goldenberg (1973) proposed another dimension that serves as a common ground for all psychotherapies. He stated that all systems of psychotherapy have adopted a set of hypothesized propositions. These propositions are concerned with human nature, a theory of abnormal behavior, a theory of psychopathology, the role of the therapist, time orientation for treatment (past, present, and future), the influence of automatic or unconscious processes, role of insight versus action, and treatment goals.

Goldfried and Davison (1976) firmly believe that behavior therapy has much to offer in the way of added effectiveness to clinicians of other orientations. On the other hand, they acknowledge that treatment procedures derived from nonbehavioral orientations have important applications to the clinical practice of behavior therapy. As examples, they cite the work of Sullivan on interview procedures, Roger's client-centered techniques for the establishment of rapport, and Perls's Gestalt therapy procedures for facilitating awareness and open expression of "here-and-now" feelings.

Most important, Goldfried and Davison see behavior therapy as employing the same fundamental principles and practices of the client–therapist relationship as established in psychoanalytic, gestalt, client-centered, and related approaches. They state that the therapeutic relationship between behavior therapist and client is indistinguishable from that observed in other approaches. While behavior therapists may have different rationales for what they are saying or doing, their interpersonal actions are experienced by clients as quite similar to the actions of nonbehavioral therapists. Furthermore, research evidence suggests that the therapeutic relationship in the context of behavior therapy can enhance the effectiveness of behavior change techniques (Goodstein, 1971; Morris & Suckerman, 1974). Specifically, Morris and Suckerman found that systematic desensitization proved more effective in reducing fear of snakes when the therapy was conducted by a "warm" therapist (in terms of good eye contact, soft voice, supportive comments) than by a "cold" therapist (e.g., impersonal, unconcerned, distant in posture).

Now let us put the shoe on the other foot. It may come as a surprise to some nonbehavioral clinicians that they are actually using behavioral interventions in their clinical work. One common behavioral intervention is social reinforcement. Whether through verbal means ("That was a good effort," or "I am pleased with your progress") or through nonverbal means (smiles, head-nods, leaning forward) therapists convey their approval and satisfaction of client's insights, congruent expectations and language, and behavior change. Nearly all dynamic therapists also employ a variation of a behavioral procedure known as systematic desensitization. Therapists are faced with clients who are initially fearful of revealing themselves in individual or group situations. Without realizing it, therapists create a nonpunitive atmosphere in the sessions which is paired with the client's initial attempts at self-disclosure. The pairing of a facilitating environmental condition (one incompatible with the experience of anxiety) and client statements low on a fear hierarchy of self-disclosure is the first basic step in desensitization. Slowly, clients are encouraged to disclose more sensitive material about their lives (going up the hierarchy) while each occurrence of self-disclosure is paired with the facilitating relationship condition.

Other behavioral procedures have common referents in psychodynamic practice. In one or another form all therapists employ assertion training, cognitive restructuring, prescription for change, and shaping. What therapist has not discussed and/or role-played ways by which clients could gain interpersonal competencies (assertiveness training)? What therapist has not pragmatically suggested to clients new ways to label and evaluate problem experiences (cognitive restructuring)? What therapist has not directed clients as to where, when, and how to handle reality life stress situations (prescriptions for change)? What therapist has not structured or encouraged client change in small steps, slowly approximating the change necessary to reach a major treatment goal (shaping)?

It is apparent from the discussion thus far that considerable overlap exists between behavioral and nonbehavioral orientations in that they share some similar assumptions and clinical practices. Yet, at the same time, behavior therapy is a distinctly different approach to clinical assessment and treatment. Basically, behavior therapy distinguished itself by selecting specific symptoms of behaviors for treatment, by using concrete, systematically planned procedures to bring about behavior change, and by continuously monitoring progress through quantitive means (Kanfer & Phillips, 1970).

Rimm and Masters (1974) offer a number of issues and dimensions that separate behavior therapy from more traditional treatment approaches. They claim that in behavior therapy the emphasis is placed on behavior as opposed to presumed underlying causes. In other words, behavior therapists are not hesitant to treat symptoms, because they equate symptoms with clinical problems worthy of treatment. Behaviorists are unconcerned with the warning issued by some that removing symptoms, especially while neglecting the underlying cause, will lead to symptom recurrence or substitution. A large body of research tends to support the behavioral position on symptom substitution (Bandura, 1969).

Sophisticated behavior therapists do not automatically treat presenting behaviors or symptoms. They may wait and treat other behaviors that become more apparent as a careful behavioral assessment proceeds. Furthermore, they view people as having problems, sometimes many, that functionally interrelate with one another in the present and yet do not have an underlying cause. As an example, one of us treated a man who complained that he couldn't concentrate at college and was receiving poor grades as a result. It turned out that he couldn't concentrate because he was was unprepared for tests and woefully behind in classwork. He was unprepared at school because he couldn't stop obsessing about his girlfriend toward whom he could not be assertive. He couldn't be assertive because he feared her rejection if he stepped out of a subordinate role and also he lacked assertive skills, had he chosen to take that step. His lack of success with his girlfriend caused him to drink excessively, which retarded his ability to cope with the demands made by girlfriend and school. All these behaviors or symptoms functionally relate to one another as a chain of stimuli and responses. All human behavior problems coexist in this sort of chain; problems do not functionally underlie one another, although some behavioral problems may be more central to treatment. That is, more behaviors are correlated or associated with these than with other behaviors.

Another hallmark of behavior therapy is that it makes available to clients a wide array of pragmatic and experimentally validated techniques that are tailored to their unique problems and needs. The great majority of techniques are concrete and systematically conducted (e.g., systematic desensitization, modeling, behavior rehearsal, operant conditioning, the token economy, extinction procedures, aversive therapy, and cognitive strategies). This allows for scientific investigations of their utility. In fact, it is safe to say that no other major treatment approach has subjected itself to such close experimental scrutiny. One of the reasons why behavioral technologies have grown in numbers and effectiveness is that the adoption of methods shifts back and forth between the laboratory and the clinic for hypothesis testing and clinical applications.

The advantages of techniques being concrete and pragmatic are numerous. First, they lend themselves to experimental investigation. Second, behavior therapists can learn these procedures and achieve a high level of proficiency with a minimum of distortion or trial and error. Third, some procedures are sufficiently concrete for paraprofessionals, parents, and other parties to use them under professional guidance to help change people in their social system.

Perhaps the most important aspect of behavioral techniques is that the therapist is freed from practicing an "all purpose, single method" therapy (Bandura, 1969, p. 89) such as found in most psychodynamic and humanistic approaches. Instead, behavior therapists employ different procedures and combinations thereof to deal with varying clinical problems. A depressed person may receive cognitive restructuring, assertiveness training, and self-reinforcement training. A person fearful of lightning may be simply desensitized. An exhibitionist may be treated with aversive conditioning, systematic desensitization, and bibliotherapy, for fears of sexual intimacy; and with assertiveness training for increased interpersonal effectiveness with women. A chronic hospitalized schizophrenic may participate in a ward-wide token economy program conducted by psychiatric attendant staff. The program might be designed to foster awareness of the environment, self-care skills, motivation to participate in rehabilitation activities, and so forth. A business executive suffering from stress may be given instruction in music relaxation and positive imagery, in effective communication tactics with subordinates, and in decision-making skills. A woman with a hand-washing compulsion may be offered response prevention procedures, thought stopping, covert sensitization, and relaxation training. An agoraphobic may receive behavioral marriage counseling (including exchange contracts, communication training, and caring days), *in vivo* desensitization, assertion training, and child management training. Lastly, a person with a chronic pain disorder could be offered biofeedback training, hypnosis, transcutaneous nerve stimulation, thought stopping, as well as social reinforcement for increased activity level and nonpain behaviors. Thus, it can be asserted that behavior therapy is one of the most flexible and truly individualized forms of psychotherapy. We wonder how many forms of psychotherapy can offer such diverse treatment procedures in the context of flexible treatment planning to such an array of problem areas!

A few unique features of behavior therapy remain for discussion. First, tools of treatment include apparatus and instrumentation generally not available or used in other orientations. Behavior therapists make ample use of biofeedback equipment, videotape and other recording equipment, aversive conditioning apparatus, slide projectors, bug-in-the-ear devices, automated desensitization devices, and telemetry instrumentation. These and other types of instrumentation have been used to automate select behavioral procedures, to extend behavioral procedures outside the office, to give feedback to clients on the process of therapy, and to evaluate the effectiveness of ongoing behavioral activities in sessions. Because of their experience in this realm, therapists have learned how to introduce, time, and structure the use of apparatus in ongoing therapy without sacrificing or diminishing emotional learning experiences.

Second, behavior therapy has extended its applications into the natural environment and has often used mediators including the client himself to conduct behavior change programs (Tharp & Wetzl, 1969) Operant conditioning incentive programs have been the most widely applied. Although a behavior therapist might design and/or consult on such programs, the programs are generally conducted by nonprofessionals outside of the office. With careful training in the application of operant conditioning, psychiatric attendants have treated hospitalized patients (Hollander, 1973, 1976; Hollander & Plutchik, 1972); teachers have better managed students in the classroom (O'Leary & O'Leary, 1972; Wolf, Giles, & Hall, 1968); parents have learned to communicate better and relate with their children (Becker, 1971; Browning, 1980; Patterson, 1975); and clients themselves have overcome weight problems, smoking problems, study problems, and common fears (Goldfried & Merbaum, 1973).

In our professional interaction and communication with colleagues of other therapeutic persuasions, some specific integrations and contrasts have become evident. We share a family tie with rational–emotive therapists. In fact, a large part of the cognitive behavior therapy we practice includes most, if not all, rational–emotive therapy (RET) techniques. Theoretically, we accept Ellis's assumption that psychological disorders arise from irrational thinking, but see this as an incomplete explanation. Therefore, in therapy, we may be altering overt behavior and thinking processes independently. A RET therapist would most likely begin by changing cognitions. Ellis and other RET therapists are trying to teach their clients new ways to think so as to eliminate self-defeating behavior, while we are likely to teach our clients how to change their overt social behavior and, consequently, act their way into new patterns of thinking.

In contrast to our psychoanalytic colleagues, we take a more active teaching role with our clients. If, by chance, transference reactions occur, we de-emphasize them unless therapy has reached a stalemate. Even when dealing with transference, we behave differently. We focus on the current manifestations and implications of transference reactions and do not dwell on the past. Furthermore, we role play more effective ways for clients to relate to us as therapists.

We are less likely to blame our clients for therapy stalemate and failures. We assume the largest part of the problem rests in our own failure to assess the problem situation completely and/or design the most appropriate treatment program. We tend to have more realistic goals for our clients and see them for therapy less often. We do as much for our clients outside of the office as within the walls of our offices. Specifically, we give clinical homework assignments, audio cassette tapes to listen to at home, apparatus to practice with outside, and so forth, to our clients.

With our humanistic and Gestalt colleagues, we feel a philosophical kinship of sorts. We dislike psychopathology labels and avoid using them. In large part we all reject the medical model, and our respective approaches grew out of this dissatisfaction. We accept for our clients the goals of self-actualization and personal freedom set forth by the humanists. However, because we are behaviorists, we specify behaviors necessary to reach them and achieve these goals for our clients through the humanistic application of the technology of behavior therapy (Thoresen, 1974). Thus, we may use vastly different methods, but our view of clients as people and our goals for them are shared by many humanistic therapists.

The rich achievements and unique nature of all people is in no way detracted from when we or others practice behavior therapy with groups or individuals. The American Humanistic Association shares this view somewhat and not long ago awarded B. F. Skinner the "Humanist of the Year" award.

THERAPY

Theory

As has been pointed out earlier, it is our opinion that there is very little theory related to behavioral group therapy in the sense of a systematic set of theoretical principles and concepts which provide a framework for understanding this approach in its entirety. Rather than such a theory, what has evolved is the application of a variety of theoretical and conceptual systems, in part or in whole, in order to gain an understanding of what behavioral group therapy is about. As one would expect, the result has been a patchwork with little coherence or agreement as to which theoretical systems or concepts are critical to the understanding of behavioral group therapy. What we have found is that workers in this area have approached their subject matter principally from an empirical and applied perspective. Reliance upon theoretical and conceptual matters occurred as a secondary consideration, if such matters were considered at all. What is usual is a more or less simple focus upon a particular intervention or set of interventions for a particular population or set of populations. Indeed, practically no work has focused specifically upon theoretical and/or conceptual issues. Due to this lack of a systematic theoretical and conceptual framework, we found that we were faced with the task of selecting those theoretical and conceptual materials which we felt were most germane to the subject of behavioral group therapy. This choice clearly means that we excluded as well as included materials which touch upon the general subject area, and thus it represents our bias rather than an exhaustive attempt at presenting all relevant theoretical and conceptual materials.

Without question the single most important source of theoretical and conceptual materials has been the general area of behavior theory. As we see it, practically all of the theoretical and conceptual materials drawn from behavior theory and integrated into the area of behavior therapy are germane to the work of behavioral group therapy. Thus, texts such as Bandura (1969, 1977), Nay (1977), Meichenbaum (1977), Mahoney (1974), Gambrill (1977), and Rimm and Masters (1979) discuss the entirety of behavioral theory and concepts from operant to respondent, radical behaviorist to neobehaviorist, experimental–clinical to clinical–experimental, and all attest to the extent to which behavior therapy as well as behavioral group therapy leans upon the empirical and theoretical fruits of general behavior theory.

In addition to the more general contributions of general behavior theory, there are several specific contributions which are worthy of note. Specifically, these are: (a) portions of the literature related to the social psychology of groups (Cartwright & Zander, 1968; Maccoby, Newcomb, & Hartley, 1958; Rose, 1977; Sherif & Sherif, 1956); (b) the recent work of Patterson and his colleagues on reciprocity and coercion (Patterson, 1976; Patterson & Reid, 1970); (c) the application of equity theory to groups by Thibaut and Kelley (1961); (d) the application of social systems analysis within a behavioral framework (Wahler, Berland, Coe, & Leske, 1977); and (e) social learning theory, with particular reference to the work of Bandura (1977).

Of the extensive literature related to the social psychology of groups, the following topic areas and related research would appear to be particularly relevant to the conduct of behavioral group therapy; (a) social factors related to perception, memory, and motivation; (b) person perception; (c) attribution theory; (d) communication and opinion change; (e) interpersonal influence; (f) role and role conflict; (g) attitude development and change; (h) leadership, group structure, and process; and (i) attraction. Indeed, these nine areas probably do not exhaust the areas in social psychology which would be relevant to the conduct of behavioral group therapy. Suffice it to say that, in the opinion of the present authors, it is probable that the entire body of work in social psychology should and could serve as a source of material for the behavioral clinician who is interested in behavioral group therapy.

Patterson and his colleagues, beginning with the seminal paper appearing in 1970 (Patterson & Reid), have investigated the relationship of reciprocity and coercion as it relates to the family as well as to couples. It is their thesis that the viability of a social system, in particular small groups including dyads, lies in the nature of the distribution of reinforcers and punishers within that system. In order for the system to survive, there must be an equitable distribution of reinforcers among and between the members of the group with the use of punishers occurring at some acceptable minimum. This basic notion of reciprocity has been modified and expanded while being applied to a variety of phenomena related to families and couples (Jacobson & Margolin, 1979; Miller, 1975; Patterson, 1975).

The work of Patterson and his colleagues mentioned above owes much to the pioneering work of Thibaut and Kelley (1961) who were the first to apply the notion of equity theory to social systems. Their work was principally concerned with the functioning of the dyad; however, they also discussed the possibility of generalizing their model to larger systems such as a triad. They did not extend their notions beyond the triad, except to speculate how their concepts might be generalized to larger groups. The difficulty of moving beyond the triad is obvious and remains to be accomplished at this juncture.

Social systems analysis assumes that behavior is a function of systems which themselves are composed of subsystems, and that each must be understood as a whole. Wahler et al. (1977) point out that there are various levels of analysis which must be comprehended. At the first level, there is the system of behaviors within the individual. At the second level, there is the system related to the individual's primary group. Finally, at the third level, the primary group functions as a subsystem of a larger system such as the community. With reference to the issue of behavioral group therapy, it is reasonable to suppose that the behavioral clinician must be aware of the interactions occurring within and among all three levels. This interaction of systems and subsystems occurs simultaneously within and among all levels and results in phenomena of such complexity that current technology is notably unable to investigate such systems in a meaningful way. This may, in part, account for the dearth of research relevant to these complex group phenomena.

There is also the work related to social learning theory, and most appropriate here would be the work of Bandura (1969, 1977, 1979). The most powerful influence growing from this work has been that related to observational learning. Bandura and his colleagues have amassed an impressive body of data demonstrating that vicarious learning is a major mode of human learning, and much of what is learned occurs in the context of a group. In addition, Bandura (1969) has proposed a view of human beings as active agents in constructing their realities through the reciprocal interaction of persons and environment. If this is the case, what more powerful avenue of change is there than the social environment within which a person is embedded, including the group?

In their reviews of group therapies, Shaffer and Galinski (1974) and Korchin (1976) make the assumption that the behavioral group is merely a context for applying individualized techniques, rather than a means in itself for promoting behavior change. These reviewers further assume that behavioral group therapy is essentially multiple individual therapy. According to Korchin, and using the group classification system of Parloff (1968), the behavioral group approach is intrapersonalistic (emphasizing the client–therapist dyad in the group). Most other group approaches are said to fall into the transactionalistic category. Here, groups focus more on interpersonal relationships between diverse client dyads or subgroups. The remaining group approaches are classified as integralistic, meaning that the group is treated as a unit and the focus of therapy is on the problems of the group rather than the problems of the individual (Bion, 1959).

We find the above assumptions and classifications to embody certain misconceptions. Behavioral group therapy does, in fact, recognize the importance of the group in its own right as a vehicle for change. Behavior therapists have discovered ways to manipulate and guide dyad interactions, implicit norms, cohesiveness, feedback processes, reinforcement contingencies, developmental phases, and status patterns of a group. We see these attributes of a group, often called group process phenomena, as environmental influences on the behavior of individual participants. Because they are environmental influences, these group attributes can be systematically manipulated and structured in ways that produce therapeutic change in individual members. In other words, behavior group therapists work to attain interactive group goals and see this as a means of achieving select individual treatment goals. Using Parloff's classification system again, we conceptualize behavior group therapy as a transactional approach rather than an interpersonalistic one.

Certainly, there are some forms of behavioral group therapy practiced today that do not take into account the group process and client–client interactions. Usually these groups are heavily instructional, with sessions structured well in advance. Clients tend to be homogeneous with respect to presenting problems, and treatment goals of the group are synonymous with the treatment goal of each member. Furthermore, goals are highly specified and selected because they may be realized in a short period of time. Usually these goals center on issues of self-management and basic skills training.

Examples of this type of group include: weight-control groups, parent-training groups, daily-living skills groups, stress immunization groups, smoking cessation groups, public-speaking groups, and study skills groups. There is ample documentation of the clinical effectiveness of such types of groups (Rose, 1977). Although it is not often stated in the research literature, we suspect an important part of the reported success of these groups depends on the therapist's ability to provide a meaningful group atmosphere, to control deviance and nontherapeutic group norms, and to allow some leadership behavior to emerge from clients in the group.

In contrast, behavioral psychotherapy groups place a strong emphasis on group attributes and processes. Groups of this nature accept more heterogeneous clients and adopt broad, yet specifically delineated treatment goals, usually of an interactional form. The group therapist has a more flexible repertoire of techniques available, and changes roles as the developmental process of the group changes. Behavioral strategies are not necessarily limited to those contracted for at the beginning of the group. The therapist may purposely vary leadership and consultation roles with the clients to make the group experience more reinforcing, to teach clients to be more assertive, and to make the transition easier from depending on the group to terminating from the group.

Behaviorally oriented group therapy commonly deals with problems that involve unsuccessful interactions with others. Clients in behavioral psychotherapy groups present problems in establishing or holding on to friendships, giving affection to others, refusing the insensitive demands of others, enjoying the presence of other people, to name a few. Furthermore, nearly all problems suitable for individual behavior therapy are equally amenable to behavioral group therapy, because these problems are likely to have social problem components. Even uncomplicated phobias are partially maintained by interpersonal consequences, such as attention from others through the expression of sympathy, encouragement, and pressure to change. Furthermore, "habit" problems such as smoking or obesity are often under the influence of and occur in the presence of significant others.

Because of the social-interactional nature of most client problems, behavioral group therapy offers some distinct advantages over its individual therapy counterpart. In general, it provides clients with a broader range of social stimuli, behavioral repertoires, and reinforcement mechanisms. The group approach affords clients the opportunity to develop and systematically practice many newly learned skills with and on other clients in the protective setting of the group. The behavioral group is construed as a social learning laboratory that simulates the real social world of the client. We agree when traditional group therapists say that the relationship between therapist and individual client does not approximate the true realities of the client's diversified world.

Because a behavioral group is also a community of sorts, clients can use the group as an intermediate step in making significant personal changes in their lives. Client changes are first tested out in the group for reaction and, hopefully, peer reinforcement before these changes are transferred to the outside community. Behavior group therapists, perhaps more than others, consistently structure group situations so that clients have numerous opportunities for peer reinforcement, encouragement, instruction, and corrective feedback as they attempt to change.

Of equal importance, clients learn to reinforce others in behavioral groups. The ability to help and assist others is a significant behavior that can be shaped and practiced. The beneficial results of having learned how to reinforce others in the group are numerous. Clients tend to diminish the exaggerated, self-centered features of their problems when they begin to help others. Clients also find that their relationships improve as they develop the ability to mediate social rewards for people (Lott & Lott, 1961; Patterson, 1975). Specifically, they see themselves as having positive effects on other people and in turn receiving positive, caring exchanges. In Patterson's terms this reinforcement exchange illustrates the principle: What you give is what you get.

Thus far, the primary advantages of behavioral groups are reflected in opportunities for peer reinforcement and "safe" people on whom to practice newly developed social skills. Two other distinctive features over individual behavior therapy are: (a) the abundance of models available who have been more successful in modifying a shared problem area; and (b) peer reinforcement and the monitoring of behavior problems both within the group and outside of the group. Behavioral groups also possess the same advantages that nonbehavioral groups have over their individual therapy counterparts. Examples include: clients learning that they are not alone in suffering through personal problems; clients living out their characteristic ways of relating in the group; client self-esteem increasing through helping others; clients' distortions and deviances challenged by other group members via peer pressure.

According to Feldman and Wodarski (1975), behavioral group therapy is characterized by the convergence of three theoretical frameworks: social exchange theory, social learning theory, and social role theory. Social exchange theory was set forth by Thibaut and Kelley (1959). Their formulation of interpersonal relationships rests on the assumption that whenever people interact, they strive to maximize the rewards of the interaction, while also attempting to minimize the costs or personal penalties involved. Every behavior enacted is thought to have definitive reward and cost values to others. In psychologically healthy relationships the costs are low enough so that personal efforts can focus on maintaining or enhancing the rewards of the relationship. In dysfunctional relationships, however, efforts to have a rewarding, meaningful relationship has been abandoned. Instead, people reluctantly concentrate on keeping the aversive features (costs) at bay. Responses to minimize costs include emotional withdrawal, begrudging compliance to the demands of others, seeking alternative relationships, and coercion.

Coercion is an important response requiring brief discussion. In a coercive interaction pattern, people train each other to be more and more destructive (Patterson & Cobb, 1971; Patterson & Hops, 1972). It may begin with one or more parties requesting a change of the other group members. The aggrieved party may escalate the demands if the request is not met. If compliance does not follow, the aggrieved one(s) may present aversive stimuli in the form of nagging or threats, and continue to present these stimuli until compliance finally occurs. When the other group members comply, the aversive consequences are simply turned off. Thus, all parties feel relief, and coercion "works."

In all types of groups it is critically important to keep the development of coercive interactions under control while creating group activities that have high reinforcement value for all participants. Coercion can be curtailed by the use of peer pressure. Also, potential coercive members can be helped to avoid this self-defeating behavior by learning to achieve the same results through assertion, communication training, and social reinforcement skills. The results are compliance, recognition, and acceptance by the group.

Social learning theory is an amalgamation of operant conditioning, classical conditioning, and modeling theories as they apply to the understanding of interpersonal behavior. The concept of group contingencies and the influence they have over the behavior of group members serves to illustrate our discussion of social learning theory. By definition, group contingencies are consequences applied to an entire group or most of its members following the attainment of some goal by one or more members.

Usually, the behavioral group leader arranges that positive reinforcements are awarded to all group members, thus fostering both group integration and cohesiveness. Numerous forms of dispensing reinforcement are available to the group therapist. The group consequence easiest to dispense and most frequently used is social reinforcement. Almost as often, group behavior therapists provide the group with tangible and material rewards. In residential and institutional settings these include access to recreational activities, food, passes off the premises, and bonus tokens for use by all at the token "store." In behavioral psychotherapy groups, the reinforcement shared by the group are social praise from therapist and other members, as well as occasional refreshments, planned social activities outside of the group, and intrinsic reinforcement that is gained from the feeling of belonging to a cohesive group.

With the behavioral technique of group contingencies, the group becomes highly integrated and cohesive. This occurs primarily because each group member's reinforcement is contingent upon the performance of the entire group. This contingency also fosters cooperation. Hollander (1976) established a group contingency involving rewards shared by the group that were produced through cooperative group effort. In one group, individual members participated in the manufacture of cigarettes which were shared by all when completed. The research findings suggested that group members became more reinforcing to each other as a result of the group contingency. Also, members had more frequent and beneficial interactions within and outside of the group. Other studies on group contingencies and cooperative behavior have demonstrated similar results (Azrin & Lindsley, 1965; Lindsley, 1966).

The third theoretical framework integrated into behavioral groups is social role theory. Akin to social exchange and social learning theories, it relies on the study of observable behaviors and measurable phenomena. This theory has its greatest applicability to the assessment process in behavioral groups. In any group, people occupy certain social positions and are expected to exhibit the behavior commensurate with the position. Relevant social positions found in behavioral groups are "leader," "client," "model," "buddy-system companion," "scapegoat," and "favorite child."

When group members try to abandon roles ascribed to them by others or through their own self-perceptions, group conflict results. Conflict also arises when a member exaggerates his role behavior, as in the example of a group leader who dominates group discussion, blocks client–client interaction, or continues to use interventions regardless of the fact that the group has not contracted for them.

It is the responsibility of the astute behavioral group therapist to see to it that dysfunctional social roles do not develop or at least do not seriously interfere with group learning activities such as role playing or homework assignments. Furthermore, the astute therapist should permit maximum role flexibility in the group, identify the people in high functioning roles as models, and use group contingencies to avoid deviant roles such as "scapegoat," and "favorite child."

Process

The process of behavioral group therapy may be envisioned in a variety of ways (Flowers, 1979; Rose, 1977). Thus, any particular view of the process would be somewhat arbitrary. With this in mind, the current authors believe that a fruitful view of a behavioral therapy group would be as follows:

Step 1: Forming the Group

Rose (1977) identifies a number of organizational details which must be addressed prior to recruitment and initiation of a behavioral therapy group. He cites such questions as "the size of the group, the frequency and length of meetings, the degree of similarity of members, the number of therapists, and the comparative merit of group and dyadic treatment for each client." Rose continues, stating that " additional concerns include the type of group to be organized, recruiting policies, physical attributes of meetings, and organizational restraints to organizing a group." Of these details, the issue which we feel requires greatest elaboration is that related to the degree of similarity of members. In particular, we wish to address the issue related to the heterogeneity or homogeneity of problem behaviors of group members. It appears that this issue ranges in importance from extremely to not very, depending on the nature of the target behavior or behaviors to be addressed by the group. In the case of the behavioral group treatment of sexual dysfunction, client selection is extremely important, because clients with differing target behaviors may require completely different approaches (Lobitz & Baker, 1979). For example, the client suffering from premature ejaculation will require a considerably different program from someone who is experiencing erectile difficulties. In the case of behavioral groups designed to meet the needs of a particular group of clients who manifest a clearly distinguishable and easily specified target behavior such as smoking, it is clear that the selection of clients would occur on the basis of the presence of the target behavior. Finally, in the case of the Comprehensive Behavioral Therapy group, client selection need simply occur by meeting such loose criteria as approximate and reasonable age range, similar socioeconomic and educational background, sex, and so forth.

Step 2: Establishing the Initial Group Attraction and Identity

Step 3: Establishing the Norm of Openness and Sharing of Emotions and Experiences

Steps 2 and 3 are to some extent difficult to separate and, indeed, it is our feeling that the separation is artificial, but is made for its convenience. This view of the separation of the two steps is supported by the work of Flowers

(1979) who with his colleagues have been attempting to operationalize the concept of group cohesion. Their approach has been to attempt to arrive at an operational definition of group cohesion in terms of a set of covarying components.

> To date . . . we have identified the following eight variables as indicative (and productive when the variables are manipulated) of group cohesion:
> 1. Increased percentage of eye contact with the speaker.
> 2. Increased percentage of client–client interactions.
> 3. Decreased number of members on whom or by whom negative messages are repeatedly focused.
> 4. Increased use of negative messages by the entire group.
> 5. Increased frequency of self-disclosure.
> 6. Client change in patterns of activity from session to session (activity, role, input and output flexibility).
> 7. Increase in self-reported satisfaction with sessions.
> 8. Increased numbers of group members trusted by other group members. (p. 17)

These eight variables contributing to group cohesion are clearly related to Step 2 and in part, to Step 3. In addition to these eight variables, there are other variables which have been identified. For example, in his discussion of building group cohesiveness, Rose (1977) cites such procedures as subgroup introductions, modeling of expected behaviors, use of role playing, teaching relaxation, the use of food, requirement of subgroup interaction in the form of talking about some suggested content, differential reinforcement of positive evaluative statements, and intergroup competition. Finally, there are a number of discussions of nonspecific effects on the effectiveness of psychotherapy which would be relevant here (Coe & Buckner, 1975; Fish, 1973; Frank, 1972; Goldstein, 1962).

Step 4: Establishing a Behavioral Framework for All Participants

In a sense, the steps preceding this step can be viewed as appropriate to any group, regardless of the theoretical persuasion of the group leaders. It is in this fourth step that a clear and unequivocally behavioral event occurs: namely, the establishment of a behavioral frame of reference in all participants. This step is essential, because most clients will enter the group with a variety of points of view as to the nature of human behavior and the process of change. In fact, it is likely that the majority of participants will bring with them some variation or combination of a dynamic, usually psychoanalytically based set of theoretical assumptions, combined with some variation of a trait-theoretical approach to human behavior and change. The behavioral framework and its details favored by the present authors is based on the work of Bijou, Peterson, and Ault (1968). Bijou et al. present a method of analysis of behavioral and stimulus events which allows for the tentative identification, and later verification, of the antecedent and consequent events which are functionally related to observed responses. All participants in a behavioral therapy group must acquire the knowledge and skills necessary for defining behavior in clear and unequivocal terms, and to accept the point of view that behavior is functionally related to its antecedent and consequent events. This acceptance is crucial, for this antecedent–response–consequent model provides the basis not only for the analysis of behavioral events, but also for the planning of interventions leading to behavioral change.

Step 5: Establishing a Positive Expectancy and Placebo Effect in All Participants

The nonspecific effects referred to at the conclusion of the discussion of Steps 2 and 3 are most relevant in this fifth step. There is now a great deal of support for the power of nonspecific variables to affect the outcome of any change program (Coe, 1980; Coe & Buckner, 1975; Fish, 1973; Frank, 1972; Goldfried and Davison, 1976; Golstein, 1962; Wilkens, 1977; Wilson & Evans, 1977). If this possibility exists, then it would be foolish for the change agent to ignore what is potentially an ally in his efforts to bring about change (Meichenbaum, 1977). Thus, it is the recommendation of the authors that every effort be made by the group leaders to maximize the positive effects of expectancy and placebo by providing the participants with information about and a rationale for both the interventions which will occur and the behaviors that are expected as the group progresses.

Step 6: Establishing and Implementing a Model for Change

The model for change favored by the authors is one presented by Madsen and Madsen (1970). They viewed the process of change as being composed of four essential steps:

1. *Pinpoint*—the identification, specification and definition of the behavior or behaviors targeted for change.
2. *Record*—the establishment of a baseline record of the target behavior(s).
3. *Consequate*—the implementation of an appropriate change program based upon the information obtained in steps one and two.
4. *Evaluate*—the establishment and implementation of an appropriate data gathering system which would enable the change agent to evaluate the efficacy of the change program.

Step 7: Establishing and Implementing a Mechanism for the Generalization and Transfer of Treatment Effects to the Natural Environment

Step 8: Establishing and Implementing a Mechanism for the Maintenance of Behavior Change as the Group Ends and Is Faded Out

Steps 7 and 8 are to some extent related and will be discussed together in what follows. This is particularly appropriate because many behavioral clinicians have discussed these issues at the same time. It has become increasingly clear to behavioral therapists that the task of changing behavior entails more than simply modifying the behavior in the desired manner (Baer *et al.*, 1968; Bandura, 1969, 1976; Koegel & Rincover, 1977). Indeed, the problem of relapse and return to treatment has been identified as a major one in the treatment of individuals in need of change. Increasingly, the behavior therapy literature has come to emphasize the need for insuring the generalization and maintenance of behavior change in the natural environment as an active part of therapeutic planning (Karoly & Steffen, 1980; Koegel & Rincover, 1977). In order to accomplish this, the change agent must plan for the eventual generalization of acquired behavior to the natural environment and the provision of adequate safeguards for maintenance of that behavior. Thus, increasing emphasis is placed upon such approaches as the training of significant figures in the environment (Koegel & Rincover, 1977; Mash, Hammerlynck, & Handy, 1976) and the increasing emphasis on self-control and self-management techniques (Mahoney & Thoresen, 1974; Stuart, 1977; Thoresen & Mahoney, 1974).

Mechanisms

A variety of learning mechanisms may be identified as having relevance to the conduct of behavioral group therapy. Indeed, it would not be an exaggeration to state that at one time or another any or all of the varieties of learning mechanisms may come to play a part in behavioral group therapy. Nevertheless, there are some learning mechanisms which are more commonly seen to be involved, and these will be discussed in what follows. This discussion of the relevant learning mechanisms will assume a minimal knowledge of the language of behavioral psychology, and the authors have no intention of claiming that the discussion is at all exhaustive. The principle learning mechanisms which the present authors feel are most relevant to the conduct of behavioral group therapy are: (a) expectancy/placebo manipulations (Johnson, 1972); (b) persuasion and public commitment (Johnson, 1972); (c) group norms (Johnson, 1972; Rose, 1977); (d) contracting (Rose, 1977); (e) individual and/or group contingencies; (f) modeling (Rose, 1977); (g) role playing and behavior rehearsal (Johnson, 1972; Rose, 1977); (h) structured exercises; (i) buddy system (Rose, 1977); and (j) peer reinforcement (Johnson, 1972).

Expectancy/placebo manipulations. Expectancy/placebo manipulations refer to the variety of interventions which would enhance the positive expectancies of the clients and placebo effects of the treatment through the manipulation of nonspecific effects. Thus, for example, the group leader could discuss and emphasize the past successes and beneficial effects of the treatment procedures to be used.

Persuasion and public commitment. A variety of techniques are available to enhance the persuasiveness of the group context for behavioral change including that of public commitment. These techniques have a long history and originate in the early work of Ash (1951).

Group norms. Group norms exert a powerful effect on the behavior of individuals in groups and can be manipulated by the group leader to support behavioral change in the direction of the behavioral goals agreed upon as desirable by the group. A particularly effective technique by means of which the group leader may influence the establishment of desirable group norms would be through the differential reinforcement of appropriate norm related behaviors.

Contracting. The use of behavioral contracts has been useful in obtaining behavioral change. These contracts are usually quasi-formal, written documents which specify the behaviors targeted for change and the consequences attendant upon the occurrence of those behaviors.

Individual and/or group contingencies. Response–consequence contingencies are reliable means of obtaining behavioral change and these contingencies may be applied to particular behavior(s) of individual clients, or they may also be applied to particular behavior(s) as they are manifested by the group. The choice of individual as opposed to group contingencies or vice versa is a clinical decision and can only be made following the careful assessment of the behaviors under consideration.

Modeling. Observational learning has been demonstrated to be a powerful source of behavior change (Bandura, 1977, 1979) and the group setting provides an ideal context for the occurrence of such learning. To this end, the group leader has many opportunities to model appropriate behaviors and, in addition, the group members may also model behaviors for the other members of the group.

Role playing and behavior rehearsal. Bandura (1969, 1977) has described the process of behavior change through observational learning and has emphasized the importance of practice in the acquisition of new behaviors. Thus it is important, not only that the clients observe the appropriate behaviors, but also that they have an opportunity to practice precisely those behaviors which are targeted for change.

Structured exercises. Related to behavior rehearsal and role playing is the use of structured exercises. These exercises call for the practice of target behaviors by clients through the use of preplanned and standardized sets of exercises. These exercises range from the practice of relevant behaviors in the context of a gamelike and rather artificial activity to activities which simulate real-life situations as accurately as possible.

Buddy system. The buddy system enhances the change process by creating dyads from the group participants with the goal of mutual support and encouragement from members of each dyad. Mutual reinforcement and learning has been found to enhance the change process for each member of the dyad and for the group as a whole.

Peer reinforcement. It has been long known that varying individuals and sources have differential reinforcing effects. It has also been known that one of the most powerful sources of reinforcement has been that which originates from one's peers. The group provides an ideal context for the application of peer reinforcement and finds it to be an effective tool for change.

PRACTICE

Introduction

A review of the current work in behavior therapy reveals that there does not appear to be a workable classification system for categorizing the varieties of behavioral groups that have appeared in the literature. Flowers points out that behavioral group therapy can be defined in three ways (1979): (a) the application of an established behavioral technique in a group setting (e.g., desensitization); (b) the use of a behavioral intervention for a particular purpose on a particular occasion in the context of an ongoing group which is nonbehavioral in character (e.g., modeling); and (c) a group where "the interventions must be matched to the client's problem, executed by the entire group, and based on learning principles" (Flowers, 1979, p. 7). He then concludes that only the third definition describes what he believes to be a true behavioral group. The authors' earlier definition of behavioral group therapy would also be relevant here and differs from Flowers's mainly in its emphasis on data collection. Upper and Ross (1979) have generalized an earlier distinction regarding group therapy made by Goldstein, Heller, and Sechrest (1966) to the conduct of behavioral therapy groups: namely, that groups may be distinguished by "the process of doing therapy in groups and that of doing therapy through groups" (p. 1). These distinctions provide some basis for a rational classification system for distinguishing between behavioral groups and nonbehavioral groups, principally that a behavioral group is characterized by the fact that change occurs through the group in a context where specific interventions are designed to meet specific target problems; where specific interventions are implemented by the group; and where the interventions are based upon learning principles and the collection of data. However, this sort of distinction fails to provide us with a system that allows for the classification of varieties of behavioral groups which have been conducted, and which to some extent or another fulfill the various definitions of behavioral group therapy. Thus, the present authors believe that it would be worthwhile for them to present a classificatory schema which would allow for a tentative classification of the major types of behavioral groups appearing in the literature.

It is our belief that a useful classification schema would identify at least three distinct types of behavioral groups. First, there are those groups which have as their major goal the modification of specific behaviors which would minimize the difficulties and maximize the ease with which individuals negotiate their environment, both physical and social. Groups which fall within this class we will label as *Skills-Training Groups*. Second, there are those groups which have as their major goal the modification by the person him- or herself of specific behaviors inimical to the welfare of the individual. Groups which fall within this class we will label as *Self-Management* and/or *Self-Control Groups.* Third, there are those groups which have as their major goal the modification of behaviors related to broader life goals or those related to the more subtle and complex issues which are not capable of simple translation into one or even several discrete behaviors. Groups which fall within this class we will label as *Comprehensive Behavior Therapy Groups.*

Practice I: Skills-Training Group

The major types of skills-training groups are those related to interpersonal skills training, assertion training, behavioral-skills-training groups for specific populations, communication training, and training in activities of daily living. Because it would be cumbersome to present each of these types of groups in detail, we decided to present some examples of the groups in detail. This strategy was arrived at based on the assumption that these groups had much in common and that familiarity with some of the available programs would provide the reader with an appreciation as to the nature of the programs as a whole. With this in mind, the *Skills-Training Groups* will be discussed by presenting in some detail two particular programs: an interpersonal skills-training program and an assertion-training program. Finally, the remainder of the skills-training groups will be discussed in more general terms, with only a cursory attempt to represent their content.

Interpersonal Skills Training

An interpersonal skills-training group attempts to teach individual participants a series of specific interpersonal skills which would enhance their functioning in their social environment and maximize their ability to negotiate that environment and maximize their ability to negotiate that environment in ways which are satisfactory to them and those around them. One of the most detailed and best designed of these programs is that of Goldstein and his colleagues (Goldstein, 1973; Goldstein, Sprafkin, & Gershaw, 1976). Goldstein *et al.* designed a program for clients who are returning to their natural environment and who lack the skills necessary to remain out of the mental health care delivery system by successfully coping with the demands of that environment. This program and its implementation are referred to as Structured Learning Therapy and the particular program for clients returning to the natural environment following hospitalization or other contact with the mental health system is known as Skills Training for Community Living (STCL).

The STCL program has incorporated two specific methods for evaluating clients and their progress. The initial evaluation is by means of a skills inventory and alternate forms are provided making it possible to obtain an overall evaluation of a person's skill repertory by the person him- or herself and by the trainer. These measures may then serve as pre- and posttraining measures to evaluate overall client progress. In addition to these inventories, the STCL program also relies upon a series of Homework Reports, which are self-report devices designed to provide information as to the client's performance between sessions. These homework reports are keyed to specific homework assignments made in relation to the skill goals identified for each session. Thus, the homework reports provide an index of a client's progress from session to session.

Each training session is divided into four distinct phases designed to teach behaviors through observation, practice, reinforcement, and transfer of training. In Phase 1, specific skills are presented to the group either through the use of audio tapes or by means of live models; in Phase 2, each member of the group is given the opportunity and, where necessary, the aid required for them to practice the skills observed; in Phase 3, each person receives corrective feedback necessary for improvement of his or her performance and is reinforced for their appropriate behaviors; and, finally, in Phase 4, each person discusses the results of their homework completed between sessions and every effort is made to arrange for the transfer of training through whatever means are appropriate.

A particularly effective characteristic of this training program is the presentation of concrete models of desired behaviors in a systematic format designed to maximize the observational learning of the individual client. Due to its unique character the organization of the modeling tapes will be presented in some detail. Each modeling tape follows a standard format that begins with a narrator's introduction, followed by the modeled behavior, and ending with a narrator's summary.

The components are described by Golstein *et al.* (1976) as follows:

I. Narrator's Introduction
    1. Introduction of self
        (a) Name and title
        (b) High status position—e.g., Hospital Director
    2. Introduction of skill
        (a) Name
        (b) General (descriptive) definition
        (c) Behavioral (learning points) definition
    3. Incentive statement—How and why skills-presence may be rewarding
    4. Discrimination statement—Examples of skill-absence, and how and why skill-absence may be unrewarding
    5. Repeat statement of learning points and request for attention to what follows
II. Modeling Displays: Ten brief vignettes of the learning point behaviors, each vignette portraying the complete set of learning points which constitute the given skill. A variety of actors (models) and situations are used. Situations portray a mix of in-hospital and community settings and events. Model characteristics (age, sex, apparent socioeconomic level, etc.) are similar to typical trainee characteristics. The displays portray both overt model behaviors, as well as ideational and self-

instructional learning points. Models are provided social reinforcement for skill enactment.

III. Narrator's Summary
  1. Repeat statement of learning points
  2. Description of rewards to both models and actual trainees for skill usage
  3. Urging of trainees to enact the learning points in the Structured Learning Therapy session which follows and, subsequently, in their real-life environments

Goldstein *et al.* have identified a series of 37 specific skills which they have converted into this teaching format, with an additional 22 so-called Application Tapes which use the same format but portray a model using some combination of several or more of the identified skills to illustrate the fact that the skills are not isolated behaviors but form the basis of an entire repertory of skills necessary to cope with the natural environment.

Clients for this group are selected from those persons who have demonstrated a clear deficit in the skills which are to be taught in the group. Information for making such judgments come from the Skills Inventory which are completed by clients and staff. Goldstein *et al.* recommend that, where possible, clients also be grouped with reference to the degree of impairment in the skill or skills to be taught. The optimal size of a group is seen as consisting of 6 to 12 clients and 2 trainers. This number was arrived at based upon the need for intensive involvement of each client in every session and the finding that client learning suffered if sessions were to exceed 2 hours in length. Thus, in order for each client to maximize his or her learning, they must have sufficient time alloted for that learning and this places an automatic ceiling as to number of clients who can be trained in any 2-hour session. In the event that the individual clients in a group demonstrate a shortened attention span, a recommendation is made that the session length be shortened to as little as 30 minutes if necessary. In the event that this is done, the number of sessions per week would be increased proportionately. The STCL program consists of from 3 to 15 sessions, depending upon the nature of the group and the specific skills taught. Goldstein *et al.* caution that in planning sessions the spacing of the sessions is crucial, due to the emphasis on the transfer of training which necessitates activity by the clients between sessions. Thus, following any given session clients must be given the opportunity for sufficient practice of those skills which have been learned.

The interpersonal skills-training approach appears to be a promising one and is being carried out by others as well as Goldstein and his colleagues (e.g., Bedell & Weathers, 1979). However, the efficacy of this approach still awaits verification through further research, because the bulk of the work has been done by Goldstein and his colleagues without the additional replication and extension needed to establish the validity of such an approach. In addition, there are various issues which require further work and, perhaps most important of all, a thorough going components analysis is needed to identify those specific components which are contributing to change and in what fashion.

Assertion Training

Assertion training in recent years has seen a proliferation of recommended programs originating with a variety of investigators and designed for a variety of populations ranging from institutionalized psychiatric patients to college students. One of the best of these programs is described by Lange and Jakubowski in their book *Responsible Assertive Behavior* (1976). They identify assertion training as being composed of four basic procedures:

(1) Teaching people the differences between assertion and aggression and between nonassertion and politeness; (2) helping people identify and accept both their own personal rights and the rights of others; (3) reducing existing cognitive and affective obstacles to acting assertively, e.g., irrational thinking, excessive anxiety, guilt, and anger; and (4) developing assertive skills through active practice methods. (p. 2)

Thus, the goals of assertion training involves discrimination training to enable clients to distinguish between aggression and assertion; education with regards to personal rights and the rights of others; persuasion and other more traditional therapeutic interventions related to a therapeutic dialogue in order to change cognitions and affect as well as more behavioral approaches to changing affect; and skills training to ensure the acquisition of the necessary assertion-related skills.

The evaluation of initial, terminal and ongoing behaviors is based upon a variety of data sources including interview, paper-and-pencil tests, questionnaires, behavior sampling in simulated situations, and the use of homework assignments and reports. Lange and Jakubowski (1976) thus include a Discrimination Test on Assertive, Aggressive, and Nonassertive Behavior in their Book, as well as discussing a variety of other measures, including assertiveness questionnaires, behavioral tests, paper-and-pencil scales and inventories, and more global personality measures. Thus, they clearly feel that measures are necessary and discuss them in the context of initial evaluation, measures of progress, and measures of change.

Among other suggested assertion groups, Lange and Jakubowski (1976) refer to a program which they describe as appropriate for a group with the objective of personal growth rather than therapy as such. This program occurs in 9 weeks and its basic format is illustrated by Session 1 which is described below.

Session 1 begins with a lecture which provides "(1) a brief overview of the nine sessions, describing the focus of exercises and the general nature of cognitive restructuring and behavior rehearsal, (2) a clear definition of assertive behavior as contrasted with nonassertive and aggressive behavior, and (3) some generalizations about reasonable expectations as a result of being in the group" (pp. 202–203). The recommendation is that this lecture be no longer than 10 minutes at the most, in order to avoid the loss of attention. Following the lecture, the remainder of the session is made up of a series of behavioral structured exercises designed to: (1) maximize participant learning and use of skills, (2) help the members become more comfortable and involved in the group, (3) focus on specific aspects of assertive behavior, and (4) prepare participants for the cognitive and behavioral procedures which come later in the group sessions. Each of the exercises described. . . includes the procedure, specific outcome goals, the issues to be raised while conducting the exercise, and some nuances for conducting the exercise. (pp. 69–70)

Included also is a recommended interval of time to be devoted to each of the exercises as well as homework for participants and trainers. The specific exercises recommended for Session 1 are as follows:

Introductions—round-robin introductions [take place].

Inane topics—each person is asked to talk for about a minute and a half on some inane topic.

Yes–No exercise—dyads are asked to say yes and no to each other matching loudness levels with one another while varying loudness from one occasion to the next.

Giving and receiving compliments—each person is asked to give a genuine compliment to another person in the group and then they are asked to state one way in which the person receiving the compliment reacted that they found pleasing.

Social conversations—dyads are asked to practice a social conversation focusing on three components of communication skills: "asking open-ended questions, responding to free information, and paraphrasing."

Whip—each person simply makes a statement regarding any thing he/she wishes and the group simply attends to the statement with no discussion. (p. 77)

Prior to the conclusion of the session homework assignment is made relevant to the exercises. For example, related to "Introductions," each person is asked to

1. Introduce yourself three times this week. Assess what you liked about how you came across and what you liked about how the other person responded. (Do not assess what happened after the introductions, that is a separate interaction!)
2. Notice how other people introduce themselves to strangers.
3. Ask someone to repeat his name shortly after you have been introduced; assess how direct and assertive you were; if you were nervous, identify clearly what the worry was. (pp. 71–72)

The format of each exercise consists of a description of the exercise, identification of the goals of the exercise, homework suggestions for participants, and homework suggestions for trainers. It can be seen that the structured exercises provide the backbone of this program and afford a context for modeling, behavior rehearsal, feedback, and practice.

Sessions 2 through 5 continue a series of structured exercises designed to teach specific assertion skills and then, during Session 5, group participants identify and begin to define a set of exercises relevant to their idiosyncratic needs. The remainder of the sessions, from Sessions 6 through 9, are devoted to working with the individual needs of each participant as they have presented them in the group.

In the selection of clients for an assertion training group, Lange and Jakubowski (1976) recommend that the group leader pay attention to the following:

1. Specific situations in which a person experiences difficulty in acting assertively.
2. Specific conditions that prevent the occurrence of assertive behaviors.
3. Situational versus general problems in assertion.
4. Motivation to change.
5. Commitment to work.
6. Willingness to self-disclose.
7. Ability to talk in groups.
8. Realistic expectations.
9. Triadic factors—low anxiety related to being in the group, marked vulnerability and low self-esteem, and intense motivation to change. All factors related to identifying individuals likely to experience an adverse reaction to such a group.
10. Prior bad experience in a group.
11. Other issues—"Individuals who see the trainer as a power figure to be rebelled against, whose obvious anger is denied and covered by a thin veneer of sweetness, who are highly manipulative, who have a borderline hold on reality, who are paranoid or psychopathic, who deny their obvious anger, who are overadaptive and take the position, 'Just tell me exactly what I should do in the group and I'll do it,' are generally poor candidates for group assertion training." (pp. 278–279)

In terms of group composition, they report that single-sex groups are probably the most effective. However, they do not preclude the use of mixed-sex groups, and recommend that in these groups that there be an equal number of males and females. They also recommend that group members be relatively homogeneous in age, level of assertiveness, and the situational or general nature of their assertiveness. Each session is about 2 hours in length and sessions are scheduled once a week enabling participants to carry out their homework assignments between sessions.

Rimm and Masters (1979) and Rose (1977), following reviews of the literature related to the efficacy of assertion training in groups, conclude that there is good evidence to demonstrate that such training is effective and worthwhile. However, as noted earlier, there are many different approaches to assertion training, and the details of the many intervention packages which have come about differ. It would be desirable to establish if, indeed, these differing programs are equally effective or not. If not, then obviously the most effective package should be identified. If these programs are equally effective, then it would be important that the choice of intervention be made on the basis of issues other than efficacy, for example, convenience, ease of implementation and cost. Finally, although the various components of the different packages were chosen for the most part because of their demonstrated effectiveness, the most effective combination of such components and the possible impact of including components in one or another configuration are still not known. Thus, it would seem that the most pressing research question deals with the most effective implementation of assertion training, rather than whether assertion training is possible.

Behavioral-Skills-Training Groups for Specific Populations

Groups of this type seek to train persons in the implementation of behavioral programs in order to modify the behavior of a particular target group.

Thus, included here would be training programs for such populations as parents, teachers, nurses and ward staff. These programs have it as their goal to train change agents to modify the behavior of a selected target population. In the main, the basic model for training is a didactic one, where the trainer is seen as an instructor and the members of the group as students/learners rather than recipients of a service. Within this didactic model, it is usual to have training materials available in the form of a manual, and the training proceeds from session to session on the basis of the program described and presented in the manual. Training programs are so structured that the typical program may extend anywhere from several weeks to as many as 15 weeks, with individual sessions lasting from 1 to 2 hours, (90 minutes) being the most usual. Entrance into the group is usually predicated on being a member of the population being trained, with little screening beyond some assurance of the homogeneity of the group on such variables as education, socioeconomic level, level of sophistication, level of knowledge of behavioral psychology, and so forth.

The two groups for which there are training programs with the most empirical support are parents and teachers. There are a variety of parent-training programs, depending upon the population targeted for change. Of the available parent-training programs, the best of these are represented by the Patterson, Reid, Jones, and Conger program (1975) developed for use with families with aggressive children; Kozloff's program (1974) developed for use with developmentally disabled children; and the programs by Rettig (1974), Miller (1975) and Becker (1971) for less disturbed or disabled children. Each of these parent-training programs places an emphasis on the behavior of children. Each emphasizes obtaining actual behavioral samples of parent behavior as they demonstrate their acquisition of the necessary skills. Thus, the emphasis is on data and data collection, with the use of charting to provide information to the parents as well as to the trainer.

Of the variety of teacher-training programs, the best of these are represented by the Project Follow Through program (Jackson, Hazel, & Saudargas, 1974), the Rettig and Paulson program (1975) and the CORBEH program (Greenwood, Hops, Delquadri & Walker, 1977). Each of these programs is designed to provide the teacher with a series of well-planned steps entailing specific behavioral objectives which are to be attained by the teacher. The Project Follow Through and the CORBEH programs are particularly well done since they provide the teacher with a great deal of support materials in the form of both observational and teaching devices. The Project Follow Through program is unique in that it has incorporated a teacher certification device which is carried out on an annual basis, ensuring the maintenance of skills acquired in the initial training.

Communication Training Groups and Groups for Training ADL Skills

It is not our intention to imply that these groups have any particular feature in common simply because they are discussed in the same section. To the contrary, we view them as having quite different and well discriminable goals, and they are being discussed together only as a matter of convenience. There are basically two types of communication training programs which have been developed: one for use with families and the other for use with couples. Representative of the former are those programs developed by Patterson (1975) and Brownstone and Dye (1973). Representative of the latter are those programs developed by Thomas (1977) and Gottman, Notarius, Gonso, and Markman (1976). Each of these programs has had as its main thrust the teaching of a basic theoretical and conceptual framework, a means of assessment, and a set of exercises/lessons which teach the necessary communication skills to the persons involved. Again, as with all good behavioral training programs, there is an emphasis on data and data collection as the basis for evaluation and decision making.

Of the many programs for teaching Aid to Daily Living (ADL) skills, perhaps the most comprehensive is that developed by a team at Harvard University in the Behavioral Education Projects (Baker, Brightman, Heifetz, & Murphy, 1978). This program presents a detailed set of step-by-step instructions for teaching ADL skills to a developmentally disabled population. Included are not only instructions for training but also appropriate recording forms and procedures to ensure proper data collection and monitoring of progress.

Comprehensive Skills-Training Groups

Finally, there are the Comprehensive Skills-Training Programs which are designed for application to the more disabled psychiatric populations such as those persons who have a life-long history of contact with the mental health system and are often described with the label of "career patient." Representative of this type of program are the Behavior Analysis and Modification (BAM) Project at the Oxnard Community Mental Health Center (Liberman, King, & DeRisi, 1976) and the Community Training Center of the Palo Alto VA Hospital (Spiegler & Agigian, 1977). The Community Training Center provides a comprehensive model of this type of program and provides what the authors term "an educational-behavioral-social systems model for rehabilitating psychiatric patients." This program is based upon an educational model and, more specifically, uses the school model as its base. Thus, the clients are expected to attend a series of classes designed to teach them the varieties of skills necessary for successful adjustment to the community at large. Classes are taught in such skill areas as (a) the Interpersonal and Cognitive Skills area, which includes classes in Social Communication, Social Relations, Thinking Straight, and Problem Solving; (b) the Community Survival Skills area, which includes classes in Community Interaction, Money Management, Driving, and Telephone Usage; (c) the Health-related Skills area, which includes classes in Relaxation, Exercise, and Self-medication; (d) the Socialization Skills area, which includes classes in Humor, Social Customs, Current Events, and Social Dancing; and (e) a Miscellaneous category, which includes Academic Subjects and a specialized predischarge group called the Graduate Seminar.

This final class, the Graduate Seminar, is designed specifically to review and assess the status and progress of an individual client in order to determine whether she or he has met the criteria for graduation from the program. If the client requires further work in a particular skill or skill area, she or he will be provided with guidance in developing his or her own individualized program for improving the necessary skills. Thus, it can be seen from this cursory description that the Community Training Center does indeed provide a comprehensive program for clients and practically all learning occurs in a group context.

Practice II: Self-Management and/or Self-Control Groups

Self-management and/or self-control groups are characterized by the fact that their explicit goal is to provide the individual client with a set of skills which would enable them to gain control over behaviors which are troublesome to them. Unlike the other types of groups, the specific goal is to provide the client with the skills necessary for him or her to modify his or her own behaviors. Thus, the target persons are the clients themselves, and the focus is upon individual behavior problems and the variety of skills and techniques which are necessary to deal with the target problems. Examples of groups in this category would be stress immunization groups, including those designed for anxiety management, anger control, and pain control; self-control groups (impulse control); study skills groups; sexual dysfunction groups; text anxiety/math anxiety groups; the varieties of groups designed to deal with the addictive behaviors, such as alcohol and drug abuse, weight control, and smoking control; and life-style groups.

Early attempts to teach self-control skills to clients were from an operant framework (Ferster, Nurnberger, & Levitt, 1962; Goldiamond, 1965) and the operant approach continues in the more current work of operant behaviorists (Goldfried & Merbaum, 1973; Mahoney & Thoreson, 1974; Stuart, 1977; Thoreson & Mahoney, 1974). However, there has recently been increased interest in more cognitively based strategies which represent quite a departure from the early operant approach (Foreyt & Rathjen, 1978; Kendall & Hollan, 1979; Mahoney, 1974; and Meichenbaum, 1977).

The defining characteristics of self-management–self-control groups based upon operant principles is the modification of target behaviors through environmental manipulation and control. Thus, emphasis is placed on antecedent and consequent events which are related to and may control the occurrence or nonoccurrence of the target behaviors. Included here then would be such strategies as the direct manipulation of environmental S^D (ess-dee) and S^Δ (ess-delta), as well as the contingencies of reinforcement including formational feedback. The emphasis is clearly, as it should be in an operant approach, on events outside the skin of the client. The teaching task is to provide the clients with the knowledge of operant principles necessary to manipulate the environment in such ways as to modify their target behaviors in the desired directions.

In contrast to the operant approach, the more recent cognitive behavior therapy approach places its emphasis clearly upon events occurring under the client's skin. Meichenbaum's (1977) identification of the components common to a variety of coping-skills programs is illustrative of the type of model used:

> (1) Teaching the client the role of cognitions in contributing to the present problem, through both didactic presentation (often in the form of Socratic dialogue) and guided self-discovery; (2) training in the discrimination and systematic observation of self-statements and images, and in self-monitoring of maladaptive behaviors; (3) training in the fundamentals of problem solving (e.g., problem definition, anticipation of consequences, evaluating feedback); (4) modeling of the self-statements and images associated with both overt and cognitive skills; (5) modeling, rehearsal, and encouragement of positive self-evaluation and of coping and attentional focusing skills; (6) the use of various behavior therapy procedures, such as relaxation training, coping imagery training, and behavioral rehearsal; (7) *in vivo* behavioral assignments that become increasingly demanding. (p. 147)

Finally, as with the discussion of the skills-training groups, two examples of self-management–self-control groups will be presented in some detail with a cursory discussion of the remaining groups. The two will be chosen to represent an operant program and a cognitive behavior therapy program. The operant based program to be described will be the behavioral program for weight control developed at the Stanford Eating Disorders Clinic (Ferguson, 1976) and the cognitive behavior therapy program to be described will be the Anger Control Program designed by Novaco (1978).

The behavioral program for weight control developed at the Stanford Eating Disorders Clinic (Ferguson, 1976) is a treatment package designed to be administered by "relatively untrained individuals" in a group context. The program occurs over two 20-week therapy periods designed in such a way as to provide five weekly therapy meetings focusing on maintenance and practice. The composition of the groups has been mixed (age, sex) and includes from 6 to 13 persons. Groups meet each week for 90 minutes and are led by a group leader with a coleader who helps in the weighing and in the checking of homework. The maintenance mettings are not required, but clients are "advised" to attend. Focus is on troubleshooting the issues brought to the meetings as a result of behavioral practice during the week. The program as described by Ferguson (1976) is as follows:

1. Introduction to the behavioral control of weight: An overview of the principles of behavior modification and the first ten weeks of instruction.
2. Cue elimination: Exercises in stimulous narrowing, e.g., eating in one place, eliminating other activities while eating, removing food cues from the environment, etc.
3. Changing the act of eating: Slowing down the act of eating by putting eating utensils on the table between bites.
4. Behavioral chains and alternate activities: Substitution of alternate activities for antecendent behaviors.
5. Behavioral analysis, feedback, and maintenance: An introduction to problem solving.
   M1 to M5: Five weeks of maintenance or practice, with optional weekly weighings at the Clinic.

6. Preplanning: Thinking ahead about meal content to take impulse out of eating.
7. Cue elimination part two, and energy use part one; Stimulus narrowing associated with food, e.g., leaving food behind, throwing away leftovers, taking serving dishes off the table, etc. An activity baseline is obtained for one week with a pedometer.
8. Energy use part two: Systematic increase of energy expenditure.
9. Snacks, cues, and holidays: Hints for dealing with snacks and social situations, and a discussion of the caloric content of snacks.
10. Environmental support—family and friends: A discussion of family interactions and the need for support at home. Families are requested to attend this meeting. *M6 to M10:* Five weeks of maintenance or practice, with optional weekly weighings at the clinic.
11. Progress, maintenance, feedback, and review: A session designed to provide feedback about maintenance, and review the first ten weeks.
12. The behavioral diet: An introduction to the Stuart and Davis (1972) food exchange diet.
13. Self Instruction I—becoming aware of internal dialogue: A baseline week of exercises to increase the awareness of cognitive processes.
14. Self Instruction II—rescripting and reward: Instruction on how to change internal dialogue, and the principles of and need for self-reward.
15. Self Instruction III—rescripting, reward, self-image, and maintenance: Self-image is presented as a key to maintenance, the need for systematic change of this image is stressed, and the use of self-reward to help make this change is introduced. *M11 to M15:* Five weeks of maintenance or practice with optional weekly weighings at the clinic.
16. Review, reattribution, and negative self-instruction: Introduction to positive attribution to hunger, negative attribution to satiety, and covert sensitization for problem foods.
17. Contingency contracting—making a deal with yourself: Contingency contracting on a day-to-day basis with practice specifying goals and rewards.
18. Contingency contracting with others: Long-term goals and rewards, and social involvement.
19. Social cues to eating—how to avoid them: Attribution of hunger to external cues, and dealing with social situations more directly with nonfood related behaviors.
20. Final review, and discussion of maintenance.

As can be seen from this description, the weight control program is a combination of a variety of treatment components, and reflects the trend toward inclusion of several types of interventions in a treatment package (Azrin, 1979; Davidson & Davidson, 1980; Jacobson & Margolin, 1979; Kendall & Hollon, 1979; Meichenbaum, 1977; Sjoden, Bates, & Dockens, 1979; Williams, Martin, & Foreyt, 1976). A word needs to be added as to the inclusion of the Stanford program as an examplar of an operant based program, when there are obvious cognitive components. The overriding consideration was to present a current program which appears to be representative of the work that is occurring now. Thus, as noted above, the trend is away from simple operant models and toward maximizing treatment effects through a shotgun approach (Meichenbaum, 1977). However, the Stanford Program retains a clear operant emphasis, and for this reason it was chosen to represent the operant approach.

Novaco (1978) presents a program for aiding clients in dealing with their anger problems in the form of an initial assessment followed by the treatment intervention. During the assessment, he notes the objective as determining the persons and situations related to the anger behaviors, with particular attention being paid to the following characteristics: (a) frequency, (b) intensity, (c) duration, (d) mode of expression, (e) effect on performance, (f) effect on relationships, and (g) effect on health. Novaco recommends the use of the Novaco Anger Scale which was comprised of 80 items for which the respondent rates the level of anger on a 5-point scale. In light of the retrospective nature of such scales, it is probably desirable, if not necessary, to obtain corroborative data in the form of self-monitoring and/or observations by trained observers. Novaco does not explicitly recommend such observations but refers to the possibility of "other behavioral measures."

The intervention begins following the initial evaluation, and is designed to be used with individuals or groups. With individuals, the sessions are designed to be 1 hour in length; this increases to 90 minutes with groups. In all, the program is designed to include 10 sessions. A brief description of the sessions follows.

Session 1: The results of the rating scale and any other data or observations are discussed with the client. Then an interview ensues with the following steps:

1. Obtain information from the client regarding (a) the degree to which he believes he experienced a problem with anger; (b) the greatest concern he has about his anger; and (c) how working on this problem will make his life different.
2. Conduct a situation – person – mode of expression analysis of the anger problem.
3. Assess the deficits in anger control through examining the related external events, internal factors (cognitive and effective), and behavioral factors.
4. Present a rationale for the treatment.
5. Assign homework:
   a. An anger diary which includes frequency and ratings of degree of anger; and proficiency in managing anger.
   b. Provide with index cards to note a hierarchy of anger incidents from minor annoyance to intense anger.
   c. Track internal dialogue through informal self-monitoring.

Session 2: Focus on relaxation and desensitization.
1. Review homework assignments.
2. Use anger diary to continue assessment of anger problem.
3. Establish a hierarchy of seven items using homework cards as point of departure.
4. Introduce Jacobsonian relaxation training.
5. Desensitize client to first anger-hierarchy scene using coping imagery and relaxation.
6. Review experience with desensitization procedure.
7. Assign homework.

    a. Practice relaxation.
    b. Continue to monitor internal dialogue.
Session 3: Introduction of Antecedent, Behavior, Consequences (*ABC*) model and continued work on anger hierarchy.
    1. Review diary, refine assessment, and reinforce for completing homework.
    2. Introduce the Ellis *ABC* model.
    3. Using diary, begin discrimination training for distinguishing anger which is positive from anger which is negative, in terms of appropriateness and functional consequence.
    4. Introduce relaxing imagery in relaxation procedures and relax the client.
    5. Desensitize to next hierarchy scene.
    6. Review relaxation and cognitive coping process.
    7. Assign homework:
        a. Anger diary.
        b. Practice relaxation.
Session 4: Introduce thought modification, tracking physiological and behavioral signs of anger, and staging strategy.
    1. Review anger diary and focus on *in vivo* experience with hierarchy items already dealt with.
    2. Using an actual anger incident, modify thoughts about anger situation. Focus on assumptions and "should" statements.
    3. Focus on physiological and behavioral cues related to anger and their relation to each other.
    4. Introduce staging strategy through examples of:
        a. Preparing for provocation.
        b. Impact and confrontation.
        c. Coping with arousal and agitation.
        d. Think back when conflict is either unresolved or resolved.
    5. Have client rehearse steps of staging strategy.
    6. Desensitize to next two hierarchy items.
    7. Continue anger diary.
Sessions 5–10: Introduce and implement behavioral interventions.
    1. Review anger diary and evaluate progress to date.
    2. Focus on anger as a cue for coping strategies and adaptive use of arousal.
    3. Introduce and implement behavioral interventions.
        a. Communication of feelings.
        b. Assertion.
        c. Remaining on-task and goal-oriented.
    4. Continue desensitization of anger hierarchy using abbreviated relaxation procedure.
In general, groups labeled as self-management or self-control groups emphasize either the operant model or the cognitive behavior therapy model or both, with some programs embedding these in a context of other approaches

such as family therapy, medical treatment and individual therapy. Increasingly it is becoming obvious that many behaviors previously approached from a narrow base do not yield to such an attack, particularly over the long run. Indeed, there is every indication that behavior change programs must attend as much to the maintenance of behavior change as they have to behavior change (Davidson & Davidson, 1980; Stuart, 1977). Thus, investigators are moving in the direction of treatment packages such as Novaco (1976, 1977) where a variety of components are combined to enhance change and the maintenance of change.

Practice III: Comprehensive Behavior Therapy Groups

In this section, we will present the topic outline used in the other chapters to facilitate your comparison of the comprehensive behavior therapy group with the other types of nonbehavioral groups discussed in this volume.

Problems

Any problem that is interpersonal in nature is suitable for comprehensive behavior therapy groups. Individuals whose primary difficulties are self-management problems (i.e., overeating, smoking, stress) may be appropriate for this type of group, provided they see the interpersonal ramifications of their problem and are willing to work on them. The main treatment goals are far broader than those of the two groups discussed thus far.

Targets for change are ones that ultimately lead to major life-style and self-image modifications. Through the group experience, someone afraid to sleep alone in their room at their parents' home may not only overcome the problem, but may move out on his or her own and also secure a better job. Someone who can't complete job responsibilities may not only become more self-disciplined at work, but may set and achieves higher goals for him- or herself: goals such as developing intimate relationships with members of the opposite sex learning to live alone, cultivating many avocations, and having fun without feeling guilty.

There are, in our judgment, three categories of problem-focus groups. First, the mixed group in which the emphasis is on individual problems that may not be common to other group members. Second, the situational group where members are facing a common situational difficulty in their own ways, say, as found in a single parents' group. Third, the developmental group, where people face common difficulties because of similar age or stage of life, such as in adolescent or geriatric therapy groups.

Problems treated in comprehensive therapy groups are not addressed in terms of conventional diagnostic categories—neurosis, psychosis, character disorder, and so forth. Instead, the behaviors that lead to the label are the focus of group interventions. At the relationship level, behavioral problems lead to goals such as: (a) feeling more secure, (b) reducing dependencies on others, (c) expressing genuine affection, (d) letting go or holding on to relationships, and (e) reducing emotions that interfere with sound interpersonal relations (social anxiety, explosive anger, depression).

Some people exhibit problems that would interfere with the therapeutic process of the group. Such problems may lead to a decision to exclude these clients. Severe antisocial problems such as child abuse and rape may well threaten the integration of a heterogeneous group and must be addressed to minimize such impact. Finally, involuntary referrals to the group should be discouraged, because they present special problems regarding motivation to change.

Evaluation

As mentioned earlier in this chapter, evaluation is the hallmark of behavior therapy. Once individual problems are identified in the group through discussions, completing checklists, and self-observation, baselines can be taken. That is, before treatment, one records the frequency, intensity, and/or duration of the identified problems. Recordings are generally made on a daily basis for 1 to 3 weeks. Progress toward reaching treatment goals is also charted and recorded weekly. Usually the results of weekly homework assignments serve as data to judge progress. The concepts of baseline, taking weekly change measures, self-observation, and filling out problem checklists are evaluation features which are all unique to behavior therapy groups. Some other forms of group therapy take pre- and postgroup measures, but only behavior therapy groups have the technology and the commitment to evaluate change precisely and continually throughout the life of the group. It is also important to assess client expectations in order to determine if they are consonant with the met goals of the group. Do they see interpersonal problems as being helped through the group? Do they anticipate and accept sharing problems, doing homework assignments, being of help and encouragement to others, and trying on new behaviors in the group? These are important expectations for comprehensive behavioral groups. All expectations must be present for a client to have a successful behavioral group experience.

We also evaluate whether goals have been well formulated. Criteria include specifying who is going to change and what behaviors in that person will be worked on? Under what social conditions or settings will the behaviors be changed? How long is the estimate of time necessary to change? How will one know when the goal is achieved?

From a general clinical perspective, it is important also to know if group members are taking any significant medication, have been in group therapy before, or are currently in any other therapy.

Arnold Lazarus (1976) proposed a behavioral problem framework he has called the BASIC ID. This is a way to target interventions to individual group members based on the evaluation of seven areas of individual functioning. They are: behavior, affect, sensation, imagery, cognition, interpersonal relationships, and drugs. Let us look at an illustration of a male participant who comes to the group and complains that he is afraid to travel alone after a car accident.

- Behavior: Avoids driving alone, encourages others to drive him places.
- Affect: General anxiety in cars; high anxiety when alone in cars. Depression over inability to change.
- Sensation: Tension in stomach in car; dizziness when travel by car.
- Imagery: Recalls accident vividly; frightening pictures of his injury or death if he drives alone.
- Cognition: Believes that he is helpless; thinks there is a catastrophic danger in driving alone.
- Interpersonal: Many people who previously did not associate with him much now are chauffeuring him to and from work.
- Drugs: Taking occasional prescribed tranquilizers; drinks scotch before going into a car.

Treatment

There is no formal and well-established way to conduct comprehensive behavior therapy groups at this time. Step-by-step programs where problems and treatment plans are clearly delineated in advance are more characteristic of skills training and self-management-type groups.

In the comprehensive type of group, technical eclecticism is an important doctrine (Lazarus, 1971). We feel it appropriate to use whatever techniques work, in order to produce interpersonal change. This includes promising techniques from other schools of therapy—psychodrama, Gestalt awareness exercises, transference analysis, reflection, transactional analysis procedures. For admission into behavioral practice, these techniques must be parsimonious, clearly delineated, and addressed to relatively specific observable interpersonal problems.

Comprehensive behavior therapy groups progress through certain informal stages. In the beginning or orientation stage, the members and leaders get acquainted. Group members are asked to introduce themselves and are expected to learn each other's name. Each gradually gives the group background information on his or her life experiences before coming to the group. The group leader encourages members through structured exercises to become more relaxed in the group, learn to self-disclose personal information, respect the beliefs and life-styles of others, as well as give and accept constructive criticism and praise.

The behavioral group leader sets down certain expectancies and guidelines for conduct. We emphasize that group members must do things in order to change themselves and their life. They shouldn't expect that more intellectual understanding or feeling better will automatically lead to change without effort. We further emphasize the value of cooperation and the philosophy that everyone in the group can be of help to everyone else. Each member has certain knowledge, skills, or contacts that can be of use to fellow group members.

Four rules of conduct are laid down: (a) Group discussions are strictly confidential; (b) criticism must be constructive and helpful (directed at what the person does, not at the person him- or herself); (c) members should not discuss reactions outside the group that they are unwilling to share in the group; and (d) holding back of expressing feelings, or observations about oneself and/or the group diminishes the usefulness of the group for all.

In the second or problem-focus stage, the assessment work of the group begins. In the group conducted by Lazarus (1976), multimodal BASIC ID profiles are obtained for each group member, whether formally or informally. Members look for problems in terms of behavior, affect, sensation, imagery, cognition, interpersonal relations, and drugs. We also have our members doing home observation and baseline recordings of identified problems.

In the third or treatment stage, behavioral techniques are applied to individuals in the group and to the group at large. Some of the techniques are leader-directed. Examples include the leader teaching members to relax successfully, structuring and guiding assertion/communication exercises, and giving guided images to the members to control guilt, anger, and fear. Other techniques are introduced and demonstrated by the leader but directed and conducted by group members. They include cooperation trading (coping with knowledge or skill deficiencies by trading off expertise), giving constructive feedback and encouragement, and modeling roles for assertive training vignette.

One important facet of this stage is continuity. Certain theme issues for individuals (examples: getting a new job or reducing reliance on other people) and for the group (working cohesively and learning to rely less and less on the leader) are tracked week after week. The group leader maintains some reasonable control of the process in sessions so that new behavior problems or issues are brought up and dealt with thoroughly only after issues from prior sessions have gotten considerable therapeutic attention. Also some meetings have structured review periods, where progress is reported on from the perspective of the group members and of the leader.

Problems treated in the group are looked at from as many angles as possible. Treatments are mutually agreed upon and revised as necessary. Many sorts of treatment interactions may go on within any one session. For example, everyone may be asked to practice relaxation exercises and role play how to disagree with respected authorities. The entire group helps Diane clarify her misperceptions of mature boyfriend–girlfriend relations. The leader teaches Frank a technique called blow-up in which he imagines absurd comical consequences should he fail to do his checking ritual. Tim and Louise are role playing the put-downs and hostility of Norma's parents. Norma tries to communicate effectively with them. All group members discuss strategies for making new friends. With the assistance of the leader, everyone is given a homework assignment in the friendship area, assignments being commensurate with their motivation and skill deficits.

In the last or consolidation stage, many interpersonal changes have already taken place. Two major remaining group tasks are to review all the strategies used to produce the behavior changes and to develop a self-motivating plan to insure future use of these strategies if necessary when the group terminates. The supports of the group are slowly faded out as members become more self-reliant and learn to maintain the new self-image, behavior changes, and life-styles on their own.

Application

Group Selection and Composition

Groups are organized in large part to provide clients with a wide range of social interaction and feedback experiences. To further facilitate this goal, group members are recruited and selected with heterogeniety in mind. That is, group members tend to vary in age, sex, range of life experiences, strengths, and problem areas. Such a group composition more nearly approximates the real social world.

Most often, these groups are co-led by a male and a female therapist. An advantage of this arrangement is that they would tend to demonstrate and model a coequal relationship. They can show group members how two people with different personalities, gender, and so forth, can work together in relative harmony. They also can provide approximately twice the amount of leader-directed feedback and social reinforcement to the group.

Group Setting

Learning theory tells us that behavior is a function of the environment and, in this particular case, the physical environment. Because we want group members to feel comfortable, relaxed, and well provided for, we simply try to find a setting that will promote these feelings.

We prefer to use a room that has the comfortable look of an informal den or family room, in contrast to that of a busy professional office with a large desk, file cabinets, and so forth. The room should be carpeted and the chairs should be upholstered and of equal size. Also, chairs should be very portable, because many behavioral exercises require moving chairs about the room. Further, it would be helpful to have some floor pillows for relaxation and guided imagery training.

Chairs or pillows are best arranged in a circle to promote more meaningful interactions. We recommend having a refreshment table available somewhere in or near the room and to offer members coffee, tea, and food tidbits. Good insulation and soundproofing are urged. Last, the room should have some warm personal touches reflected in choice of paintings, room colors, and other miscellaneous decorations.

Group Size

There are no fixed prescriptions for group size. Groups we have conducted vary from 6 to 12 members. We have found that with over 12 people we cannot address the therapeutic needs of everyone at each session. This becomes significant when all group members have behavior change assignments and are expected to report on results in the next session. An additional problem for a group therapist is to keep aware of the multitude of interactions and dynamics that occur in such a size group.

If the group were to have fewer than six members, other problems would be expected to arise. The discussions would be somewhat more limited in range, there would be fewer coping styles and social skills to model, and the group might temporarily lose its identity and therapeutic benefit if two or more people were absent or perhaps dropped out.

Therapy Frequency, Length, and Duration

Commonly, comprehensive behavior therapy groups meet no more often than 1 day per week for approximately 1½ to 2 hours per session. Marathon sessions of many hours or days are discouraged. Instead, the emphasis is on systematic step-by-step learning, practicing, and changing—all of which requires time to be integrated into new perceptions and life-styles.

The life or duration of this kind of group varies with therapist and group preferences, schedule availabilities, goals of therapy, to name just a few variables. Most often groups last 8 months to 1 year, with some extending well beyond 1 year. Groups of very long duration tend to be open-ended, with new members being added as appropriate.

Media Usage

The use of media, particularly videotape recording and playback, is encouraged in our group practices. Videotape is thought of as a tool that yields objective feedback on verbal and nonverbal events that occur between people in groups.

Videotape feedback is used in several ways. Group members may receive immediate playback on their attempts to practice the group leader's recommendations. Examples include speaking louder, trying to interview for a job, and giving another person constructive criticism. They notice any performance deficits in the playback and try to improve their verbal and nonverbal performance skills. Sometimes playback is used merely to make group members more aware of themselves—how they sit, their facial reactions, style of communication, and defensive/avoidance patterns. Occasionally, we play back tapes from earlier sessions to help clients objectively see the progress that has been made since then, the promises that have not been kept, and the changes in group focus over time.

One must remember to secure permission to use videotape from all members of the group. Also, careful thought should be given to the question of who will operate the equipment during the recording and/or the playback phases of the session. Persons outside the group may be called in for this sole purpose, or the leader may select group members to take turns operating the equipment.

Leader Qualifications

The preference we have is for group leaders to be duly licensed to practice their mental health profession in the state of their residence and practice. The expectation is that such a leader would have an advanced degree in psychology, psychiatry, or social work.

Inasmuch as most graduate schools offer very few, if any, graduate courses in behavior therapy, we urge that behavior group leaders complete at least two years of formal supervised postdoctoral training in behavior therapy. For example, at the Center for Behavioral Psychotherapy postdoctoral trainees first complete 1 year of advanced seminars, workshops, and practicums. They also participate in a didactic behavior therapy group, an important prerequisite, in our judgment, to becoming a seasoned group leader. In the second year, trainees receive intensive supervision with individual clients, with all three types of groups, and with serving as a consultant to psychiatric hospitals, rehabilitation centers, schools, and corporations.

Ethics

Group leaders are obligated to follow the code of ethics established by the state licensing boards of their professions, as well as to adhere to the standards of practice and conduct established by their national professional organization.

RESEARCH

Behavioral group therapy has now reached the point where it may be considered as having concluded its infancy, and is now emerging as a rather healthy and vigorous youngster. As evidence we can cite such trends as (a) the inclusion in reference texts of articles or chapters focusing on behavioral group therapy as a treatment modality and phenomenon worthy of investigation in and of itself, rather than merely as a convenient context in which to apply interventions developed for the treatment of individuals (cf. Liberman & Teigen, 1979); (b) the publication of texts dealing solely with the subject of behavioral group therapy (cf. Rose, 1977); and (c) the publication of an annual review of behavioral group therapy (Upper & Ross, 1979, 1980). A review of the literature of behavioral group therapy reveals that much of the research pertinent to behavioral group therapy is devoted to those issues which have perplexed research scientists for many years in their investigations of the general subject of psychotherapy. This is not surprising, because behavioral group therapy is simply another approach to changing human behavior and, as such, must deal with all the issues which have faced change agents throughout the history of psychotherapy, for example therapy outcome, the process of therapy, and the theory of change.

In addition to these familiar issues, however, behavior therapy has emphasized two issues which have not received their due in earlier research. These have to do with components research and the generalization and maintenance of treatment effects. Components research refers to the increasing emphasis by behavioral researchers upon the need for investigating the unique contributions of individual treatment components as they are used in total treatment packages. An excellent example of such a recommendation is Meichenbaum's (1979) call for what he terms "dismantling" research. This sort of research becomes especially appropriate for behavioral therapy groups, because most such groups encourage the use of treatment packages for maximizing behavioral change. The issues of the generalization and maintenance of treatment effects has become an equally timely and appropriate research focus, because there is general agreement that behavioral interventions have been successful in helping people change (Bergin & Suinn, 1975). However, the generalization and maintenance of that change has been problematic, to say the least (Marholin, 1976). Nowhere is this clearer than in the literature of behavioral interventions with families, career psychiatric patients, and persons with addictive behaviors. (Conway & Burcher, 1976; Davidson & Davidson, 1980; Gambrill, 1977; Johnson, Bolstad, & Lobitz, 1976; Koegel, Glahn, & Nieminen, 1979; Lovaas, Koegel, Simmons, & Long, 1973; and Mash, Hammerlynck, & Handy, 1976). These latter populations have clearly been the focus of behavioral group therapy interventions and the issues of generalization and maintenance of treatment effects have been no less important in the group context as in the case of individual behavior therapy.

Finally, there is increasing attention to the specific research issues related to behavioral group therapy (see earlier discussions of such issues in each section) and a number of investigators are beginning to develop a body of data aimed at clarifying the what and how of behavioral group therapy (Liberman & Teigen, 1979; Upper & Ross, 1979, 1980). Clearly this kind of research is necessary and as increasing interest leads to the accumulation of empirical data it is the hope of the present writers that there will ultimately be a translation of such data into theory and practice.

GROUP SESSION ILLUSTRATION

For purpose of illustration, we present Dr. B, a fictitious behavioral group therapist who conducts groups at his private office suite in the New York area. Currently, he leads a 2-hour evening group consisting of eight members: Frank, Norma, Mary, Jim, Diane, Louise, Susan, and Bob. Two members of the group are also seeing Dr. B privately for individual psychotherapy. The remaining group members are only in group therapy and were referred to Dr. B from family agencies, psychiatric outpatient departments, and other private therapists.

The group was organized with the metagoal of improving interpersonal relations at home, at work, and at play. Dr. B screened each potential group member, hoping to rule out deviant-type individuals and to select those with diverse social competencies and deficits. Contracts were set up specifying the number of sessions, member and leader responsibilities in the change process, and fees, to name a few contract issues.

This is the eighth session, with everyone present. In the prior seven sessions group members introduced each other; slowly began to disclose personal information; established individual and within-group interpersonal goals; learned how to give constructive feedback; learned how to use reinforcement principles to motivate oneself; became aware of irrational cognitions that created emotional and behavioral problems; and came to realize their assertive bill of rights.

As the group enters the room slowly each sits in a comfortable chair, all arranged in a circle. The members occasionally vary whom they sit next to, in part, encouraged by Dr. B to stimulate new patterns of interaction.

The session opens with no one having any pressing or critical problem. Dr. B gives ample time and support to allow even the shyest member to express him- or herself if such a problem exists. Dr. B moves on and asks the group to review the results of last week's homework assignment: practicing ways of being reinforcing to others. Surprisingly, the group shows that cohesiveness is evolving; all members attempted the homework assignment. Dr. B makes sure that the same people do not start the reporting phase week after week. Members listen attentively to each other and, with Dr. B's guidance, give positive feedback for any demonstration of effort or small success in the homework assignments. Members discuss the various ways used to be reinforcing to others. Each learns vicariously from the others' efforts. Some members used praise, listening, remembering, cooperating, joking, and related behaviors to be reinforcing to key people in their lives.

Still in the opening phase, Dr. B has the group practice an assertive self-disclosure exercise with each member telling the group calmly and without guilt about some important mistake made in life.

Dr. B now reviews some individual member problems addressed in past sessions. Diane appears interested to pursue a problem with her boyfriend that was introduced last week. Diane says that, with the group support, she has stood up for herself and he has stopped teasing her. However, she is still jealous and cannot stop thinking of him. "Nothing else matters in my life," says Diane. The group carefully challenges Diane's irrational thought that she can't live without him. Several members, especially Jim, urge her to expand her social relationships. Suggestions were given for going on group dates, making girl friends (Diane had none), where to meet other men, and so forth. Dr. B intervened, stating that Diane might be anxious about making these changes unless she attempted these changes in small, planned steps, and also learned how to relax or desensitize her social contact fears away.

The group appears quiet and contemplative for a few moments after assisting Dr. B in breaking down into small components Diane's goals for more social contacts. Dr. B looks around the room and then Frank begins to speak up. He says, "You know we've been working on my concentration problem at my job in the Bronx. But maybe I have a bigger problem now. I keep checking things around the house for many hours before I can go out. It drives me nuts."

Dr. B, Jim, and Susan complement Frank on his self-disclosure. Dr. B reflects that Frank may now feel more comfortable with the group and possibly the cooperation trading and assertion self-disclosure exercises over the past few sessions may have given Frank the necessary skills and self-confidence to do it. Frank listens and, following some thought, agrees with Dr. B and accepts the group's feedback and social reinforcement. Frank continues to describe his rituals. The group takes pains to understand Frank's "strange" behavior. Dr. B explains briefly some of the behavioral dynamics of compulsive behavior and introduces Frank to a technique called "blow-up." Frank is guided by Dr. B to imagine a sequence of absurd consequences for his imagined failure to check the doors, stove, and so forth. Absurdities include being locked out forever, house and having the neighborhood destroyed by his stove being on fire. Frank actually begins to smile and relax as he goes through the blow-up procedure. He is now less serious and more relaxed about his problem. Dr. B indicates that this technique is but a first step in treatment of the ritual and encourages Frank to practice the image at home. A brief group discussion follows about how others can use this technique on related but less severe worries and impulses in their lives.

Mary responds to the issue of using the blow-up procedure by focusing on her continuing concern with her difficulty in controlling her 3-year-old son. It is obvious to the group that she has simply taken Dr. B's comments about using the blow-up procedure to deal with other worries and impulses and has used it to reintroduce her continuing complaints about her son, Billy. Bob, with an impatient tone of voice, responds to Mary by remarking, "Here we go again." Nancy looks at him and he glances around the group for support. Louise lends her support to Bob by commenting on the fact that Mary's complaints are old hat and that the group has helped her to problem-solve the issue of her son many times in the past. She continued by accusing Mary of being the problem, in that she was just unable to get herself to follow a structured program. At this point, the remainder of the group is in obvious agreement. Dr. B, aware of the scapegoating that is in process, intervenes by picking up on the issue of Mary's difficulty in implementing a structured program as suggested by the group. He refocuses the issue from "Mary's difficulty" to the challenge of creating a program which would provide Mary with the support necessary to successfully implement a program. Dr. B reiterates the point that when behavior change does not occur, the source of difficulty must be sought not in the person, but in the program of change. He helps the group adopt a problem-solving attitude by first assisting the members to focus on the feelings aroused in them by Mary's repetitive inability to follow through with their suggestions. The issue of persons not responding to help and the reasons for the failure to respond are discussed and analyzed according to a strict problem-solving approach. Specifically, the group is prompted through the process of generating a number of possible reasons why Mary is not responding. During this process, emphasis is shifted from Mary's not responding because she doesn't want to or doesn't care, to other reasons which are less emotionally loaded, such as that she doesn't know what to do or how to do it. Thus the issue is redefined as a teaching–learning problem, rather than as a "person-ality" or "emotional" problem on Mary's part. With this focus, the group is able to return on task and generate a series of suggestions, which Nancy accepts. These suggestions are then incorporated into a new program, its major difference lying in the area of how Mary will follow more consistently a realistic schedule of positive reinforcement for appropriate behaviors. The specific suggestion is that Mary is to carry a kitchen timer in her apron pocket and randomly set the timer to intervals under 5 minutes. Each time the timer rings Mary is to check Billy, and if he is behaving appropriately she is to provide him with a token and a social reinforcer. Mary appears comfortable with this suggestion snd promises to do her best in the next week to follow the program. Dr. B then reinforces all for their "good behaviors" and asked what else is new.

Norma responds by reporting that during the week past she has had a great deal of difficulty at home. Dr. B asks what was happening, and Norma complains that she just can't handle her parents' hostility toward her. Dr. B then asks Jim and Louise if they would role play Norma's parents, and asks Norma to set up the scene for them. Norma, Jim, and Louise go to the side of the room to set up the scene. Meanwhile, Dr. B asks the remainder of the group to share whether they have had problems with hostility from their own parents. Several group members relate that they have had such experiences in the past, and Dr. B universalizes the experiences for them by saying that it is common for persons to have experienced such difficulties. He then asks the group to think about how they would handle such a situation with their own parents. At this time, Norma, Louise, and Jim return to the group, indicating that they are ready to begin. Dr. B shares with them what has transpired in the past few minutes. Then he asks them to go on with their role playing. Jim and Louise begin the role playing by belittling Norma for not being married at her age. They refer to her shortcomings and focus directly on her lack of social skills and her physical appearance. During this harangue by Jim and Louise as her parents, Norma is silent and looks at them only occasionally with her eyes downcast for the most part. After 2 minutes of this, Dr. B interrupts and asks Norma if this was an accurate representation of what usually happened. Nor-ma confirms that it is. Dr. B then turns to the group and asks them what their observations are as to what was happening and asks for suggestions as to how Norma could behave differently in order to handle the situation better.

The group agrees that Norma's silence and unassertive physical demeanor simply exacerbates the situation and they tell her to speak up and look her parents in the eye. Dr. B asks for several specific suggestions as to how Norma could act and what specifically she could say. The next few minutes are spent in modeling the suggested behaviors by the group members and shaping Norma's attempts to imitate the behaviors through feedback and reinforcement. When Norma is able to emit the suggested behaviors, Dr. B then asks Jim and Louise to share their experience as they acted out the roles of Norma's parents. They both agreed that they were initially a little uncomfortable in berating Norma but when they saw how sheepish Norma looked and how passively she behaved, it made it easier to do the role playing. Dr. B then relates this experience to the possibility that Norma's parents were experiencing a similar reaction to her passivity and submissiveness; that, indeed, they were being reinforced for their hostility by Norma's passive acceptance of their behaviors. Dr. B then asks that Jim and Louise repeat the earlier scenario and instructs Norma to handle it in her newly learned way. Jim and Louise begin role playing in the same way that they had earlier, but this time with a visual prompt by Dr. B. After about 15 seconds, Norma is able to interrupt and, looking Jim and Louise in the eye, to tell them that they are out of line for talking to her in the way that they do, and that she is not going to allow that to happen. Norma is able to do this with some degree of proficiency and Dr. B reinforces her for her effort, noting the good part of her performance and then asking the group to give her feedback. The group members are reminded that they are to give the positive feedback first and then make suggestions for change in how to do it better, if they had any such suggestions.

The group picks up the cue and everyone is able to praise Norma about some aspect of her performance, and the general consensus of the group is that in order to improve, she has to act out the behaviors with greater intensity and sense of confidence in the form of firmness of voice and posture. Norma then role plays the situation again with Jim and Louise and is reinforced for her improvement. Norma is then instructed to practice these new behaviors on her own with someone she trusts until she feels comfortable with them. However, she is also instructed not to try the behaviors with her parents until she comes back and shares her improvement in practice with the group.

With the exception of the opening phase where homework achievements were reported and warm-up assertion exercises were practiced, most effort and focus has been on clinical problems of a few group members—Frank, Diane, Norma, and Mary. Dr. B wants more unity and cohesiveness as the end of the session draws near. He reviews common complaints expressed by all group members in past sessions. The one that creates the most interest is learning to be more relaxed.

Dr. B spends considerable time differentiating relaxation and tension for the group. He explains that one cannot be both relaxed and tense at the same time. The group also hears Dr. B saying that being relaxed is a skill that can be learned by anyone willing to practice. This makes the group excited and eager to begin. One group member, Jim, expresses doubts, but says he will try with the group.

All bring out floor pillows to the center of the room for relaxation training. Dr. B begins. Step by step he tells the group to tense a muscle group such as the forehead and to study that tension for 7 to 10 seconds. He then cues the group to relax that muscle quickly and uses autogenic phrases such as "Your forehead is now heavy, relaxed, very warm." The group practices alternately tensing and relaxing all major muscles. They are becoming more aware of tension in their bodies and are beginning to learn how to create feelings of body relaxation. Some group members are more successful than others at relaxing but, regardless, all receive praise and encouragement to practice at home from Dr. B. All members report feeling much more calm after the exercise and seem eager to practice. Dr. B then fields several questions such as, "How long will it take until I feel relaxed at will?" "Where should I practice?"

STRENGTHS AND LIMITATIONS

The application of behavior therapy to groups is relatively new. We have stated that in its short history the approach has already proven effective, as demonstrated by research studies. Certainly, Gestalt, RET, encounter, and psychoanalytic groups also have research and clinical studies to support their effectiveness. What, then, further separates behavioral groups from its counterparts?

For one, it can be safely stated that behavioral groups have the widest applicability. Such diverse populations as overweight people, parents, tense business executives, "garden variety" neurotics, alcoholics, mentally retarded/developmentally disabled persons, sex offenders, shy people, smokers, math anxiety sufferers, chronic pain patients, families, marital couples, and students with poor study skills have been helped successfully through behavior therapy groups. Most other approaches to group therapy do not offer the technology sufficient to serve such diverse people and problems.

In a similar vein, the self-management and skills-training-type groups have an educational as well as therapeutic emphasis and focus. The advantages of a dual focus are many. These groups attract people who are not in need of formal in-depth counseling or psychotherapy. Other people who need more formal therapy, but are afraid, can approach these groups as a first step toward comprehensive therapy, since these groups pose little threat or stigma. These groups are often perceived as "fun" and many constructive social networks evolve after the group has terminated. In these groups, most members are high functioning in areas other than the target problem of the group. This means opportunities for a great deal of vicarious modeling and skill building among group members.

Many groups create unnecessary dependencies on the leader. This is less so in behavioral groups. The leader is part coach and part educator in life skills. The group members are responded to on an adult level. Members are encouraged to model, guide, and practice with each other, thus quickly weaning some of the power and authority away from the leader onto the group itself.

Behavioral groups are noted for the flexibility of their treatment programs. If an idea or a technique does not work, others are available to be tried. Clients are not forced to conform to a single method or technique, nor blamed if the therapy does not work for them.

There are also economic and practical strengths in behavioral groups. Many can be effectively structured as short-term groups, say 6 to 10 weeks. This condition attracts people who are legitimately busy and/or wish to limit therapy costs. Short-term groups help to mobilize client motivation to change. The groups are direct, action-oriented, and highly structured, conditions that facilitate fast clinical change in everyday problems.

Last, another strength of behavioral groups is the adherence to research and accountability. Especially in the skills-training and self-management groups, several treatment programs have been experimentally validated. If these programs are later applied to a client group comparable to the experimental population and by a group leader comparable to the experimenter, chances of continued success are high. In all three type groups, success is not merely judged on client statements that they "feel better" or "like the group." Standardized tests, problem checklists, observation groups, and so forth, are also used to evaluate group effectiveness.

With all these strengths can behavioral groups have any limitations? Certainly. As previously mentioned, there is no unified behavioral theory of group process to guide a group leader in designing and conducting groups. Also, as with the other group modalities, only reasonably well-motivated clients whose expectations are appropriate for the group experience can be helped with reasonable assurance. Another limitation is the novice status of behavioral group therapy. Most behavioral clinicians and researchers have invested their energies in other areas, thus depriving behavior group therapy of needed support and expertise. Hopefully, change is on the way.

SUMMARY

We have presented behavioral group therapy as a historically recent and promising addition to the group therapies. Behavioral therapy makes available a wide array of pragmatic and experimentally validated techniques to the group context. As such, different procedures and combinations thereof are employed to varying clinical problems in the individual group members and also to the group at large. The emphasis is on "doing" and learning to change behavior affect and cognitions. The leader and other group members are used for modeling, practice, feedback, and support, all in structured ways. Insight and self-awareness are encouraged in behavioral groups, but most emphasis is placed on learning how to make significant personal and interpersonal changes.

Although there is no consistent, unified behavioral theory of group dynamics, we have offered a tentative formulation. It includes reformulated theoretical constructs from individual behavior therapy, as well as from the more general field of social psychology. Examples include social exchange theory, group contingency, theory, social role theory, placebo effect, *ABC* model, contracting, persuasion, and modeling.

Our review of the work in behavior therapy reveals that there does not appear to be a workable classification for the varieties of behavioral groups in the literature. In an attempt to remedy this situation, we have proposed a classification schema, identifying three distinct types of behavioral groups. First, there are those groups which focus on treating specific skill problems which we label as *Skills-Training Groups*. There are assertion-training groups, couples communication groups, parent-training–teacher-training groups, daily living skills-training groups for institutional populations, and shyness groups.

Second, there are those groups where individuals learn to modify specific problem behaviors and habits that are necessary only for the welfare of the person himself or herself. We label groups in this class as *Self-Management–Self-Control Groups*. In such groups problems of obesity, smoking, stress, chronic pain, and test anxiety are treated.

Third, there are those groups that focus on subtle and complex interpersonal issues and subscribe to broad life goals such as changing one's life-style and self-image. This type of group is called a *Comprehensive Behavior Therapy Group*. The mechanisms and procedures used in these groups are presented.

References

Aiken, E. G. Changes in interpersonal descriptions accompanying the operant conditioning of verbal frequency in groups. *Journal of Verbal Learning and Verbal Behavior*, 1965, *4*, 243–247.

Ash, S. E. Effects of group pressure upon the modification and distortion of judgments. In H. Guetzkow (Ed.), *Groups, leadership, and men*. Pittsburgh: Carnegie Press, 1951.

Azrin, N. H. The present state and future trends of behavior therapy. In P. Sjoden, S. Bates, & S. W. Dockens (Eds.), *Trends in behavior therapy*. New York: Academic Press, 1979.

Azrin, N. H., & Lindsley, O. R. The reinforcement of cooperation between children. *Journal of Abnormal and Social Psychology*, 1956, *52*, 100–102.

Baer, D. M., Wolf, M. M., & Risley, T. Some current dimensions of applied behavior analysis. *Journal of Applied Behavior Analysis*, 1968, *1*, 91–97.

Baker, B. L., Brightman, A. J., Heifetz, L. J., & Murphy, D. M. *Steps to independence*. Champaign, Ill.: Research Press, 1978.

Bandura, A. *Principles of behavior modification*. New York: Holt, Rinehart & Winston, 1969.

Bandura, A. Behavior theory and the models of man. *American Psychologist*, 1974, *12*, 859–869.

Bandura, A. *Social learning theory*. Englewood Cliffs, N.J.: Prentice-Hall, 1977.

Bandura, A. The self system in reciprocal determinism. *American Psychologist*, 1978, *33*, 344–358.

Bavelas, A., Hastorf, A. H. Gross, A. E., & Kite, W. R. Experiments on the alteration of group structure. *Journal of Experimental Social Psychology*, 1965, *1*, 55–70.

Becker, W. C. *Parents are teachers*. Champaign, Ill.: Research Press, 1971.

Bedell, J. R., & Weathers, L. R. A psycho-educational model for skill training: Therapist-facilitated and game-facilitated applications. In D. Upper & S. M. Ross (Eds.), *Behavioral group therapy*, 1979. Champaign, Ill.: Research Press, 1979.

Bennet, P. S., & Maley, R. F. Modification of interactive behaviors in chronic mental patients. *Journal of Applied Behavior Analysis*, 1973, *6*, 609–620.

Bergin, A. E., & Suinn, R. M. Individual psychotherapy and behavior therapy. In M. R. Rosenzweig & L. W. Porter (Eds.), *Annual review of psychology*, 1975, *26*. Palo Alto, Cal.: Annual Review, 1975.

Bijou, S. W., Peterson, R. P., & Ault, M. H. A method to integrate descriptive and experimental field studies at the level of data and empirical concepts. *Journal of Applied Behavior Analysis*, 1968, *1*, 175–191.

Bion, W. R. *Experiences in groups*. New York: Basic Books, 1959.

Bowers, K. S. Situationism in psychology: An analysis and a critique. *Psychological Review*, 1973, *80*, 307–336.

Braginsky, B. M., & Braginsky, D. D. Schizophrenic patients in the psychiatric interview: An experimental study of their effectiveness at manipulation. *Journal of Consulting Psychology*, 1967, *31*, 543–547.

Browning, R. M. *Teaching the severely handicapped child*. Boston: Allyn & Bacon, 1980.

Browning, R. M., & Stover, D. O. *Behavior modification in child treatment*. Chicago: Aldine-Atherton, 1971.

Brownstone, J. E., & Dye, C. J. *Communication workshop for parents of adolescents*. Champaign, Ill.: Research Press, 1973.

Cartright, D., & Zander, A. (Eds.), *Group dynamics: Research and theory*. New York: Harper & Row, 1968.

Coe, W. C., Expectations, hypnosis, and suggestion in behavior change. In F. H. Kanfer & A. P. Goldstein (Eds.), *Helping people change* (2nd ed.). New York: Pergamon Press, 1980.

Coe, W. C., & Buckner, L. G. Expectation, hypnosis, and suggestion methods. In F. H. Kanfer & A. P. Goldstein (Eds.), *Helping people change*. New York: Pergamon Press, 1975.

Conway, J. B., & Bucher, B. D. Transfer and maintenance of behavior change in children: A review and suggestions. In E. J. Mash, L. A. Hamerlynck, & L. C. Handy (Eds.), *Behavior modification and families*. New York: Brunner/Mazel, 1976.

Davidson, P. O., & Davidson, S. M. *Behavioral medicine: Changing health styles*. New York: Brunner/Mazel, 1980.

Dinoff, M., Horner, R. F., Kuppiewski, B. S., Rickard, H. C., & Timmons, E. O. Conditioning the verbal behavior of a psychiatric population in a group therapy-like situation. *Journal of Clinical Psychology*, 1960, *16*, 371–372.

Dollard, J., & Miller, N. E. *Personality and psychotherapy*. New York: McGraw-Hill, 1950.

Feldman, R. A., & Wodarski, J. S. *Contemporary approaches to group treatment*. San Francisco: Jossey Bass, 1975.

Ferguson, J. M. A clinical program for the behavioral control of obesity In B. J. Williams, S. Martin, & J. P. Foreyt (Eds.), *Obesity: Behavioral approaches to dietary management*. New York: Brunner/Mazel, 1976.

Ferster, C. B., Nurnberger, J. I., & Levitt, E. B. The control of eating. *Journal of Mathetics*, 1962, *1*, 87–109.

Fiedler, F. E. A comparison of therapeutic relationships in psychoanalytical, non-directive, and Adlerian therapy. *Journal of Consulting Psychology*, 1950, *14*, 436–445.

Fish, J. M. *Placebo theory*. San Francisco: Jossey-Bass, 1973.

Flowers, J. V. Behavioral analysis of group therapy and a model for behavioral group therapy. In D. Upper & S. M. Ross (Eds.), *Behavioral group therapy*, 1979. Champaign, Ill.: Research Press, 1979.

Foreyt, J. P., & Rathjen, D. P. (Eds.), *Cognitive behavior therapy: Research and application*. New York: Plenum Press, 1978.

Frank, J. D. *Persuasion and healing*. Baltimore: Johns Hopkins Press, 1972.

Gambrill, E. D. *Behavior modification*. San Francisco: Jossey-Bass, 1977.

Garfield, S. L. Research on client variables in psychotherapy. In S. L. Garfield & A. E. Bergin (Eds.), *Handbook of psychotherapy and behavior change* (2nd ed.). New York: Wiley, 1978.

Gazda, G. M. (Ed.). *Basic approaches to group psychotherapy and group counseling* (2nd ed.). Springfield, Ill.: Charles C Thomas, 1975.

Goldenberg, H. *Contemporary clinical psychology*. Monterey, California, 1973.

Goldfried, M. R., & Kent, R. N. Traditional versus behavioral personality assessment: A comparison of methodological and theoretical assumptions. *Psychological Bulletin*, 1972, *77*, 409–420.

Goldfried, M. R., & Davidson, G. C. *Clinical behavior therapy*. New York: Holt, Rinehart & Winston, 1976.

Goldfried, M. R., & Merbaum, M. (Eds.), *Behavior change through self control*. New York: Holt, Rinehart & Winston, 1973.

Goldiamond, I. Self-control procedures in personal behavior problems. *Psychological Reports*, 1965, *17*, 851–868.

Goldstein, A. P. *Therapist–patient expectancies in psychotherapy*. New York: Pergamon Press, 1962.

Goldstein, A. P. *Psychotherapeutic attraction*. New York: Pergamon Press, 1971.

Goldstein, A. P. *Structured learning theory*. New York: Academic Press, 1973.

Goldstein, A. P., Heller, K., & Sechrest, L. *Psychotherapy and the psychology of behavior change*. New York: Wiley, 1966.

Goldstein, A. P., Sprafkin, R. P., & Gershaw, N. J. *Skill training for community living*. New York: Pergamon Press, 1976.

Goodstein, L. D. & Lanyon, R. I. *Adjustment, behavior, and personality*. Reading, Mass.: Addison-Wesley, 1979.

Gottman, J. M., & Leiblum, S. R. *How to do psychotherapy and how to evaluate it*. New York: Holt, Rinehart & Winston, 1974.

Gottman, J. M., Notarius, C., Gonso, J., & Markman, H. *A couple's guide to communication*. Champaign, Ill.: Research Press, 1976.

Greenwood, C. R., Hops, H., Delquadri, J., & Walker, H. M. *PASS: Consultant manual*. Eugene, Oregon: University of Oregon, Center at Oregon for Research in the Behavioral Education of the Handicapped, 1977.

Hardy, R. E., & Cull, J. G. (Eds.), *Modification of behavior of the mentally ill*. Springfield, Ill.: Charles C Thomas, 1974.

Heckel, R. V., Wiggins, S. L., & Salzberg, H. C. Conditioning against silences in group therapy. *Journal of Clinical Psychology*, 1962, *18*, 216–217.

Hollander, M. A. Programs for drug abuse prevention and treatment in a suburban community. *Group Process*, 1973, *5*, 47–61.

Hollander, M. A. *Comprehensive behavioral assessment and treatment of marital problems*. Paper presented at the 82nd Annual Meeting of the American Psychological Association, New Orleans, 1974.

Hollander, M. A. A behavior therapy approach to frigidity: The case of June. In C. Loew, H. Grayson, & G. Loew. (Eds.), *Three psychotherapies: A clinical comparison*. New York: Brunner/Mazel, 1975.

Hollander, M. A. Cooperative responses in schizophrenics. *Behavior Therapy*, 1976, *7*, 696–697.

Hollander, M. A., & Plutchik, R. A reinforcement program for psychiatric attendants. *Behavior Therapy and Experimental Psychiatry*, 1972, *2*, 297–300.

Jackson, D. A., Hazel, M. M., & Saudargas, R. A. *A guide to staff training*. Lawrence, Kansas: University of Kansas Support and Development Center for Follow Through, Department of Human Development, University of Kansas, 1974.

Jacobson, N. S., & Margolin, G. *Marital therapy*. New York: Brunner/Mazel, 1979.

Johnson, D. W. *Reaching out: Interpersonal effectiveness*. Englewood Cliffs, N.J.: Prentice-Hall, 1972.

Johnson, S. M., Bolstad, O. D., & Lobitz, G. K. Generalization and contrast phenomena in behavior modification with children. In E. J. Mash, L. A. Hamerlynck, & L. C. Handy (Eds.), *Behavior modification and families*. New York: Brunner/Mazel, 1976.

Kanfer, F. H. & Phillips, J. *Learning foundations of behavior therapy*. New York: Wiley, 1970.

Kanfer, F. H., & Saslow, G. Behavioral diagnosis. *Archives of General Psychiatry*, 1965, *12*, 529–538.

Kaplan, H. I., & Sadock, B. J. (Eds.). *The evolution of group therapy* (Vol. 2). New York: Jason Aronson, 1972. (a)

Kaplan, H. I., & Sadock, B. J. (Eds.). *New models for group therapy* (Vol. 5). New York: Jason Aronson, 1972. (b)

Karoly, P., & Steffen, J. J. (Eds.). *Improving the long-term effects of psychotherapy.* New York: Gardner Press, 1980.

Kendall, P. C. (Ed.). Mini-series on integrationism in psychotherapy. *Behavior Therapy,* 1982, *13,* 559–623.

Kendall, P. C., & Hollon, S. D. (Eds.). *Cognitive-behavioral interventions: Theory, research, and procedures.* New York: Academic Press, 1979.

Koegel, R. L., & Rincover, A. Research on the difference between generalization and maintenance in extra-therapy responding. *Journal of Applied Behavior Analysis,* 1978, *10,* 1–12.

Koegel, R. L., Glahn, T. J., & Nieminen, G. S. Generalization of parent-training results. *Journal of Applied Behavior Analysis,* 1979, *11,* 95–110.

Korchin, S. *Modern clinical psychology.* New York: Basic Books, 1976.

Kozloff, M. A. *Educating children with learning and behavior problems.* New York: Wiley, 1974.

Krasner, L., & Ullmann, L. P. *Behavior influence and personality.* New York: Wiley, 1974.

Lange, A. J., & Jakubowski, P. *Responsible assertive behavior.* Champaign, Ill: Research Press, 1976.

Langner, T., & Michael, S. *Life stress and mental health.* New York: Free Press, 1963.

Lazarus, A. Group therapy of phobic disorders by systematic desensitization. *Journal of Abnormal and Social Psychology,* 1961, *63,* 504–510.

Lazarus, A. *Behavior therapy and beyond.* New York: McGraw-Hill, 1971.

Lazarus, A. *Multi-modal behavior therapy.* New York: Springer, 1976.

Liberman, R. Behavioral group therapy, 1. *Behavior Therapy, 1,* 1970, 141–175.

Liberman, R. P., & Teigen, J. Behavioral group therapy. In P. Sjoden, S. Bates, & W. S. Dockens, III (Eds.), *Trends in behavior therapy.* New York: Academic Press, 1979.

Liberman, R. P., King, L. W., & DeRisi, W. J. Behavior analysis and therapy in community mental health. In H. Leitenberg (Ed.), *Handbook of behavior modification and behavior therapy.* Englewood Cliffs, N.J.: Prentice-Hall, 1976.

Lieberman, M. A. Group methods. In F. H. Kanfer & A. P. Goldstein, (Eds.), *Helping people change.* New York: Pergamon Press, 1975.

Lindsley, O. R. Experimental analysis of cooperation and competition. In T. Verhave (Ed.), *The experimental analysis of behaviors: Selected readings.* New York: Appleton-Century-Crofts, 1966.

Lobitz, W. C., & Baker, E. L. Group treatment of sexual dysfunction. In D. Upper & S. M. Ross (Eds.), *Behavioral group therapy.* Champain, Ill.: Research Press, 1979.

Lott, A. J., & Lott, B. E. Group cohesiveness, communication level, and conformity. *Journal of Abnormal and Social Psychology,* 1961, *62,* 408–412.

Lovaas, O. I., Koegel, R., Simmons, J. Q., & Long, J. S. Some generalization and follow-up measures on autistic children in behavioral therapy. *Journal of Applied Behavior Analysis,* 1973, *6,* 131–166.

Maccoby, E. E., Newcomb, T. M., & Hartley, E. L. Readings in social psychology. New York: Holt, Rinehart & Winston, 1958.

Madsen, C. H., Jr., & Madsen, C. K. *Teaching/discipline.* Boston: Allyn & Bacon, 1970.

Mahoney, M. J. *Cognition and behavior modification.* Cambridge, Mass.: Ballinger, 1974.

Mahoney, M. J., & Thoresen, C. E. *Self-control: Power to the person.* Monterey, Cal.: Brooks-Cole, 1974.

Marholin, D., Siegel, L. J., & Phillips, D. Treatment and transfer: A search for empirical procedures. In M. Hersen, R. M. Eisler, & P. M. Miller (Eds.), *Progress in behavior modification,* 1976, *3.* New York: Academic Press, 1976.

Mash, E. J., Hammerlynck, L. A., & Handy, L. C. (Eds.), *Behavior modification and families.* New York: Brunner/Mazel, 1976.

Mash, E. J., Handy, L. C., & Hammerlynck, L. A. (Eds.), *Behavior modification approaches to parenting*. New York: Brunner/Mazel, 1976
Meichenbaum, D. *Cognitive-behavior modification: An integrative approach*. New York: Plenum Press, 1977.
Meichenbaum, D. Cognitive-behavioral modification: Future directions. In P. Sjoden, S. Bates, & W. S. Dockens, III (Eds.), *Trends in behavior therapy*. New York: Academic Press, 1979.
Miller, W. H. *Systematic parent training*. Champaign, Ill.: Research Press, 1975.
Mischel, W. *Personality and assessment*. New York: Wiley, 1968.
Mischel, W. Toward a cognitive social learning reconceptualization of personality. *Psychological Review*, 1973, *80*, 252–283.
Mischel, W. Processes in delay of gratification. In L. Berkowitz (Ed.), *Advances in experimental social psychology*. New York: Academic Press, 1974.
Morris, R. J., & Suckerman, K. R. Therapist warmth as a factor in automated systematic desensitization. *Journal of Consulting and Clinical Psychology*, 1974, *42*, 244–250.
Nay, W. R. *Behavioral intervention*. New York: Gardner Press, 1977.
Novaco, R. W. Treatment of chronic anger through cognitive and relaxation controls. *Journal of Consulting and Clinical Psychology*, 1976, *44*, 681.
Novaco, R. W. Stress inoculation: A cognitive therapy for anger and its application to a case of depression. *Journal of Consulting and Clinical Psychology*, 1977, *45*, 600–608.
Novaco, R. W. Anger and coping with stress. In J. Foreyt & D. Rathjen (Eds.), *Cognitive behavior therapy: Therapy, research and practice*. New York: Plenum Press, 1978.
Oakes, W. F. Reinforcement of Bales categories in group discussions. *Psychological Reports*, 1962, *11*, 425–535.
Oakes, W. F., Droge, A. E., & August, B. Reinforcement effects on conclusions reached in group discussion. *Psychological Reports*, 1961, *9*, 27–34.
O'Leary, K. D., & O'Leary, S. G. *Classroom management: The successful use of behavior modification*. New York: Pergamon Press, 1972.
Parloff, M. B. Analytic group psychotherapy. In J. Marmor (Eds.), *Modern psychoanalysis*. New York: Basic Books, 1968.
Patterson, G. R. *Families: Applications of social learning to family life*. Champaign, Ill.: Research Press, 1975.
Patterson, G. R. The aggressive child: Victim and architect of a coercive system. In E. J. Mash, L. A. Hamerlynck, & L. C. Handy, (Eds.), *Behavior modification and families*. New York: Brunner/Mazel, 1976.
Patterson, G. R., & Cobb, J. A. A dyadic analysis of "aggressive" behaviors: An additional step towards a theory of aggression. In J. Hill (Ed.), *Minnesota Symposia on Child Psychology, 5*. Minneapolis: University of Minnesota Press, 1971.
Patterson, G. R., & Hops, H. Coercion, a game for two: Intervention techniques for marital conflict. In R. Ulrich & P. Mountjay (Eds.), *The experimental analysis of social behavior*. Englewood Cliffs, N.J.: Prentice-Hall, 1972.
Patterson, G. R., & Reid, J. B. Reciprocity and coercion: Two facets of social systems. In C. Neuringer & J. L. Michaels (Eds.), *Behavior modification in clinical psychology*. New York: Appleton-Century-Crofts, 1970.
Patterson, G. R., Ray, R. S., & Shaw, D. A. Direct intervention in families of deviant children. *Oregon Research Institute Research Bulletin, 8* (9), 1968.
Patterson, G. R., Reid, J. B., Jones, R. R., & Conger, R. E. *A social learning approach to family intervention*. Eugene, Oregon: Castalia Publishing, 1975.
Piper, W. E., Montvila, R. M., & McGihon, A. L. Process analysis in therapy groups: A behavioral sampling technique with many potential uses. In D. Upper & S. M. Ross, *Behavioral group therapy*, 1979. Champaign, Ill.: Research Press, 1979.

Rettig, E. G. *ABC's for parents*. Van Nuys, Cal.: Associates for Behavior Change, 1973.

Rettig, E. B. & Paulson, T. L. *ABC's for teachers*. Van Nuys, Cal.: Associates for Behavior Change, 1975.

Rimm, D. C., & Masters, J. C. *Behavior therapy: Techniques and empirical findings*. New York: Academic Press, 1974.

Rimm, D. C. & Masters, J. C. *Behavior therapy*. New York: Academic Press, 1979.

Rose, S. D. *Treating children in groups*. San Francisco, Cal.: Jossey-Bass, 1972.

Rose, S. D. *Group therapy: A behavioral approach*. Englewood Cliffs, N.J.: Prentice-Hall, 1977.

Rotter, J. B. *Social learning and clinical psychology*. Englewood Cliffs, N.J.: Prentice-Hall, 1954.

Sansbury, D. L. The role of the group in behavioral group therapy. In D. Upper & S. M. Ross, *Behavioral group therapy*, 1979. Champaign, Ill.: Research Press, 1979.

Shaffer, J., & Galinsky, M. D. *Models of group therapy and sensitivity training*. Englewood Cliffs, N.J.: Prentice-Hall, 1974.

Shapiro, D. The reinforcement of disagreement in a small group. *Behavior Research and Therapy*, 1963, *1*, 267–272.

Shapiro, D., & Birk, L. Group therapy in experimental perspective. *International Journal of Group Psychotherapy*, 1967, *17*, 211–224.

Sherif, M., & Sherif, C. W. *An outline of social psychology*. New York: Harper & Row, 1956.

Sjoden, P., Bates, S., & Dockens, W. S. (Eds.). *Trends in behavior therapy*. New York: Academic Press, 1979.

Spiegler, M. D., & Agigian, H. *The community training center*. New York: Brunner/Mazel, 1977.

Stuart, R. B. (Ed.). *Behavioral self-management: Strategies, techniques, and outcome*. New York: Brunner/Mazel, 1977.

Stuart, R. B., & Davis, B. *Slim chance in a fat world*. Champaign, Ill.: Research Press, 1972.

Tharp, R. G., & Wetzel, R. J. *Behavior modification in the natural environment*. New York: Academic Press, 1969.

Thibaut, J. W., & Kelley, H. H. *The social psychology of groups*. New York: John Wiley, 1961.

Thomas, E. J. *Marital communication and decision making*. New York: Free Press, 1977.

Thoresen, C. E. Behavioral humanism. In M. J. Mahoney & C. E. Thoresen (Eds.), *Self-control: Power to the person*. Monterey, Cal.: Brooks/Cole, 1974.

Thoresen, C. E., & Mahoney, M. J. *Behavioral self-control*. New York: Holt, Rinehart & Winston, 1974.

Thoresen, C. E. & Potter, B. Behavioral group counseling. In G. M. Gazda (Ed.), *Basic approaches to group psychotherapy and group counseling* (2nd ed.). Springfield, Ill.: Charles C Thomas, 1975.

Ullman, L. P. The behavioral treatment of existential problems. In H. E. Adams & I. P. Unikel (Eds.), *Issues and trends in behavior therapy*. Springfield, Ill.: Charles C Thomas, 1973, 28–42.

Ullman, L. P., & Krasner, L. *A psychological approach to abnormal behavior*. Englewood Cliffs, N.J.: Prentice-Hall, 1969.

Upper, D., & Ross, S. M. (Eds.). *Behavioral group therapy, 1979: An annual review*. Champaign, Ill.: Research Press, 1979.

Upper, D., & Ross, S. M. (Eds.). *Behavioral group therapy, 1980: An annual review*. Champaign, Ill.: Research Press, 1980.

Wahler, R. G., Berland, R. M., Coe, T. D., & Leske, G. Social systems analysis: Implementing an alternative behavioral model. In A. Rogers-Warren & S. F. Warren (Eds.), *Ecological perspective in behavior analysis*. Baltimore: University Park Press, 1977.

Wallace, J. An abilities conception of personality: Some implications for personality measurement. *American Psychologist*, 1966, *21*, 132–138.

White, R. W. Motivation reconsidered: The concept of competence. *Psychological Review*, 1959, *66*, 297–333.

Wilkins, W. Expectancies in applied settings. In A. S. Gurman & A. M. Razin (Eds.), *Effective psychotherapy*. New York: Pergamon Press, 1977.

Williams, B. J., Martin, S., & Foreyt, J. P. (Eds.). *Obesity: Behavioral approaches to dietary management*. New York: Brunner/Mazel, 1976.

Wilson, G. T., & Evans, I. M. The therapist–client relationship in behavior therapy. In A. S. Gurman & A. M. Razin (Eds.), *Effective psychotherapy*. New York: Pergamon Press, 1977.

Wolf, M. M., Giles, D. K., & Hall, V. R. Experiments with token reinforcement in a remedial classroom. *Behavior Therapy and Research*, 1968, *6*, 51–64.

Wolpe, J. *Psychotherapy by reciprocal inhibition*. Stanford: Stanford University Press, 1958.

Wolpe, J. *The practice of behavior therapy*. New York: Pergamon Press, 1969.

GLOSSARY

Aversive Stimulus. A stimulus that has the effect of decreasing a behavior when it is presented as a consequence of that behavior. A stimulus that the individual will work hard to avoid. A stimulus which functions such that its removal will increase the behavior leading to that removal.

Back-up Reinforcer. An effective reinforcer which is made available in exchange for tokens or other generalized reinforcers.

Baseline. The frequency of occurrence of a behavior in its natural environment prior to intervention of any kind. Also referred to as operant level and base rate.

Base Rate. See Baseline

Behavior. Any observable and measurable external or internal act of the organism. See Response.

Behavior Modification. Changing behavior through the *systematic* application of the methods and experimental findings of behavioral science.

Behavioral Chain. A sequence of behaviors that occurs semiautomatically in a determined order.

Behavioral Contract. The specification of the goals and procedures of a behavior modification program. Reached through agreement between the change agent and the target person and modifiable through negotiation.

Behavioral Dimensions. Measurable descriptive characteristics of a behavior such as frequency, intensity, duration, and topography.

Behavioral Goal. The specification of the set of responses to be emitted by the target person at the completion of a given behavior modification program. Usually the criteria for achievement of the goals and conditions under which the responses are to be emitted are also specified. When limited to academic instruction, this is often referred to as the instructional objective. See Target Behavior and Terminal Behavior.

Behavioral Repertoire. The total set of behaviors an organism is capable of emitting at any given point in time.

Chain. Two or more performances combined into a more complex behavioral sequence which occurs in a determined order.

Complex Behavior. A behavior consisting of two or more subsets of responses.

Conditioned Aversive Stimulus. An initially neutral stimulus that acquires aversive characteristics as a result of being paired repeatedly with (1) the absence or withdrawal of reinforcement; or (2) the delivery of primary or other conditioned aversive stimuli.

Conditioned Reinforcer. An initially neutral stimulus which acquires reinforcing properties as a result of repeated pairings with an effective primary or strong conditioned reinforcer.

Contingencies. The relationships between a given response and its environmental consequences. Contingencies may have the effect of strengthening, maintaining, weakening, or eliminating a behavior.

Contingency Control. The ability to manipulate the environmental consequences of a given behavior in order to achieve a specific behavioral goal.

Continuous Reinforcement (CRF). A schedule of reinforcement in which each occurrence of a response is reinforced.

Continuous Response. A response that does not have a clearly discriminable beginning or end. Pouting, smiling, and so forth.

Criterion. A specification of an acceptable level of performance that the person is to achieve.

Direct Observation. A method of obtaining behavioral data which records the data as it occurs. Event and time sampling are both methods of direct observation.

Discrete Response. A response that has a clearly discriminable beginning and end. Sneezing, coughing, written answers to mathematics problems, and so forth.

Discriminate. Respond differentially to different stimuli.

Discrimination. An event that has occurred when a discriminative stimulus controls the frequency of behavior.

Discriminative Stimulus. A stimulus which sets the occasion for the occurrence or nonoccurrence of a given response. Ess-D is a discriminative stimulus which sets the occasion for the occurrence of a response and ess-delta is a stimulus which sets the occasion for the nonoccurrence of a response.

Extinction. The deceleration and eventual nonoccurrence of a response due to the discontinuance of reinforcement.

Fading. The gradual removal of a discriminative stimulus, such as cues and prompts.

Fixed Interval Schedule (FI). A schedule where reinforcement is made contingent upon the passage of a given interval of time.

Fixed Ratio (FR). A schedule where reinforcement is made contingent upon the occurrence of a given number of responses.

Functional Relationship. A lawful relationship between two variables.

Generalized Reinforcer. A conditioned reinforcer that is effective over a wide variety of deprivation conditions as a result of having been paired with a variety of previously established reinforcers.

Imitation. Matching the behavior or response of a model.

Incompatible Behavior. A behavior that is mutually exclusive with a response such that the two responses cannot occur simultaneously.

Intensity of a Response. The physical force of a response.

Intermittent Reinforcement. A schedule of reinforcement in which some, but not all, of the occurrences of a response are reinforced.

Negative Reinforcement. The removal of a negative reinforcer or aversive stimulus as a consequence of a response.

Negative Reinforcer. A stimulus that, when removed or reduced as a consequence of a response, results in an increase or maintenance of that response.

Operant Behavior. Behavior that is controlled by its consequences.

Operant Level. See Baseline.

Operational Definition. A definition of a term involving its relevant operation or operations.

Positive Reinforcement. The delivery of a positive reinforcement contingent upon a response.

Positive Reinforcer. A stimulus that, when presented as a consequence of a response, results in an increase or maintenance of that response.

Premack Principle. A principle that states that contingent access to high-frequency behaviors serve as reinforcers for the performance of low-frequency behaviors.

Primary Aversive Stimulus. A stimulus that is aversive in the absence of any prior learning history.

Primary Reinforcer. A reinforcing stimulus that is effective in the absence of any prior learning history.

Prompt. A stimulus which aids the occurrence of a response.

Punishing Response. See Aversive Stimulus.

Punishment. A procedure in which the contingent presentation of a stimulus reduces the rate of the occurrence of the target behavior.

Reinforcement. A procedure where the contingent use of a stimulus results in an increase or maintenance of a target behavior.

Reinforcement Density. Frequency or rate with which responses are reinforced.

Respondent Behavior. Behavior that is elicited or controlled by its antecedents.

Response. See Behavior.

Response Cost. A procedure in which there is contingent withdrawal of specified amounts of available reinforcers.

Response Differentiation. A procedure that involves reinforcing a behavioral subset that conforms to clearly specified behavioral dimensions.

Satiation. The reduction in performance or reinforcer effectiveness that occurs after a large amount of reinforcement has been delivered.

Schedule of Reinforcement. The rule governing which of the many occurrences of a response will be reinforced.

Shaping. A procedure through which new behaviors are developed by means of the systematic reinforcement of successive approximations toward the behavioral goals.

Social Reinforcer. A conditioned reinforcing stimulus mediated by another individual within a social context.

Spontaneous Recovery. The reappearance of a response that has been eliminated by means of an extinction procedure following a time interval without any intervening reinforcement.

Step Size. The number of new responses in a subset required for a particular successive approximation in a shaping procedure.

Stimulus. A physical object or event that may have an effect upon the behavior of an organism.

Stimulus Control. Stimulus control is demonstrated when the stimuli that were present during the modification of an emitted rsponse begin to control the emission of that response.

Subset of Behavior. The group of simpler response components that compose a more complex behavior.

Successive Approximations. Behavioral elements or subsets each of which more and more closely resemble the specified terminal behavior.

Target Behavior. A behavioral goal, terminal behavior.

Terminal Behavior. See Behavioral Goal.

Timeout. A procedure in which access to the sources of various forms of reinforcement are removed for a particular period contingent upon the occurrence of a response.

Token Reinforcer. A stimulus object that can be exchanged at a later time for another reinforcing item or activity.

Topography of a Response. The shape, configuration, or form of a response.

7

The Six Group Therapies Compared

SAMUEL LONG

To this point, each of the six group therapies described in this book has been thoroughly elaborated as regards its history, goals, theoretical tenets, therapeutic processes and mechanisms, practice, and application. Certain key structural and technical features of the six therapies have not been considered, however; nor have the therapies been compared by these structural and technical dimensions.

Numerous evaluative categories and classification schemes have been outlined in the literature which might be employed in this context (Bascue, 1978; Goldenberg, 1983; Hjelle & Zeigler, 1981; Klein, 1983; Korchin, 1976; Mandanes & Haley, 1977; Marmor, 1984; Prochaska, 1979; Ryckman, 1982; Wolberg, 1977; Yalom, 1970). Because the selection of appropriate categories must remain somewhat arbitrary, the variables considered must pertain to all six therapies, and discriminating comparisons must result from usage of the categories.

The 12 structural and technical dimensions utilized in comparing the six group therapies deal with general therapeutic objectives, aspects of treatment content and style, change mechanisms, and structural factors.

Two caveats must be recognized. First, none of the group therapies has been described in its pure form, because the authors were requested to describe their own therapeutic approaches as they actually practiced them. Second, even the descriptions of the therapies as practiced exhibit considerable variation on many central dimensions. Therefore, in making comparisons of the therapies on the following categories, compromises will be made where deviations occur between pure theory and actual practice, and general patterns of practice will be relied on where variation in practice is conveyed by authors.

One continuum on which group therapies might be compared concerns the degree to which a given therapy is oriented toward problem solving or counseling, in contrast to an orientation more concerned with fundamental personality change.

Samuel Long • Empire State Poll, Inc., 154 East 29th Street, New York, New York 10016.

Clearly, behavior therapy groups, with their emphasis on the selection of specific symptoms of behaviors for treatment, as well as the utilization of metagoals for group organization, fall on the problem-solving end of this continuum.

By way of contrast, encounter group therapy, stressing both behavioral and cognitive change, resulting in an increased quality of interpersonal relationships and an increased competency in managing these relationships, would seem to fall toward the personality change end of the continuum.

Similarly, Gestalt group therapy would seem to be oriented toward personality change, particularly regarding its goals of awareness, integration, maturation, responsibility, and authenticity.

Transactional analysis groups probably also are more focused on personality change relative to problem solving, especially when they stress the development of personal autonomy and, particularly, script analysis and modification.

Both Adlerian and cognitively oriented group therapies would seem to apply to a greater range of problems, encompassing both problem solving and personality change. For example, Adlerian group therapy distinguishes between the ignorant and the discouraged, between people seeking counseling and people needing therapy. And cognitive group therapy describes applicable goals pertaining to the alleviation of subjective distress and maladaptive behaviors as well as to the reduction of neurotic disturbance and the solution of problems of living. Thus, both group therapies would appear to be best placed midway between the problem-solving and personality-change poles.

Group therapies vary regarding the extent to which they manifest a formal methodology, using similar techniques and procedures for all clients, regardless of the nature of the presenting problem. Conversely, some therapies are characterized by the design of a unique procedure for individual clients with unique problems.

It would appear that both behavior therapy groups and encounter groups exhibit rather systematic methods of treatment. In the case of the former, frequently used techniques would include systematic desensitization, modeling, behavior rehearsal, operant conditioning, and extinction procedures. Encounter groups often employ structured exercises to illustrate and generate group interaction, such as awareness exercises, skill-building exercises, and boundary and control-recognition exercises.

Both Adlerian and Gestalt group therapies appear at the opposite pole of this continuum, in that they both require a specific treatment plan and procedure for individual clients or groups with different problems. The Adlerian position is clear on this point: no Adlerian method of treatment exists, and different clients with similar presenting problems may well be treated in a totally dissimilar manner. Gestalt therapy groups, on the other hand, seem characterized by treatment which is improvised for individual clients in individual group sessions; the only common focus here is developing the client's awareness of the "here and now."

Being more educative in nature, cognitive therapy groups and transactional analysis groups fall between the two extremes on this continuum. Cognitive therapy groups, for instance, use a flexible, often experiential approach to the *ABC* model or the emotional episode; whereas transactional analysis groups initially teach the fundamental concepts and theory of the approach, then subsequently apply this learned material to the problems of individual group members.

A key distinguishing feature of group therapies involves the contrast between those which subscribe to a release-of-affect model and those subscribing to a cognitive restructuring model (Frank, 1961). The release-of-affect model holds that behavioral change is best effected through the experience of intense emotion (Gibb, 1971); the cognitive restructuring model suggests that behavior change is best effected through the modification of thoughts, values, beliefs, and attitudes.

Along this dimension, clear distinctions emerge, with encounter and Gestalt groups falling on the release-of-affect pole. Encounter groups encourage their members not only to accept their own feelings, whether positive or negative, but to express them as well. This focus on emotion and sensation follows from the notion that contemporary society overemphasizes the cognitive and underemphasizes the affective. Thus, personal growth follows from a reestablishment of emotions and sensations (Rogers, 1970). Gestalt groups stress emotional expression rather than cognition because the latter is assumed, in therapy groups, to be mere intellectualization that blocks full awareness of the here and now. Thus, Gestalt groups would view a cognitive orientation as a means of resisting present experience (Shaffer & Galinsky, 1974).

The cognitive restructuring model shares a common assumption about behavior change. This model asserts that cognition precedes emotion and behavior, and that lasting changes in emotions and behavior typically follow from cognitive restructuring.

Behavior, cognitive, Adlerian, and transactional therapy groups all share a common emphasis on fundamental education of their members, particularly about the faultiness of their thinking and the means by which that faulty thinking can be rectified. The stress is on cognitive self-understanding and different ways of thinking.

Interestingly, cognition, affect, and behavior are construed to play different causal roles for each of these theories. In behavior therapy theory, changes in overt social behavior result in cognitive restructuring; cognitive therapy theory posits that behavior change follows from modified cognitions; Adlerian therapy theory argues that cognition causes behavior, which, in turn, causes emotion. The important factor for this discussion, however, is the key role played by cognitions in the process of behavior change.

Most schools of group psychotherapy would argue that an individual's interpersonal behavior in the group is analogous in many ways to the individual's social behavior in the real world, and that personal problems occurring in the group also occur outside the group. Group therapies, however, differ regarding the degree to which the group context is used to address, analyze, and modify these problems. Some groups, purposely structured to facilitate interpersonal relations among members, focus on these relations to produce member change (Bednar & Kaul, 1978; Bednar & Lawlis, 1971; Goldstein & Simonson, 1971; Lieberman, 1976); other groups, although cognizant of group dynamics, typically follow a set agenda and established procedures to effect member change.

Encounter groups are especially prone to concentrate on interpersonal transactions among members in the achievement of therapeutic goals (Lieberman, Yalom, & Miles, 1973). Thus, encounter groups not only train group members in skills contributing to increased, effective relations among members, but promulgate no specified agenda so that these relations themselves are promoted and analyzed by the group. In this instance, group process, not content, is the central focus, and the ultimate objectives are the learning of interpersonal skills, increasing self-expression, producing autonomy, and gaining insight into the etiology of interpersonal problems.

The remaining groups considered here place much less emphasis on group dynamics than do encounter groups. This is not to assert that these approaches are oblivious to the dynamics of therapy groups; in each case, there is a recognition of the role of group dynamics in achieving or the failure to achieve therapeutic goals. Behavior therapy and cognitive therapy groups seem particularly sensitive to group norms and group cohesion, for example, in affecting therapeutic outcomes. But in these instances, client progress is produced with the aid of group-dynamic factors, not based on identifying and analyzing these factors as the primary goal of therapy.

It might be argued that Gestalt and transactional analysis groups are more variable on this dimension. Although the Gestalt position seems usually to discourage interaction among group members, this possibility is left open to the individual therapist, who might wish to focus on the interactive process in exploring the here and now with group members. In a similar fashion, transactional analysis therapists, in using script analysis, may find group members relating to one another based on past familial experiences and relations (Berne, 1963). In general, however, it would seem that these latter orientations more typically share the didactic foci of Adlerian, cognitive, and behavior therapy groups.

Is psychotherapeutic group treatment primarily a function of verbal or behavioral intervention? Here, the distinction is between seeking a cure through verbal communication or through action, such as behavioral rehearsal, role playing, modeling, awareness exercises, and physical contact. On this dimension, clear distinctions appear for the six group therapies.

Both encounter and Gestalt therapy groups would appear on the action pole of this continuum. Great emphasis, in encounter groups, is placed on initially learning the skills necessary for fruitful group participation; these skills center on effective communication, leadership, and conflict resolution. These skills are subsequently used to enhance the quality of the group experience for all members and the interrelationships among members. Gestalt groups eschew verbal communication *per se,* and instead develop members' awareness of and contact with their bodies, feelings, and milieu (Blumberg & Golembiewski, 1976).

Cognitive, Adlerian, and transactional analysis therapy groups fall on the verbal communication pole on this continuum. These orientations, all to varying degrees focusing on education and attitude change, place heavy reliance on talking between the therapist and group members.

Behavior therapy groups seem to share equally the action and verbal aspects of this dimension. To the extent that such groups incorporate theoretical assumptions from cognitive therapy, that is, that behavior is a function of cognition, verbal communication is used to examine and modify group members' faulty beliefs and attitudes. Conversely, behavior therapy groups also modify client behavior in both the group context and the natural environment through more action-oriented behavior modification techniques, such as operant conditioning, desensitization, and extinction.

Another important dimension differentiating the group therapies in this study relates to whether treatment is provided for the presenting problems of individual clients in groups, whether group dynamic factors and interpersonal relationships between group members are the foci of treatment, or whether the entire group is to receive treatment from the therapist. If this continuum is characterized as having three points, then the most extreme of these, that dealing with treatment of the group as a unit, obviously does not apply to the six group therapies described here.

The midpoint on this continuum, however, dealing with an examination of group dynamics, particularly those concerning interpersonal relations between group members, would seem germane to encounter groups. In this case, encounter group members are specifically trained in group skills so they will function as productive members. Moreover, encounter groups have no set agenda, and are formed with the general purpose of studying themselves over time. Finally, to accentuate a sensitivity to group dynamics, these groups are frequently requested to temporarily pause in their deliberations and attend to group process rather than to group content. Through this focus on group process, group members report what has been occurring, as well as their emotions which were associated with these occurrences. Thus, for encounter groups, attention is directed at the dynamics of the group and to specific interpersonal interactions among group participants; and it is these dynamics and interactions which offer benefits for group members and stimuli for the therapist.

Although, at times, the remaining group therapies under consideration focus on group-process factors, in general, they are all characterized by individual group members being the recipients of the therapist's attention within the group context. This individual attention and treatment would seem to follow from the fundamental educational and didactic nature of these therapies.

Among behavior therapy groups, this tendency seems most pronounced when the group has been organized around a common core issue, such as stress, smoking, public speaking, or weight control. Given the many techniques used in Gestalt therapy, especially the frequently employed "empty chair," it is clear that the emphasis here is on the individual, who interacts with the therapist as the other group members play primarily spectator roles (Perls, Hefferline, & Goodman, 1951). Again, Adlerian, cognitive, and transactional therapy groups, because of their heavy reliance on an education model of therapy, focus on the central role of the group therapist, who either relates to group members in a didactic fashion or encourages group interaction directed principally at the focal client or at the therapist.

Once a group therapy member's problem has been delineated, the therapist must decide which of two basic paths to take. If the therapist assumes that therapeutic change will result from an exploration of the problem, regardless of whether its cause is construed as occurring in the past or present, then the therapist will increase the member's understanding of the problem and its cause through further interpretation. Conversely, the therapist may reject the notion that interpretation and understanding will produce positive change, and instead may provide the group member with new experiences and directives, which ostensibly will produce change. Thus, another dimension on which group therapies might be placed focuses on causal interpretation versus action.

Three patterns appear when the six group therapies are placed on this dimension. Behavior, encounter, and Gestalt groups seem the most action-oriented, and view interpretation of causes as being either entirely irrelevant and possibly unknowable, as in behavior and Gestalt groups, or as more appropriately pursued subsequent to experiential learning, as seems the case in encounter groups. Transactional analysis groups seem the most insight- and interpretation-oriented of the therapies; while both Adlerian and cognitive therapy groups seem to incorporate both interpretation and action, particularly through the combined use of therapeutic inference and analysis, and behavior rehearsal and experiential assignments.

Group therapies can also be compared on a continuum defining acceptable content for group discussion. For some groups, life experiences outside the group are appropriate material for discussion in the group; for other types of groups, discussion is expected to be limited to occurrences from within the group itself. This latter stance, discouraging consideration of extragroup events, follows from a view of the group as replicating social reality and as an arena in which members' interpersonal problems will naturally occur in group members' interactions.

On this dimension, group therapies which encourage inclusion of extra-group life experiences as subject matter for group discussion include the Adlerian, behavior, cognitive, and transactional approaches. Perhaps the best example of a group with this type of external focus is a behavior therapy group formed for self-management or skill-training purposes. In this instance, the focus of group discussion would be almost solely devoted to extragroup matters.

Encounter and Gestalt therapy groups, on the other hand, typically exclude consideration of extragroup life experiences and concentrate on a here-and-now focus, dealing exclusively with occurrences in the group itself. What is then learned in the group setting is transferred and applied to the outside world. The material learned in these groups is usually humanistic in nature, dealing with an awareness of and concern for others, interpersonal trust, openness, and individuality. Given this internal orientation, members of these groups would argue that expanding their view to encompass matters external to the group would simply detract from the central goal of the group: expanded awareness and contact with the here and now.

In some groups, therapists address only the obvious or manifest meaning of group members' statements or overt behaviors, rejecting or ignoring the possibility that such verbalizations and behaviors might convey a less obvious but more important message about the individual. In other groups, therapists go beyond the surface meaning of members' expressions and attend to potentially latent or symbolic messages that may be representations of significant problems in the members' life experience.

Behavior therapy and encounter groups would seem to deal primarily with the manifest meaning of their members' verbal or behavior expressions. This focus is seen in the subject matter most frequently dealt with by behavior therapy groups, and especially by the techniques used in these groups to alleviate members' problems. Thus, attention is paid to the manifest content of members' communications, either verbal or behavioral, in groups focusing on interpersonal skills training, assertion training, stress immunization, pain control, impulse control, study skills, sexual dysfunction, and anxiety management. Similarly, encounter groups, even when dealing with the potentially latent implications of transference phenomena in the group context, typically remain on the conscious, rational level of communication. This is accomplished in encounter groups by the members being encouraged by the therapist to study group interactions and experiences which are palpable, which can be seen, heard, tasted, touched, and smelled. In addition, members are asked to express their feelings to other members of the group, maintaining this rational, conscious focus.

Of the six therapies considered here, Gestalt group therapy would seem the most oriented toward consideration of the latent content of members' verbal and behavioral communications. Gestalt theory includes conceptualization that elaborates on various mechanisms of defense designed to control anxiety—retroflection, introjection, confluence, and projection—which occur as latent communications in the Gestalt group (Perls *et al.*, 1951). Moreover, Gestalt group therapy places emphasis on members' dreamwork, in which the individual's personality and mechanisms of defense are explored by probing the latent meaning of dreams (Perls, 1969).

Without necessarily subscribing to the assumption that individuals possess an unconscious, as suggested by the psychodynamic school, Adlerian, cognitive, and transactional group therapies all deal, in one way or another, with the symbolic aspects of group members' verbal and behavioral communications through the investigation of ego defense mechanisms and dream analysis (Lazarus, 1981; Mosak & Dreikurs, 1973; Samuels, 1977). In each instance, however, these group psychotherapies seem to fall between the two poles of manifest and latent meaning of group members' communications.

In effecting therapeutic change in group members, the psychotherapist can concentrate on members' past experiences or those experiences in their present and future. Psychoanalytic groups typically focus on the events in the early childhoods of members in accounting for and attempting to change their problem behavior. By way of contrast, behavior therapy groups, especially when they are engaged in skill-training, self-management, and self-control tasks, seem more oriented toward the present and/or the future. A present-orientation would clearly characterize encounter and Gestalt therapy groups, which adhere to a focus on the here and now. This focus on the present is further maintained through the use of "how" and "what" questions, rather than "why" questions, which frequently foster a focus on the past.

Adlerian, cognitive, and transactional analysis groups all seem to combine past and present orientations in producing change in group members. Adlerian group therapists, for example, collect early recollections as a means of formulating members' life-styles (Ansbacher, 1977; Dinkmeyer, Pew & Dinkmeyer, 1979). Cognitive group therapists may focus on group members' pasts in order to argue that their pasts are not determiners of their present behavior (Ellis, 1962), or may explore members' pasts to further members' understanding of their developmental histories (Wessler & Hankin, 1986). Transactional analysis therapists may stress group members' pasts while engaged in structural analyses or analyses of scripts (Berne, 1966). In these instances, however, this focus on the past is neither as detailed and profound as in psychoanalytic therapy groups; nor is the focus on the present as rigid as in encounter and Gestalt therapy groups.

Another salient dimension differentiating different schools of group psychotherapy describes the role assumed by the group therapist in the group. Is the therapist very active and the focus of attention for group members, or is the therapist less active, not the center of attention, and more interested in contributing to interaction among all group members and to the functioning of the group as a whole (Goldstein, Heller, & Sechrest, 1966)?

Although group therapists' activity levels probably vary considerably over time and from one group to another, it seems probable that encounter group therapists exhibit less activity, compared to group members, than do therapists in the other five types of groups. This conclusion would seem to follow from the essential function of the encounter therapy group: increased self-awareness and increased effectiveness in interpersonal relations.

Therapists in the remaining group therapies would all seem to perform relatively active roles and generally serve as the focus of attention for other group members. This conclusion would certainly apply to Gestalt therapy groups, where the usual pattern would involve the therapist conducting experiments in directed awareness, one-on-one with individual group members. Likewise, in Adlerian, cognitive, and transactional analysis groups, the therapist usually performs a didactic, educative role among group members. In behavior therapy groups, where the therapist is engaged in executing a specific intervention designed to meet a specific target problem, whether it pertain to skills-training, self-management, or self-control, the therapist plays a very active role and probably plays this role in one-on-one relationships with group members.

Psychotherapeutic groups also differ in the range of psychological distance which occurs between the group therapist and the group members. This psychological distance might be evidenced by the degree to which the therapist engages in self-disclosure, by the use of informal group settings, by the frequency with which the leader assumes a participant role, and by the diminution of importance attributed to the therapist's expertise and status.

In comparing the six group therapies on this dimension, it would seem that compared to the other therapies, encounter groups probably are more characterized by low therapist–member distance. Again, the fundamental objectives and procedures of the different group therapies, as well as the different roles played by the group therapist, would seem to influence this relative positioning. Therefore, Adlerian, behavior, cognitive, Gestalt, and transactional analysis group therapies all probably manifest higher levels of therapist–member psychological distance.

Table 1 was constructed to aid in simultaneously comparing the six group therapies' positions along each of the 12 dimensions. Three patterns are manifest in this table. First, on the 12 dimensions, encounter therapy and Gestalt therapy appear clearly to stand apart from the remaining therapies, as well as frequently to share common placement on many of the dimensions. This pattern is most pronounced on the dimensions relating to the goal of problem-solving versus personality change, cognitive versus affective foci, verbal versus behavioral intervention, interpretation versus action/directives, emphases on external versus internal experiences, and a past focus versus a present–future focus. It is noteworthy that of these two group therapies, encounter is even more distinctive than Gestalt in that encounter groups are most frequently positioned alone on the evaluative dimensions, particularly those relating to the group versus the individual as the therapeutic change mechanism, an individual versus group focus, leader versus member activity, and low versus high psychological distance between group leaders and members.

A second pattern appearing in Table 1 shows a clear relationship among the Adlerian, cognitive, and transactional analysis group therapies, with these therapies being associated in the table even more frequently than the encounter and Gestalt positions. Interestingly, the Adlerian and cognitive therapies

Table 1. Structural and Technical Continuums of the Group Therapies[a]

Problem solving	B	AC	EGT	Personality change
Systematic method	BE	CT	AG	Individualized plan
Cognitive	ABCT		EG	Affective
Change mechanism: group	E		ABCGT	Change mechanism: individual
Verbal	ACT	B	EG	Behavioral
Individual focus	ABCGT	E		Group focus
Interpretation	T	AC	BEG	Action/directives
External experiences	ABCT		EG	Internal experiences
Manifest meaning	BE	ACT	G	Latent meaning
Past focus		ACT	BEG	Present/future focus
Leader activity	ABCGT		E	Member activity
High psychological distance	ABCGT		E	Low psychological distance

[a] A = Adlerian therapy; B = behavior therapy; C = cognitive therapy; E = encounter therapy; G = Gestalt therapy; T = transactional analysis therapy.

appear together on every dimension except that describing systematic versus individualized treatment. However, the commonality shared by these approaches is most apparent on dimensions reflecting a cognitive focus: the individual being viewed as the central mechanism of therapeutic change, a strategy of verbal intervention, concentration on the individual group member, the general relevance of experiences external to the group, a relatively high level of group leader activity, and a comparatively high psychological distance between group leader and members.

The behavior approach seems to fall between these two patterns, sometimes falling within the encounter–Gestalt pattern and sometimes falling within the Adlerian–cognitive–transactional analysis pattern. Clearly, however, behavior group therapy is more associated with the latter pattern, especially regarding cognitive versus affective foci, the group versus the individual as the therapeutic change mechanism, the individual versus group focus, emphases on external versus internal experiences, leader versus member activity, and low versus high leader–member psychological distance.

The placement of the six group psychotherapies examined along these 12 dimensions would tend to substantiate classifications of psychotherapy that, among other distinctions, differentiate among positions stressing growth of the self and enhancing interpersonal relations and communications, which would seem to characterize the encounter and Gestalt group therapies; habit change, which would apply to behavior group therapy; and concept and value change, which describes the Adlerian, cognitive, and transactional analysis group therapies (Sundberg & Tyler, 1962).

References

Ansbacher, H. Individual psychology. In R. Corsini (Ed.), *Current personality theories.* Itasca, Ill.: Peacock Publishers, 1977.

Bascue, L. Conceptual model for group therapy training. *International Journal of Group Psychotherapy,* 1978, *28,* 445–452.

Bednar, R., & Kaul, T. Experiental group research: Current perspectives. In S. Garfield & A. Bergin (Eds.), *Handbook of psychotherapy and behavior change: An empirical analysis* (2nd ed.). New York: John Wiley, 1978.

Bednar, R., & Lawlis, G. Empirical research in group psychotherapy. In A. Bergin & S. Garfield (Eds.), *Handbook of psychotherapy and behavior change: An empirical analysis.* New York: John Wiley, 1971.

Berne, E. *The structure and dynamics of organizations and groups.* New York: Grove Press, 1963.

Berne, E. *Principles of group treatment.* New York: Grove Press, 1966.

Blumberg, A., & Golembiewski, R. *Learning and change in groups.* Baltimore: Penguin Books, 1976.

Dinkmeyer, D., Pew, W., & Dinkmeyer, D. *Adlerian counseling and psychotherapy.* Monterey, Cal.: Brooks/Cole, 1979.

Ellis, A. *Reason and emotion in psychotherapy.* Secaucus, N.J.: Lyle Stuart, 1962.

Frank, J. *Persuasion and healing: A comparative study of psychotherapy.* New York: Schocken Books, 1961.

Gibb, J. The effects of human relations training. In A. Bergin & S. Garfield (Eds.), *Handbook of psychotherapy and behavior change: An empirical analysis.* New York: John Wiley, 1971.

Goldenberg, H. *Contemporary clinical psychology* (2nd ed.). Monterey, Cal.: Brooks/Cole, 1983.

Goldstein, A., & Simonson, N. Social psychological approaches to psychotherapy research. In A. Bergin & S. Garfield (Eds.), *Handbook of psychotherapy and behavior change: An empirical analysis.* New York: John Wiley, 1971.

Goldstein, A., Heller, K., & Sechrest, L. *Psychotherapy and the psychology of behavior change.* New York: John Wiley, 1966.

Hjelle, L., & Ziegler, D. *Personality theories: Basic assumptions, research, and applications* (2nd ed.). New York: McGraw-Hill, 1981.

Klein, R. Group treatment approaches. In M. Hersen, A. Kazdin, & A. Bellack (Eds.), *The clinical psychology handbook.* New York: Pergamon Press, 1983.

Korchin, S. *Modern clinical psychology: Principles of intervention in the clinic and community.* New York: Basic Books, 1976.

Lazarus, A. *The practice of multimodal therapy.* New York: McGraw-Hill, 1981.

Lieberman, M. Change induction in small groups. In M. Rosenzweig & L. Porter (Eds.), *Annual review of psychology.* Palo Alto, Cal.: Annual Reviews, 1976.

Lieberman, M., Yalom, I., & Miles, M. *Encounter groups: First facts.* New York: Basic Books, 1973.

Madanes, C., & Haley, J. Dimensions of family therapy. *Journal of Nervous and Mental Disease,* 1977, *165,* 88–98.

Marmor, J. Experiental, inspirational, cognitive/emotive, and other therapies. In American Psychiatric Association Commission on Psychiatric Therapies (Ed.), *The psychiatric therapies.* Washington, D.C.: American Psychiatric Association, 1984.

Mosak, H., & Dreikurs, R. Adlerian psychotherapy. In R. Corsini (Ed.), *Current psychotherapies.* Itasca, Ill.: Peacock Publishers, 1973.

Perls, F. *Ego, hunger and aggression.* New York: Random House, 1969.

Perls, F., Hefferline, R., & Goodman, P. *Gestalt therapy: Excitement and growth in the human personality.* New York: Dell Publishing, 1951.

Prochaska, J. *Systems of psychotherapy: A transtheoretical analysis.* Homewood, Ill.: Dorsey Press, 1979.

Rogers, C. *On encounter groups.* New York: Harper & Row, 1970.

Ryckman, R. *Theories of personality* (2nd ed.). Monterey, Cal.: Brooks/Cole, 1982.

Samuels, A. A TA approach to dreams. In M. James (Ed.), *Techniques in transactional analysis for psychotherapists and counselors.* Reading, Mass.: Addison-Wesley Publishing, 1977.

Shaffer, J., & Galinsky, M. *Models of group therapy and sensitivity training.* Englewood Cliffs, N.J.: Prentice-Hall, 1974.

Sundberg, N., & Tyler, L. *Clinical psychology: An introduction to research and practice.* New York: Meredith Publishing, 1962.

Wessler, R., & Hankin, S. Cognitive appraisal therapy. In W. Dryden & W. Golden (Eds.), *Cognitive-behavioural approaches to psychotherapy.* London: Harper & Row, 1986.

Wolberg, L. *The techniques of psychotherapy* (3rd ed.). New York: Grune & Stratton, 1977.

Yalom, I. *The theory and practice of group psychotherapy.* New York: Basic Books, 1970.

Index